Synthetic Studies of Marine Bioactive Natural Products and Analogs to Develop Novel Drug Leads

Synthetic Studies of Marine Bioactive Natural Products and Analogs to Develop Novel Drug Leads

Guest Editor

Naoyuki Kotoku

MDPI

Basel • Beijing • Wuhan • Barcelona • Belgrade • Novi Sad • Cluj • Manchester

Guest Editor
Naoyuki Kotoku
College of Pharmaceutical
Sciences
Ritsumeikan University
Shiga
Japan

Editorial Office
MDPI AG
Grosspeteranlage 5
4052 Basel, Switzerland

This is a reprint of the Special Issue, published open access by the journal *Marine Drugs* (ISSN 1660-3397), freely accessible at: https://www.mdpi.com/journal/marinedrugs/special_issues/36S7DUA914.

For citation purposes, cite each article independently as indicated on the article page online and as indicated below:

Lastname, A.A.; Lastname, B.B. Article Title. *Journal Name* **Year**, *Volume Number*, Page Range.

ISBN 978-3-7258-6634-2 (Hbk)
ISBN 978-3-7258-6635-9 (PDF)
https://doi.org/10.3390/books978-3-7258-6635-9

Contents

About the Editor

Naoyuki Kotoku

Dr. Naoyuki Kotoku received his PhD degree in Pharmaceutical Sciences from Osaka University in 2003, under the supervision of Prof. Yasuyuki Kita. He then moved to the Laboratory of Natural Products Chemistry in the same university, where he worked as Assistant Professor, starting his research into marine natural products with Prof. Motomasa Kobayashi. He was promoted to Associate Professor at the College of Pharmaceutical Sciences, Ritsumeikan University, in 2017 and to full Professor in 2024. His research covers the broad scope of natural products chemistry: structure elucidation, total synthesis, synthesis and evaluation of truncated analogs, and target identification using synthetic molecular probes. The aim of his studies is to develop promising natural-product-derived drug leads with novel modes of action for intractable diseases such as cancer.

marine drugs

MDPI

Review

Syntheses of Marine Natural Products via Matteson Homologations and Related Processes

Uli Kazmaier [1,2,3]

[1] Organic Chemistry, Saarland University, Campus Building C4.2, D-66123 Saarbruecken, Germany; u.kazmaier@mx.uni-saarland.de
[2] Helmholtz Institute for Pharmaceutical Research Saarland (HIPS), Saarland University, Campus, C8.1, D-66123 Saarbruecken, Germany
[3] Pharma Science Hub, Saarland University, Campus, Geb. A2 3, D-66123 Saarbruecken, Germany

Abstract: Matteson homologation, a successive extension of chiral boronic esters, is perfectly suited for the synthesis of complex molecular structures containing several stereogenic centers. The "classical version" allows the introduction of various functional groups in a 1,2-*anti*-configuration. The absolute configuration is determined by the choice of the chiral auxiliary, which can be used to introduce several stereogenic centers. In contrast, in Aggarwal's lithiation-borylation strategy, new chiral auxiliary reagents must be used in each reaction step, which on the other hand allows the individual insertion of the desired stereogenic centers. Both methods have their individual advantages and disadvantages and are well suited for the synthesis of marine natural products.

Keywords: boronic esters; borylation; lithiation; Matteson homologation; marine natural products

1. Introduction

Already in early human cultures, the biological activity of various natural products was recognized and used for different purposes [1]. The first records of the medicinal use of plants in China, India and the Middle East date back 5000 years [2]. Due to great advances in analytics, but at the same time also in organic synthesis, numerous active natural products have been isolated, identified and synthesized during the last century. In the years 1981–2006, for example, about 50% of all newly discovered active substances in the field of small molecules were substances derived from natural products [3]. Most of them were isolated from a wide range of plants, fungi and microorganisms [4], in which marine natural products represent a particularly important class of therapeutically interesting active ingredients [5–7]. The structures of the isolated compounds are as diverse as their producers. In addition to (cyclic) peptides and polyketides, also cyclodepsipeptides, which contain both structural elements, are well represented. Typical examples of these are lagunamide A [8], apratoxin A [9] or callipeltin A [10] (Figure 1).

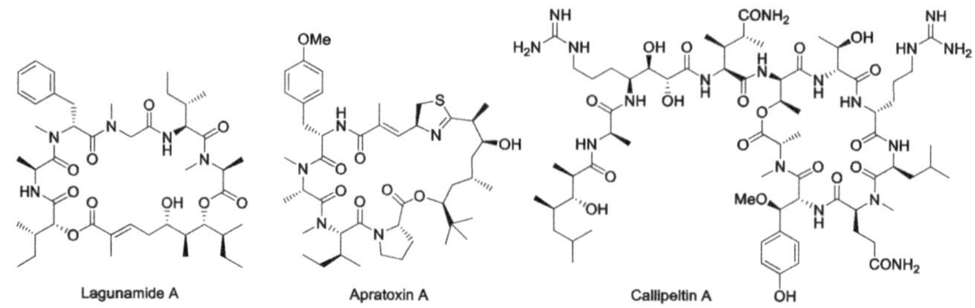

Figure 1. Marine cyclodepsipeptides.

However, isolation of bioactive substances often provides only insufficient quantities for biological studies or even complete structure elucidation, and thus the total synthesis of these compounds has been established as a valuable tool, not only to provide enough material for biological studies but often also for structure elucidation or verification [11]. There are a variety of methods for the synthesis of the often rather unusual amino acids [12–14], but asymmetric aldol reactions and related reactions are mainly used to build polyketide structures [15,16]. These methods are excellently suited for the formation of 3,5,7,... polyhydroxylated carboxylic acids, such as in lagunamide, but can only be used to a limited extent in the synthesis of polyketides with other, unusual substitution patterns, such as in apratoxin. In 1980 Matteson et al. reported an asymmetric homologation of boronic esters [17] which is also an efficient tool for total synthesis but is also much more flexible than aldol reactions with regard to the substitution pattern. In addition, not only suitable for the generation of polyketides but also for peptides and other substance classes. This review summarizes the applications of Matteson homologations and related reaction sequences [18] in the synthesis of marine natural products.

2. Homologations of Boronic Esters

2.1. Matteson Homologations

In 1963, Matteson et al. reported that the nucleophilic substitution of α-haloboronic esters is considerably facilitated by the neighboring group effect of the boron atom [19]. For example, when the α-bromoboronic acid ester **1** was reacted with phenylmagnesium bromide, the substitution product **3** was obtained in very good yield after warming the reaction mixture up to room temperature (Scheme 1). Aqueous acidic workup at low temperature, on the other hand, yielded the boric acid ester **4**, indicating that the reaction proceeded from **1** to **3** via the boronate complex **2**. From **2**, the substitution product **3** was formed via 1,2 migration of the phenyl group.

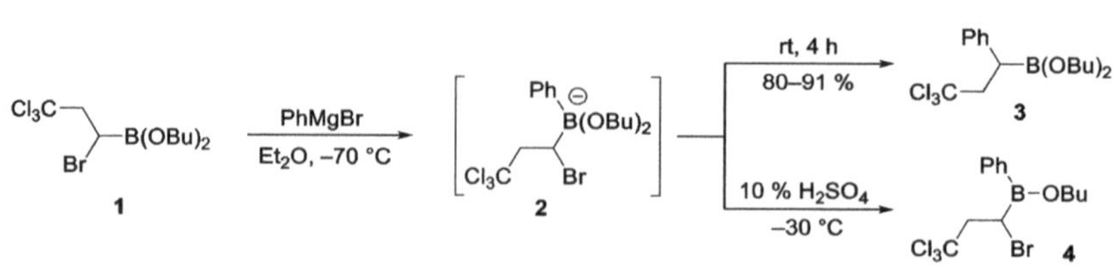

Scheme 1. Nucleophilic substitution of α-bromoboronic esters according to Matteson et al. [19].

Initially, no suitable, generally applicable routes for the synthesis of α-haloboronic acid esters were available, and therefore, the method was seldom used until Matteson et al. in 1980 reported the homologation of boronic esters to α-chloroboronic esters by using deprotonated dichloromethane [20,21]. The α-chloroboronic esters could then be reacted with a variety of nucleophiles such as alcoholates [22], enolates [23,24], organolithium compounds or Grignard reagents [18,25]. If boronic esters of chiral diols were used, highly diastereoselective reactions to chiral α-chloroboronic esters became available. In a first report in 1980 Matteson et al. demonstrated that the pinanediol ester of phenylboronic acid **5** on reaction with (dichloromethyl)lithium provides the corresponding α-chloroboronic ester which could be reacted with MeMgBr, whereby the boronic ester **6** was obtained (Scheme 2) [17].

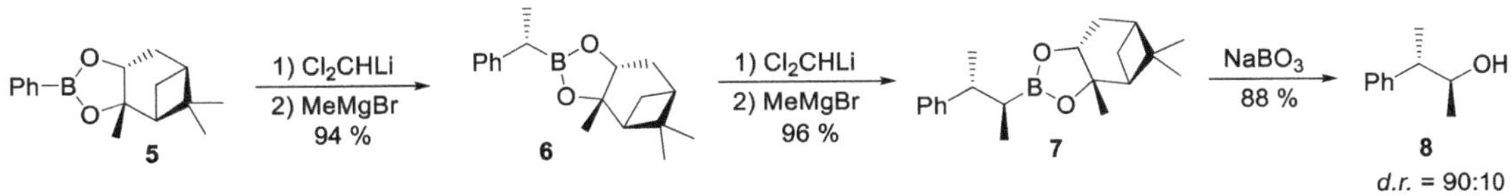

Scheme 2. Matteson homologations using pinanediol as chiral auxiliary.

Repeated homologation and reaction with the same Grignard reagent yielded the boronic ester **7**, which was oxidized to alcohol **8** with a good diastereomeric ratio (*d.r.*). The pinanediol used as a chiral auxiliary can easily be obtained in both enantiomeric forms by *syn*-dihydroxylation of either (+) or (−)-α-pinene [26].

As has been shown, the addition of zinc chloride can significantly increase both the yields and the *d.r.* values of the Matteson homologation. With pinanediol as a chiral auxiliary, diastereoselectivities of up to 98.5–99.5% can be achieved under these conditions. By using chiral, C_2-symmetric diols as auxiliaries, even better diastereoselectivities can be obtained. Excellent results can be achieved, for example, with diisopropylethandiol (DIPED) [27], which can be obtained from tartaric acid esters [28]. Dicyclohexylethandiol (DICHED) is so far the most used symmetric chiral diol, as it is relatively easy to synthesize from *trans*-stilbene [29,30].

As already illustrated with the example in Scheme 2, the Matteson homologation is perfectly suited for an iterative setup of adjacent stereocenters. The stereochemical outcome of the reaction is almost exclusively controlled by the chiral diol in a substrate-controlled manner, giving access to the 1,2-*anti*-configured product [18,25].

The generally accepted mechanism of the Matteson homologation is shown in Scheme 3 [31]. In the first step, the carbenoid (dichloromethyl)lithium is added to the chiral boronic ester **A**, forming a tetrahedral boronate complex **B**. In the presence of zinc chloride, a 1,2-migration of the substituent R′ to either **C** or ***epi*-C** takes place. This rearrangement in principle can proceed via four different transition states (TS). In all cases, an oxygen atom of the diol and a chlorine atom of the former carbenoid coordinate with the Lewis acid. In the most favorable transition state **TS1**, the coordination of zinc takes place via the free electron pair on the oxygen, which is located *anti* to the residue R′. The chlorine atoms of the (dichloromethyl) residue arrange themselves in such a way that the uninvolved chlorine atom occupies the greatest possible distance from the zinc chloride, forming the main diastereomer **C**. The transition states **TS2** and **TS3**, which each lead to the minor diastereomer ***epi*-C**, are energetically much less favorable. In the case of **TS2**, the spatial proximity of the second Cl atom of the (dichloromethyl) residue to the zinc chloride and in the case of **TS3** the proximity of R to the Lewis acid leads to steric obstruction. Particularly unfavorable and therefore negligible is **TS4**, in which steric obstruction occurs at both positions. In 1998, Midland was able to confirm by ab initio calculations that **TS1** is the most favorable transitional state [32].

If **C** and ***epi*-C** are next reacted with a nucleophile, such as a Grignard reagent, the boronate complex **D** or ***epi-D*** is formed in analogy to the first step (Scheme 4). In the subsequent 1,2-rearrangement, which is catalyzed by zinc or magnesium salts (MX_2), the chlorine atom and the newly introduced residue R″ arrange themselves antiperiplanar starting from **D** in the transition state **TS5** and the major diastereomer **E** is obtained. If C2-symmetric diols such as DICHED or DIPED are used as auxiliaries, this step further improves the diastereoselectivity, since an analogous 1,2-shift from ***epi*-D** to ***epi*-E** via the sterically hindered transition state **TS6** hardly takes place. In this case, the minor diastereomer ***epi*-D** preferentially reacts via 1,2-migration of an alkoxy residue of the chiral diol via **TS7** to dioxaborinan **F**, which is rapidly oxidized in air to the boronic ester **G** and the aldehyde **H**. Since **D** and ***epi*-D** react to different products, extremely high diastereoselectivities for the major product **E** can be achieved with such C_2-symmetrical chiral diols [33].

The (dichloromethyl)lithium commonly used in Matteson homologations can be obtained by deprotonation of dichloromethane with *n*-butyllithium at −100 °C. The carbenoid solution has to be mixed with the boronic acid ester to be homologated [20,21]. An easier method to generate (dichloromethyl)lithium was developed by Brown et al. wherein the carbenoid is produced in situ in the presence of the boronic acid ester by deprotonation of dichloromethane with *sec*-butyllithium at −78 °C [34]. Alternatively, dichloromethane can also be deprotonated with LDA at −40 °C in situ, which is more suitable for reactions on a larger scale [35].

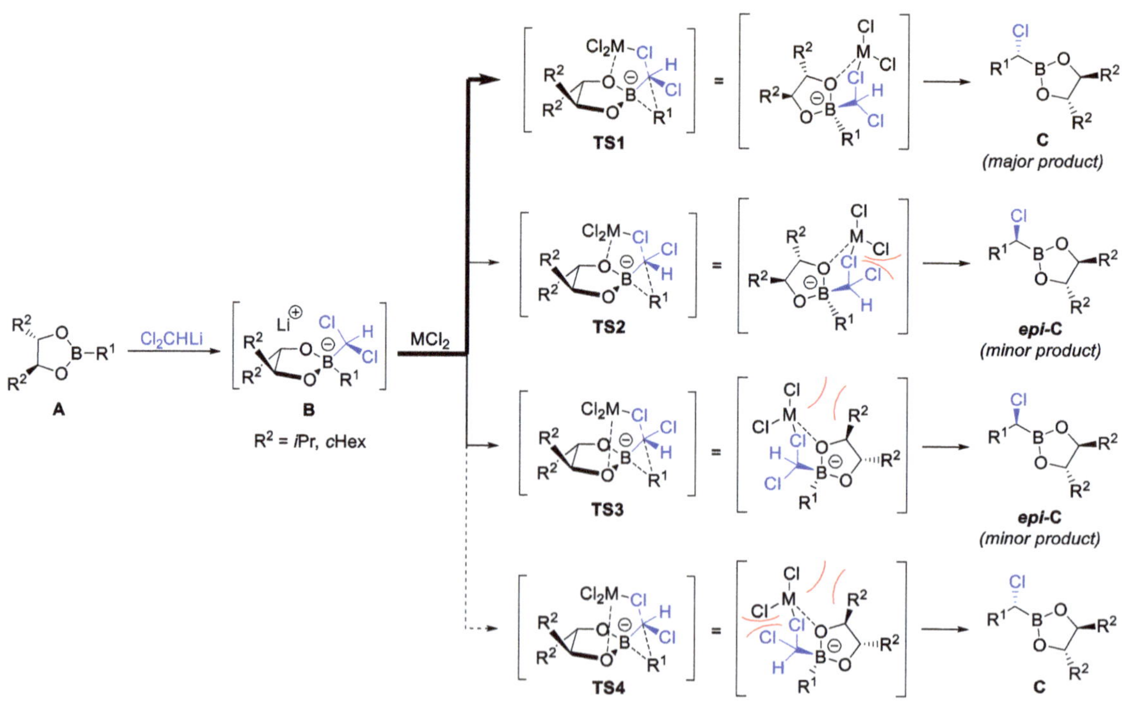

Scheme 3. Mechanism of Matteson homologation.

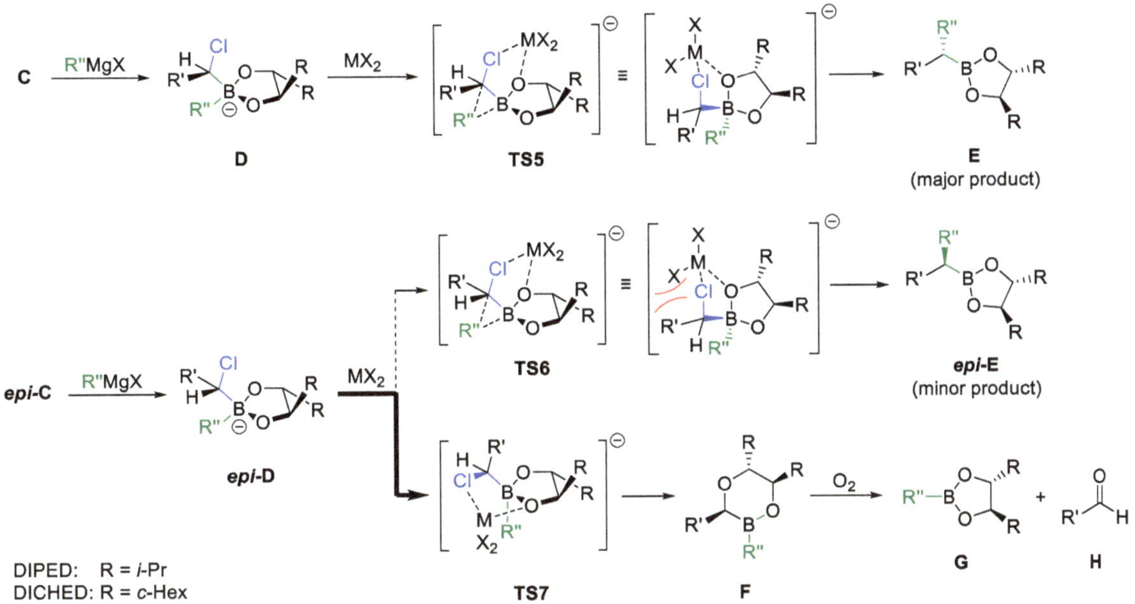

Scheme 4. Sequential double diastereo-differentiation by using C_2-symmetric diols as auxiliary according to Matteson et al. [33].

For some substitution reactions, α-chloroboronic esters are too unreactive. In these cases, the use of the appropriate α-bromoboronic esters, which can be obtained by homologation with (dibromomethyl)lithium, is recommended. This carbenoid can only be produced in situ by deprotonation with lithium diisopropylamide (LDA), as *n*-butyllithium preferentially undergoes a halogen-metal exchange to (bromomethyl)lithium [36]. α-Bromoboronic esters are more reactive than their chlorine analogs, but they are also more susceptible to epimerization, which should be taken into account in synthetic applications [37].

In addition to carbenoids of the X_2CHLi type, (chloromethyl)lithium or (bromomethyl)lithium (XCH_2Li) can also be used in Matteson homologations, whereby boronic esters can be extended by a CH_2 group. The carbenoids can be generated in situ by halogen-metal exchange with *n*-butyllithium from chloroiodomethane [38], bromochloromethane [39] or dibromomethane [40]. Alternatively, hydrides can also be used as nucleophiles in Matteson homologations, allowing for a two-stage introduction of CH_2 groups via reduction of the α-haloboronic esters. For this purpose, $KBH(i\text{Pr})_3$ [39], $LiBHEt_3$ [41,42], NaH [43] or $NaBH_4$ [44] can be used as hydride sources. The application of the corresponding deuterides enables the synthesis of asymmetrically deuterated compounds [45].

The Matteson reaction has the great advantage that with only one auxiliary any number of stereocenters can be introduced through successive homologation steps [46,47].

2.2. Reagent-Controlled Homologations

Although the Matteson homologation enables the highly diastereoselective construction of adjacent stereocenters in a 1,2-*anti*-arrangement, it is less suitable if the corresponding 1,2-*syn*-products are required. In these cases, either an exchange of the chiral diol [48] or, in the case of non-C_2-symmetric diols as an auxiliary, an inversion of the α-stereocenter is necessary [49]. Alternatively, such structures can be obtained using a lithiation-borylation strategy according to Aggarwal et al. [50] In this reagent-controlled variant of the Matteson homologation, achiral pinacol boronic esters are reacted with Hoppe's chiral lithiated carbamates (Cb) **I** [51,52]. The stereoselectivity in this case is determined by the configuration of the lithiated carbamate (**J**) (Scheme 5) [50], which is formed by deprotonation of a prochiral carbamate in the presence of a chiral auxiliary base, such as sparteine [53–55]. On reaction with a pinacol boronic ester, the borate complex **K** is formed, which delivers the elongated boronic ester **L** with good selectivity after $MgBr_2$-catalyzed 1,2-shift and substitution of the carbamate residue. Boronic ester **L** can be used again as a substrate for further homologations or converted into the secondary alcohols **M** by oxidation. Alternatively, Beak's 2,4,6-triisopropylbenzoyl ester (TIP) can be used as a directing group in such deprotonation reactions [56]. The TIB-esters are more electron-withdrawing and therefore the α-proton is slightly more acidic and easier to remove, which might be an advantage with critical substrates.

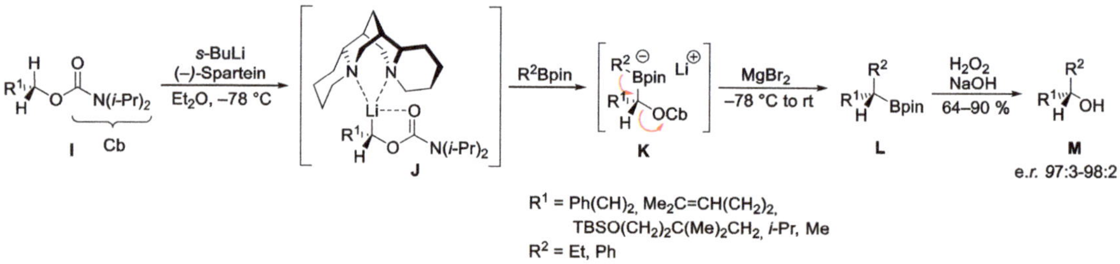

Scheme 5. Lithiation-borylation of Hoppe carbamates according to Aggarwal et al. [50].

The Aggarwal homologation allows the generation of adjacent stereocenters in both *syn*- and *anti*-constellation. However, a major disadvantage of the reaction is that stoichiometric amounts of sparteine are required as a chiral auxiliary for each homologation step. (−)-Sparteine and (+)-sparteine occur naturally and surrogates [57] are also synthetically accessible, but the availability and thus the price has fluctuated greatly in the last two decades [58]. Nevertheless, this method was used in the synthesis of a number of natural products [59,60].

In principle, the use of sparteine is not necessarily required if carbamates of secondary chiral alcohols **N** are used (Scheme 6). In 1990, Hoppe and coworkers showed that benzylic carbamates are particularly suitable for deprotonation, whereby the configuration at the chiral center is largely retained [61,62]. The lithiated species **O** can then be reacted with boronic esters with retention of the configuration to boronates **P**, which form the tertiary boronic esters **Q** with excellent chirality transfer via 1,2-shift of the residual R^3. Subsequent oxidation leads finally to the chiral tertiary alcohols **R** [63].

Furthermore, the chiral carbenoids **O** were subjected to substitution with boranes, whereby the tertiary organoboron compounds **S** were formed. Interestingly, this substitution proceeded via boronate **T** under inversion of the original configuration. After oxidation of these, the corresponding enantiomeric tertiary alcohols *ent*-**R** were obtained with excellent e.r. [64,65].

The retention in the addition step to the borate complex **P** can be attributed to an additional complexation between the lithiated carbamate and one of the *O*-atoms of the boronic ester. The corresponding boranes do not have any complexing groups, so the attack takes place under inversion from the opposite face [63].

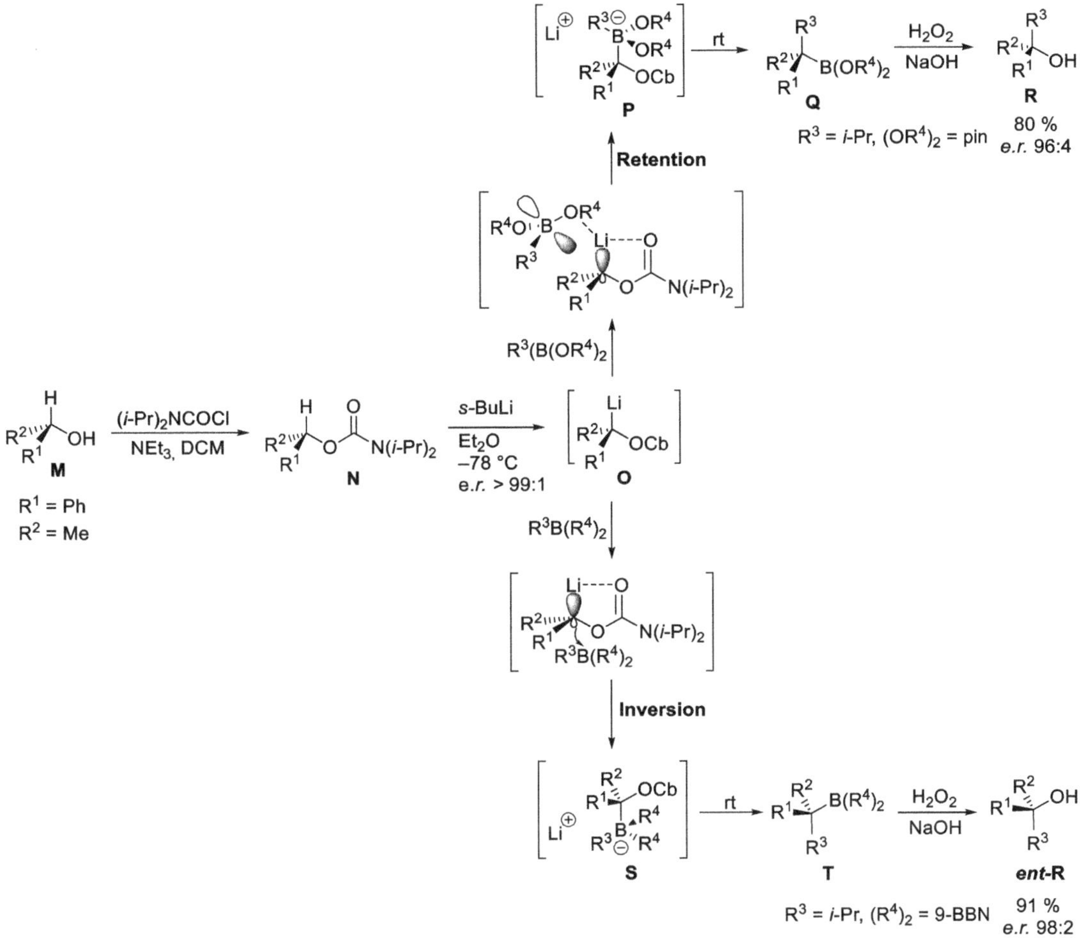

Scheme 6. Lithiation-borylation of secondary Hoppe carbamates according to Aggarwal et al. [63].

The fact that the use of sparteine is not necessarily helpful or necessary when using chiral primary esters or carbamates was shown by the work from the Kalesse group. During the synthesis of chondrochlorene, in which the chiral TIB-ester **9** had to be reacted with the vinylic boronic ester **10**, both (+)- and (−)-sparteine (sp) yielded the same product but in only very moderate yields, while without the addition of the ligand, an excellent yield of 85% and a single diastereomer could be obtained (Scheme 7) [66]. Interestingly, the Cb-carbamate **9′** provided the opposite diastereomer ***epi*-11**, albeit with poorer selectivity [67,68]. The stereogenic β-center seems to be crucial for the stereocontrolling effect of the substrate. If this substituent is missing as in **12**, the desired product **13** is formed in the sparteine-free version with an excellent yield but as a 1:1 diastereomer mixture. In contrast, in the presence of sparteine, the expected products are enantiomeric pure, but in this case, the stereochemical outcome of the reaction was solely controlled by the sparteine used.

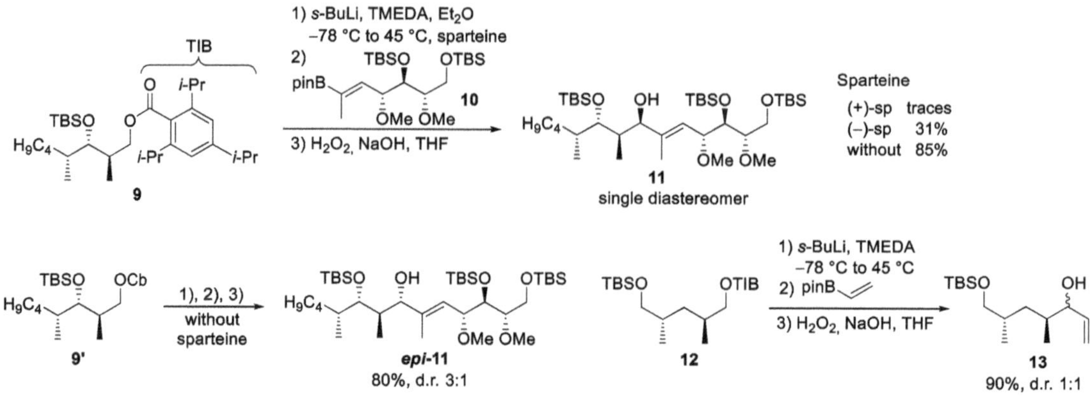

Scheme 7. Sparteine-free homologation according to Kalesse et al. [66].

Blakemore et al. were the first to describe a sparteine-free "lithiation-borylation" reaction as early as 2007 (Scheme 8) [69,70]. However, their α-sulfinyl chlorides **14** require a two-step synthesis via enantioselective Jackson–Ellman–Bolm oxidation [71–73] and Yamakawa chlorination [74] and are less stable. Also, the yields and enantioselectivities are often only moderate [75–79].

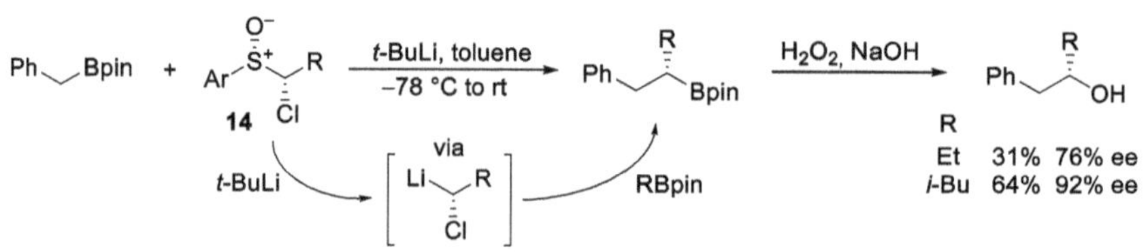

Scheme 8. Sparteine-free homologation according to Blakemore et al. [69,70].

2.3. Catalytic Homologations

A catalytic, enantioselective version of the Matteson homologation could circumvent the disadvantages of both methods. However, the first experiments on the homologation of pinacol boronic esters with chiral ytterbium catalysts were only successful in moderate enantioselectivities and required high catalyst loadings [80,81]. Jacobsen and coworkers achieved significantly better results with the lithium-isothiourea-borate complex **15** [82–84]. With this organocatalyst, various pinacol boronic esters could be homologated to α-chloroboronic esters via the corresponding boronate complex with good yield and enantioselectivity (Scheme 9). The α-chloroboronic esters could then be subjected to further homologations in the usual manner.

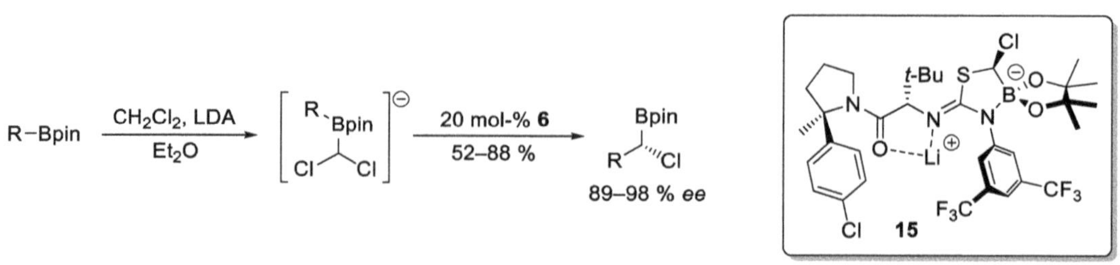

Scheme 9. Catalytic, enantioselective homologation according to Jacobsen et al. [82–84].

3. Syntheses of Marine Natural Products via Matteson Homologation

The homologation of boron esters developed by Donald S. Matteson was not only used in a variety of pharmaceutically and biologically relevant compounds [85–90], such as terpenes [91], carbohydrates [22], alkaloids [92] and pheromones [35,93–96], but also for the construction of a wide range of marine natural products.

3.1. Dictyopterene A

Dictyopterene A was isolated by Moore et al. as the main component of an odoriferous oil from seagrass of the species *Dictyopteris* [97]. It belongs to a group of sexual attractants that are found in various brown algae (*Phaeophyceae*). The various dictyopterene derivatives differ primarily in the position and in the number of unsaturations of the two substituents on the cyclopropane ring. In their synthesis of dictyopterene A, Pietruszka et al. used a Matteson homologation towards the end of their synthesis to obtain the primary alcohol **16** from cyclopropylboronic ester **16** by elongation with $LiCH_2Cl$ and subsequent oxidation (Scheme 10). Alcohol **17** was finally converted into the natural product by Dess–Martin oxidation and Wittig reaction [98].

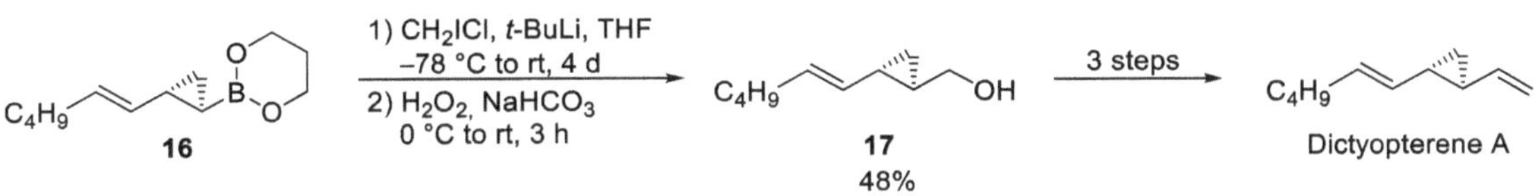

Scheme 10. Synthesis of dictyopterene A according to Pietruszka et al. [98].

3.2. Awajanomycin

Awajanomycin was extracted in 2006 from a marine fungus of the species *Acremonium* sp. AWA16-1. The compound shows moderate cytotoxicity in the mid-μ-molar range. Most conspicuous is its bicyclic structure formed by a lactone and a lactam ring [99].

To set up the (Z)-configured allyl boronic ester **20**, Koert and coworkers reacted the dichloroboronic ester **18** first with MeLi and then with the (Z)-vinyllithium derivative **19**, whereby the desired allyl boronic ester **20** was obtained with good yield and selectivity (Scheme 11). Subsequent allylation of the tricarbonyl compound **21** yielded highly stereoselective compound **22**, which could be further converted into awajanomycin [100].

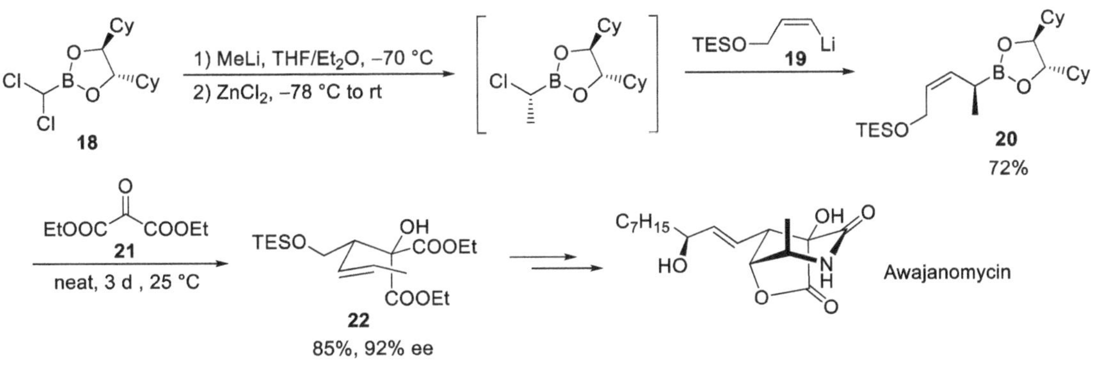

Scheme 11. Synthesis of awajanomycin according to Koert et al. [100].

3.3. Danicalipin A

Danicalipin A belongs to a group of polychlorinated natural products called chlorosulfolipids. Similar to phospholipids, sulfolipids consist of a non-polar lipophilic and a polar hydrophilic part. They are mainly found in membranes of microalgae, e.g., danicalipin A is the main component of the cell membrane of *Ochromonas danica* [101]. Sulfolipids are usually cytotoxic and often responsible for seafood poisoning. Above all, the unusual structure has aroused the interest of synthetic chemists. A key step in the synthesis of the Burns group [102] was the extension of the chlorinated vinyl boronic ester **23** to the corresponding α-chloroboronic ester **24**, which was immediately further reacted to avoid decomposition (Scheme 12). For the incorporation of the first dichlorinated side chain, the primary iodide **25** was first lithiated with BuLi and then converted into the Grignard reagent before it was reacted with **24**. Transmetalation was necessary because the lithium compound proved to be unstable and some lithium-halogen exchange with the two chlorine atoms of the side chain was observed. The second half of the molecule was also introduced in a highly stereoselective manner by reacting **26** (>99%ee) with chlorinated aldehyde **27**. For this purpose, **26** was first converted into the borinate using *n*-BuLi and trifluoroacetanhydride [103,104], which yielded significantly better yields in the subsequent allylation than **26**, so that **28** could be obtained in gram scale. Danicalipin A was finally obtained in a few further steps.

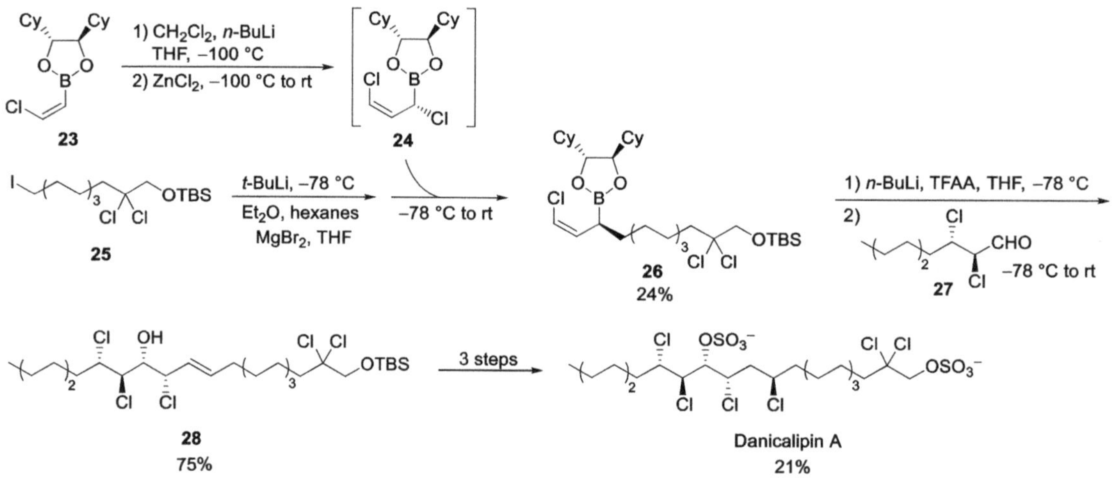

Scheme 12. Synthesis of danicalipin A according to Burns et al. [102].

3.4. Motuporin

Motuporin was isolated by Andersen and coworkers from the sponge *Theonella swinhoi Gray*, which was found around Papua New Guinea [105]. Motuporin belongs to the group of nodularins [106], very strong inhibitors of protein phosphatase 1 (PP1), and motuporin is one of the most active representatives. PP1 is inhibited at subnanomolar concentrations. In addition, motuporin also shows high cytotoxicity against various cancer cell lines. The most striking structural feature is the double unsaturated β-amino acid (2*S*,3*S*,8*S*,9*S*)-3-amino-9-methoxy-2,6,8-trimethyl-10-phenyl-4,6-decadienoic acid (ADDA), which is also found in other natural products such as microcystin [107]. Another unusual amino acid is (2*R*,3*S*)-2-methylaspartic acid. Both building blocks could be obtained by Matteson homologation via a common precursor.

To introduce *N*-functionalities either LiHMDS [108,109] or azide [110] can be used as nucleophiles. Ammonia and primary amines, on the other hand, are not suitable because the α-aminoboronic esters obtained are rather labile and decompose rapidly [111]. In contrast, reactions of α-chloroboronic acid esters with LHMDS yield stable silylated α-aminoboronic esters, which can be desilylated and acylated in a one-pot reaction. Further homologations of silylated α-aminoboronic esters are possible, but are usually slow and normally provide low yields [112,113]. In contrast, azides, generated from sodium azide under two-phase conditions in the presence of a phase transfer catalyst [23], are often tolerated in subsequent Matteson homologations.

Bauer and Armstrong used this protocol to synthesize the unusual amino acids of motuporin (Scheme 13) [114]. Starting from the PMB-protected boronic ester **29**, the α-chloroboronic ester **30** was formed under standard conditions, which was further reacted with MeMgCl to form the α-methylated boronic ester **31**. Due to the relatively low nucleophilicity of the azide, the slightly more reactive α-bromoboronic ester was prepared for further elongation, which was reacted under Matteson's phase transfer conditions. This was the only step in which some minor epimerization was observed [115]. The subsequent chain extension was carried out with $LiCH_2Cl$ to **32** before the boronic ester was finally oxidized to alcohol. The order in which the reaction components were added was of decisive importance. The hydrogen peroxide had to be added prior to the sodium hydroxide solution to obtain a reasonable yield. In reversed order, predominantly alkene was obtained, probably by elimination of the β-azidoboronate complex. After catalytic hydrogenation and Boc-protection of the free amine, the desired aldehyde **33** was obtained via Dess–Martin oxidation [116]. Aldehyde **33** was the common starting material for the synthesis of both amino acids.

For the synthesis of methyl aspartate, the aldehyde **33** was oxidized to carboxylic acid which was protected as methyl ester **34**. Subsequently, the PMB ether was cleaved with 2,3-dichloro-5,6-dicyano-1,4-benzoquinone (DDQ) [117] and the free alcohol was subjected to a Pinnick oxidation [118]. The free acid was coupled with *t*-butyl valinate to **35**. After cleavage of the Boc protecting group, the dipeptide was incorporated into the linear peptide chain.

To build up the ADDA, aldehyde **33** was subjected to a Wittig reaction with **36**, which gave the best results using LDA as a base. However, attempts to cleave the primary PMB ether of **37** with DDQ did not lead to the desired product, but to a cleavage of the *N*-Boc protecting group and oxidation of the amine to a ketone.

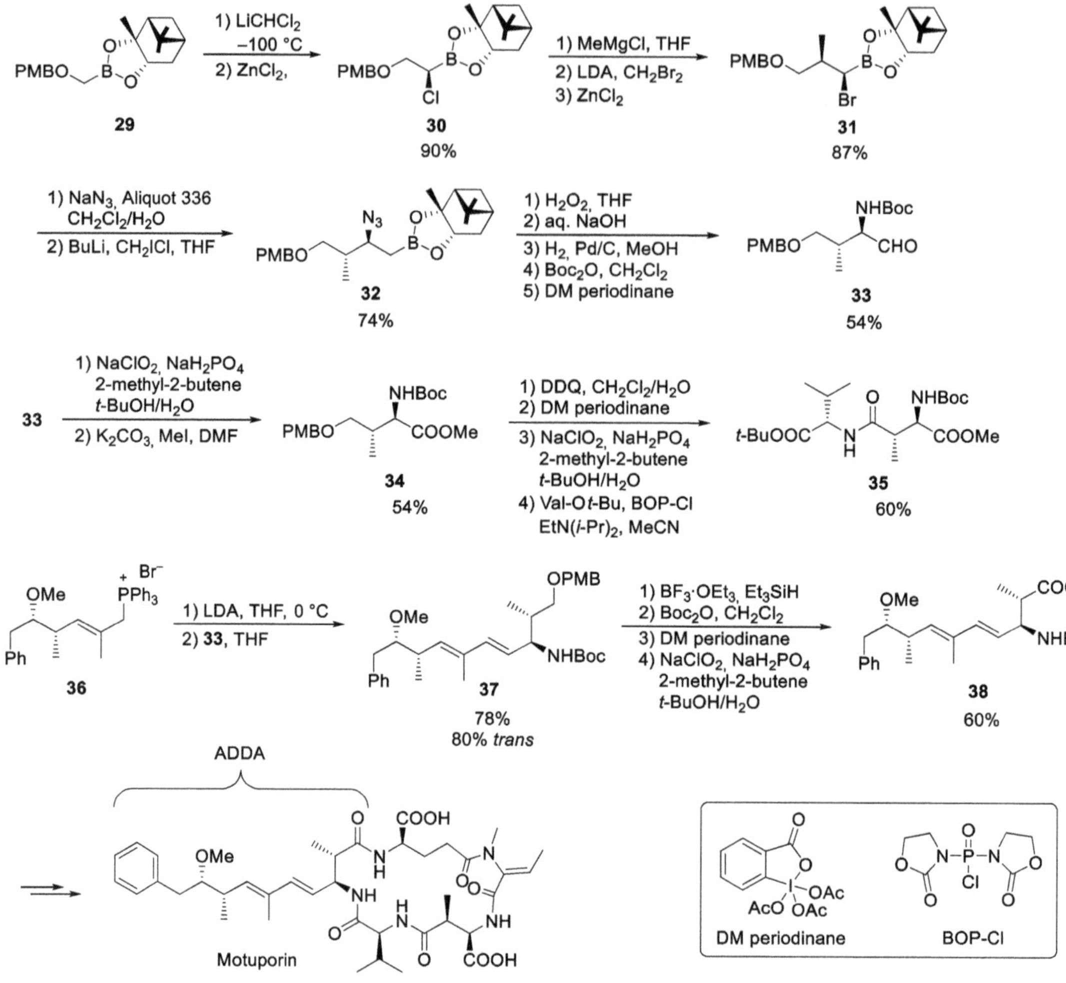

Scheme 13. Synthesis of motuporin according to Armstrong et al. [114].

Therefore, the PMB ether was cleaved simultaneously with the Boc protecting group under acidic conditions and the free amine was protected again. Subsequent Dess–Martin (DM) and Pinnick oxidation yielded the desired unsaturated amino acid **38**, which was incorporated into motuporin.

3.5. Callipeltin A

The callipeltines also belong to a group of marine cyclopeptides with unusual amino acid building blocks [119–122]. Callipeltin A, the largest representative of the family, was isolated in 1996 by Zampella and colleagues from the marine sponge *Callipelta* sp. and shows interesting antiviral, antifungal and cytotoxic properties [10]. In addition to the amino acids (2*R*,3*R*)-β-methoxy tyrosine, (2*R*,3*R*,4*S*)-4-amino-7-guanidino-2,3-dihydroxy-heptanoic acid (AGDHA), (2*S*,3*S*,4*R*)-dimethyl-glutamine (diMeGln) and (*D*)-*allo*-threonine, the natural product also contains a *N*-terminal polyketide fragment (2*R*,3*R*,4*R*) 3-hydroxy-2,4,6-trimethylheptanoic acid (TMEHA). The latter three building blocks were obtained by Horn and Kazmaier via Matteson homologation [123,124].

The *N*-benzyl-protected DiMeGln was obtained starting from boronic ester **39**, which was extended in four successive homologation steps to **40** (Scheme 14). The two methyl groups were introduced by the reaction of the corresponding α-chloroboronic esters with MeMgCl. The azide was generated here not under phase transfer conditions but using sodium azide in DMF [125,126]. Final homologation and direct oxidation of the α-chloroboronic esters under Pinnick conditions yielded the carboxylic acid which was subjected to esterification. However, the trityl residue could not be removed by catalytic hydrogenation, as spontaneous lactonization was observed. In contrast, direct Jones oxidation delivered the desired acid which was reacted with benzylamine to amide **41** in overall good yield.

The β-hydroxy acid building block TMEHA was obtained analogously from isobutyl boronic ester **42**. The protected OH functionality was introduced by using sodium *p*-methoxybenzylate as a nucleophile. The subsequent implementation with MeMgBr was extremely slow, even after 14 days no complete conversion could be achieved. In contrast, the reaction with the more reactive MeMgCl was complete after 3 days. The final homologation of **43** and Pinnick oxidation gave rise to the desired acid **44**.

The (D)-*allo*-threonine, which is commercially available but rather expensive, was obtained analogously from methylboronic ester **45**. Interestingly, the elongation of the azido boronic ester **46** had to be carried out with deprotonated dibromomethane to suppress side reactions. Subsequent oxidation yielded the desired acid in almost quantitative yields. After esterification, the azide **47** was reduced and the free amine was Alloc-protected before the methyl ester was saponified. Classical peptide coupling chemistry was used to obtain protected callipeltin A.

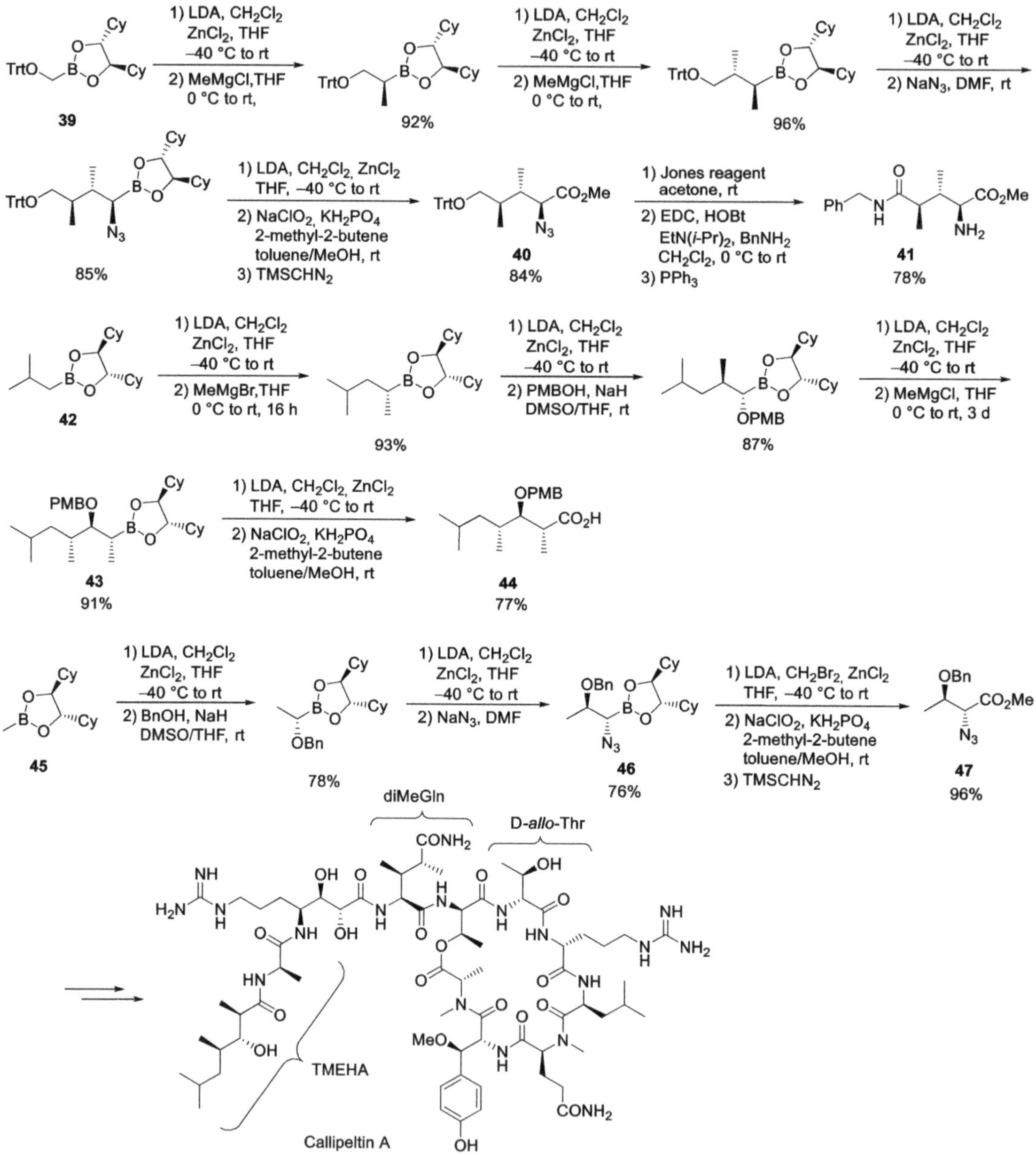

Scheme 14. Synthesis of callipeltin A according to Horn and Kazmaier [123,124].

3.6. Tautomycin

Tautomycin, which is found in various shellfish, was isolated by Isono et al. from the fermentation broth of *Streptomyces spiroverticillatus* [127]. It is a selective inhibitor of the serine/threonine phosphatases PP1 and PP2a but shows no structural similarity to motuporin, which shows a similar biological effect. Tautomycin contains an interesting spiroketal unit and a terminal unsaturated anhydride (Figure 2).

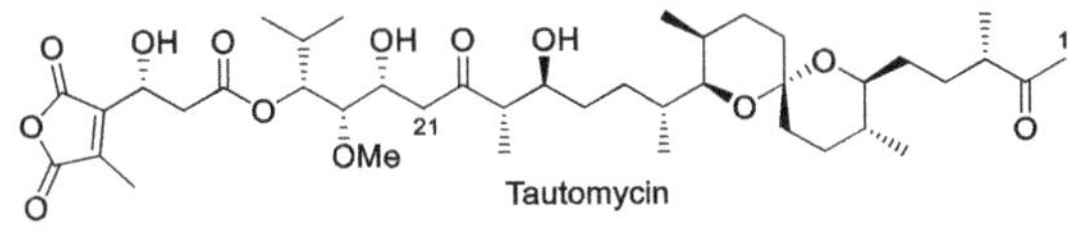

Figure 2. Tautomycin.

In connection with the synthesis of various PP1 inhibitors, Maurer and Armstrong also developed a synthesis for the right-hand C1–C21 fragment of tautomycin, based on the Matteson homologation [128]. This fragment was then to be coupled to the left half of the molecule via an aldol reaction.

The right half of the molecule was built up from two fragments, both obtained via Matteson homologations, which were then linked via a Ni/Cr coupling (Scheme 15). Starting the synthesis chiral boronic acid ester **48** was extended to the corresponding α-chloroboronic ester (61%) and further reacted with 3-butenylmagnesium bromide to **49**. The Grignard reagent was slowly added until the entire α-chloroboronic ester was consumed. The next extension to the α-chloroboronic ester **50** was unproblematic (92%), but the addition of lithium *p*-methoxybenzyl alcoholate had to be carefully controlled. The reaction was aborted after the chloroboronic ester was consumed. Longer reaction times caused a drop in the yield of **51**. In the next extension step, a TBS-protected Grignard reagent proved superior to the THP-protected derivative, which was prone to the formation of by-products. Further elongation of the boronic acid ester **52** and oxidation provided the primary alcohol **53**, which was reduced with $LiAlH_4$ after activation as a mesylate. Compound **54** was then converted into aldehyde **55** via further standard operations, which represents the C-10 to C-21 fragment of the desired building block.

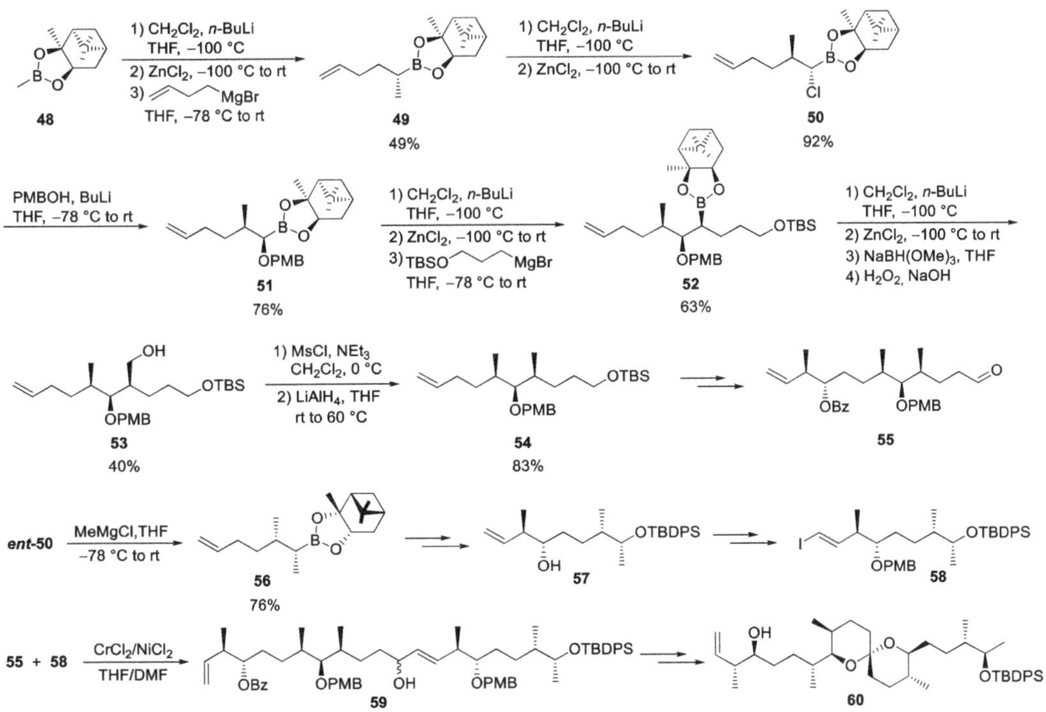

Scheme 15. Synthesis of tautomycin according to Maurer and Armstrong [128].

The second part of the fragment started from the enantiomeric boronic ester *ent*-**48**, which was converted into the enantiomeric α-chloroboronic ester *ent*-**50** as described. Reaction with methylmagnesium chloride yielded boronic ester **56**. Oxidation and protection of the secondary alcohol, ozonolysis followed by crotyl boration yielded homoallyl alcohol **57**, which gave rise to the desired vinyl iodide **58** after PMB-protection, ozonolysis and subsequent Takai reaction [129]. Kishi–Nozaki coupling [130,131] of **55** and **58** using $NiCl_2$-doped $CrCl_2$ yielded the allyl alcohol **59**, which could ultimately be converted into the desired fragment **60**.

3.7. Emericellamide A

In 2007, Fenical and co-workers described the isolation of the two cyclic lipodepsipeptides emericellamide A and B from the marine fungus *Emericella* sp. Both compounds show activity against methicillin-resistant *Staphylococcus aureus* (MRSA) strains in the low μ-molar range, with emericellamide A being the slightly more active compound (3.8 μM (A) vs. 6.0 μM (B)). The moderate cytotoxicity of both compounds is striking. For the synthesis of emericellamide A and the formation of β-hydroxycarboxylic acid **63**, Priester and Kazmaier started their synthesis from the well-known methylboronic acid ester **45** [30,37], which was reacted with hexylmagnesium bromide under standard conditions to the homologated boronic acid ester **61** (Scheme 16) [132]. The next homologation with *p*-methoxybenzylate was performed in the presence of DMSO to accelerate the 1,2-migration of the alkoxy nucleophile [22]. However, the subsequent introduction of a methyl group was very slow under the usual conditions. However, the reaction could be accelerated by isolating the α-chloroboronic acid ester and reacting with the methyl Grignard reagent. Further Matteson homologation of **62** and Pinnick oxidation yielded carboxylic acid **63**. Unfortunately, separation of the product from the auxiliary was not possible at this time, so **63** was directly linked to glycine benzyl ester (**64**). After esterification of the chiral diol with methylboronic acid (under regeneration of **45**) and PMB deprotection, the resulting alcohol could be incorporated into the peptide.

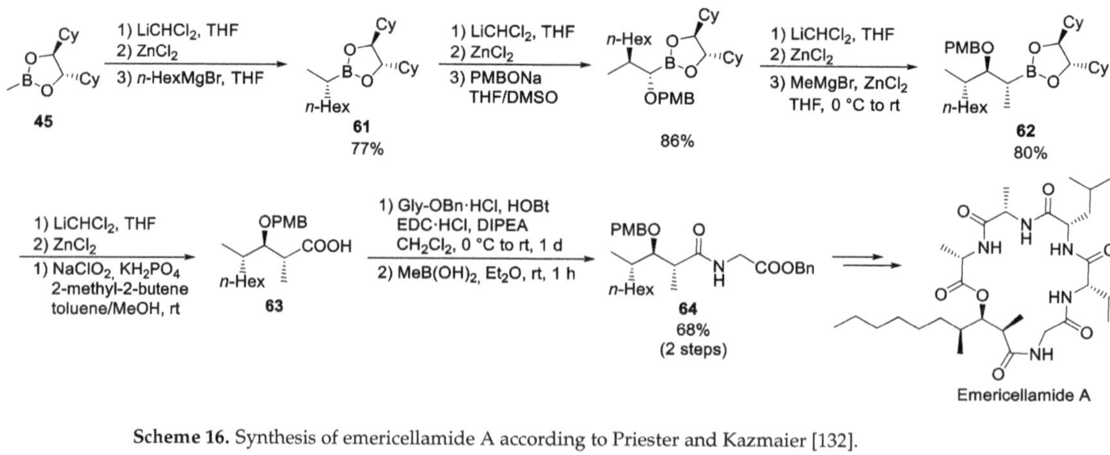

Scheme 16. Synthesis of emericellamide A according to Priester and Kazmaier [132].

3.8. Lagunamides A

Lagunamides A and B, isolated from the marine cyanobacterium *Lyngbya majuscula* [8] belong to an interesting class of structurally closely related marine cyclodepsipeptides, such as kulokekahilide-2,2 [133–135] odoamide1 [136] and aurilide [137–139]. Both lagunamides show interesting biological properties, e.g., nanomolar cytotoxicity against various tumor cell lines as well as interesting anti-malarial activity. Lagunamide A stimulates caspase-

and mitochondria-mediated apoptosis in tumor cells [140]; however, the exact target was not known until now. Very recently, based on thermal protein profiling (TPP) experiments, Sieber, Zahler and coworkers could identify EYA3 as a stabilized protein in cells upon lagunamide A treatment. Furthermore, they could show that lagunamide A sensitized tumor cells to treatment with doxorubicin, highlighting a putative therapeutic strategy [141].

In their synthesis of lagunamide A, Gorges and Kazmaier also started with methylboronic acid ester **45**, which was subjected to Matteson homologation with ethyl Grignard reagent, whereby boronic acid ester **65** was formed diastereomerically pure in almost quantitative yield (Scheme 17) [24]. In the next step, the raw chloroboronic ester formed was reacted directly with benzyl alcoholate providing ester **66**. The next homologation step with MeMgCl went smoothly but required a rather long reaction time of 14 days. The formation of the last stereogenic center was achieved by a further homologation step using *p*-methoxybenzylate. For the introduction of the CH_2 group, lithiated bromomethane was generated from dibromomethane with BuLi [40]. The final homologation from **67** to **68** was unproblematic, and the aldehyde **69** was finally obtained by oxidation of the α-chloroboronic acid ester **68**. To improve purification, the raw mixture was treated with methylboronic acid, which allowed the formation of **69** as well as the near-quantitative recovery of the initial boron ester **45**.

To complete the polyketide unit, the aldehyde **69** should be converted to the α,β-unsaturated ester in a Horner–Wadsworth–Emmons reaction. However, since the benzyl protection group could not be cleaved selectively in the presence of the α,β-unsaturated ester in the further course of synthesis, the aldehyde was first protected and the polyketide fragment was linked to *N*-methylalanine (N-Me-Ala) after cleavage of the benzyl ether (**70**). After acetal cleavage, the subsequent Horner–Wadsworth–Emmons reaction to **71** gave the best results when the lithium salt of hexafluoroisopropanol (HFIP) was used as a base. The further construction of the lagunamide A did not cause any further problems.

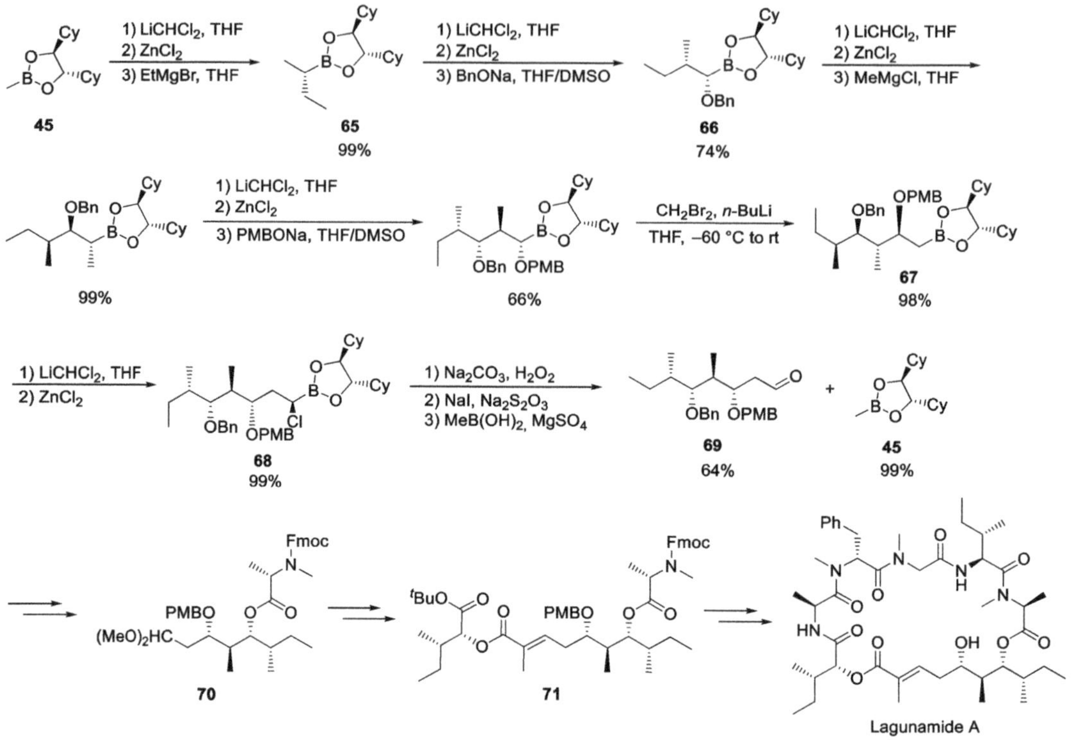

Scheme 17. Synthesis of lagunamide A according to Gorges and Kazmaier [24].

It was known from SAR studies with the structurally closely related aurimide and analogs that the hydroxyl group of the polyketide has only a minor influence on biological activity and can be removed or acylated without much loss of activity [142]. Therefore, a shortened synthesis route was developed that allowed access to a diastereomeric polyketide part, based on the use of ester dienolates as nucleophiles. Matteson had reported that deprotonated *tert*-butyl esters are suitable as nucleophiles [23,24], and Andler and Kazmaier have now extended this concept to deprotonated α,β-unsaturated esters [143]. In this case, the OH group is not generated by S_N2 reaction, but by oxidation of the boric acid ester and therefore has the opposite configuration. Starting from building block **72**, which already contains the first three stereogenic centers, homologation with $CHBr_2Li$ and the subsequent reaction with the dienolate of the ethyl tiglate yielded the extended boronic ester **73**, which was then oxidized to the desired polyketide fragment **74** (Scheme 18). However, incorporation into the isomeric lagunamide showed that in this case, an inversion of the stereocenter led to a significant drop in biological activity.

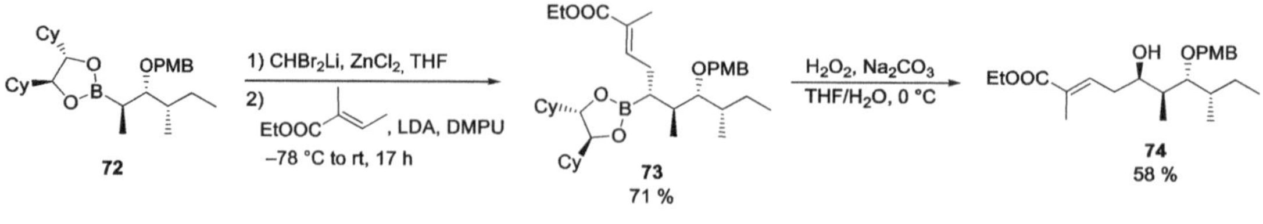

Scheme 18. Synthesis of polyketide fragment **74** according to Andler and Kazmaier [143].

3.9. Apratoxin A and B

Apratoxins are another interesting class of cyclodepsipeptides produced by marine cyanobacteria [144–147]. The first representative of this group, apratoxin A, isolated from the cyanobacterium *Lyngbya majuscula*, was described in 2001 by Moore and Paul et al. [9]. Among other activities, it showed high cytotoxicity against a number of tumor cell lines in the subnanomolar range [148–150]. In the following years, further apratoxins were isolated [146,151], some of which are shown in Figure 3. The apratoxins form a 25-membered ring consisting of a pentapeptide and a rather unusual polyketide fragment, which in most cases contains a terminal *t*-butyl group. They differ primarily in the methylation pattern and in the structure of the polyketide fragment, slight variations are also found in the peptide part.

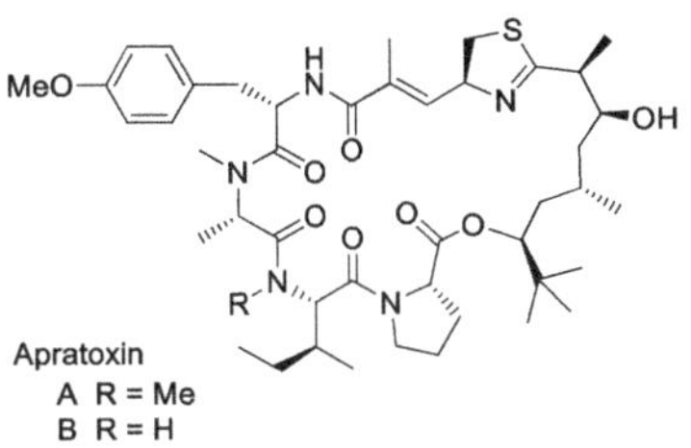

Figure 3. Selected apratoxins.

Andler and Kazmaier developed a Matteson homologation-based synthesis of apratoxin A and B starting from chiral boronic ester **75** (Scheme 19) [152]. Regardless of the steric hindrance by the *t*-butyl group, the conversion to the corresponding α-chloroboronic ester was successful, which could be reacted with an excess of alcoholate to **76**. Three further homologation steps resulted in boronic ester **77**, which was stereoselectively reacted with the Li-enolate of *t*-butylpropionate (*d.r.* 9:1) to **78** in a final extension step [8,24]. The secondary alcohol formed by oxidation was temporarily Troc-protected before the PMB protection group was removed.

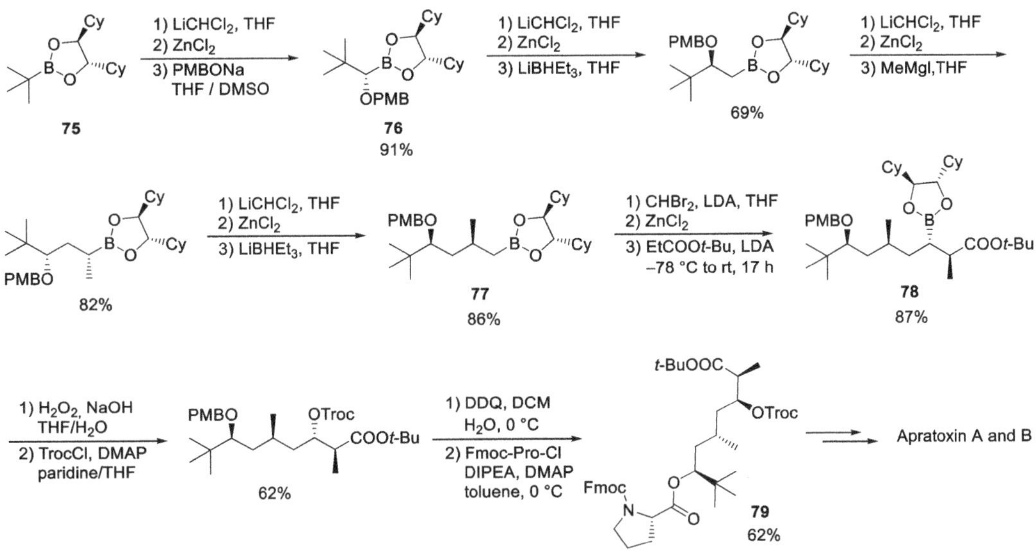

Scheme 19. Syntheses of apratoxins A and B according to Andler and Kazmaier [152].

The coupling of the alcohol formed with the acid chloride of Fmoc-proline yielded the ester **79** in excellent yield and without epimerization of the α stereocenter at the proline. The acidic cleavage of the *t*-butyl ester resulted in the free carboxylic acid, which could finally be incorporated into the desired apratoxins. During that, partial epimerization of the stereocenter adjacent to the thiazoline unit was observed, but the isomers could be separated by preparative HPLC.

3.10. Doliculide

The isolation of (−)doliculide from the Japanese seahare, *Dolabella auricularia*, was first reported by Yamada et al. almost 30 years ago, together with the pronounced cytotoxicity of this compound against HeLa-S3 cells (IC_{50} = 1 ng/mL) [153]. The nudibranch itself does not necessarily have to be the producer of this cyclic depsipeptide, as it has been shown that other metabolites isolated from *Dolabella auricularia* often come from cyanobacteria and are therefore of dietary origin [154]. Doliculide is a potent actin binder that initiates actin aggregation, resulting in inhibition of proliferation and apoptosis [155–159]. It was shown that doliculide stabilizes F-actin in a similar way to structurally related natural products such as jaspamid or miuraenamide [160–162]. Subtoxic doses of doliculide result in a transient change in reversible cytoskeletal dynamics and induction of premature senescence in p53 wild-type cells [163].

Doliculide consists of a halogenated dipeptide segment and a polyketide unit with five stereogenic centers that can be built up by Matteson homologation (Scheme 20). In order to be able to specifically vary the C-terminal end of the polyketide fragment at a late stage of the synthesis, Kazmaier and coworkers chose the sequential construction of the polyketide in the opposite direction as the natural biosynthesis [44].

Starting from the trityl-protected boronic ester *ent*-**39** [164], the reaction with deprotonated methylene chloride and subsequently with the Grignard reagent in a one-pot reaction yielded the extended boronic ester **80**. The next extension step was carried out with lithiated dibromomethane and the α-bromoboronic ester was reduced with $NaBH_4$ to **81**. The repetition of these steps led to the boronic acid ester **82**, which was homologated with *p*-methoxybenzylate to **83**. The next CH_2 insertion to **84** went well, while the introduction of the final isopropyl group required some optimizations. In this case, the direct reaction of the α-chloroboronic ester resulted in a mixture of several products. Better results were obtained when the α-chloroboronic ester was isolated before further conversion.

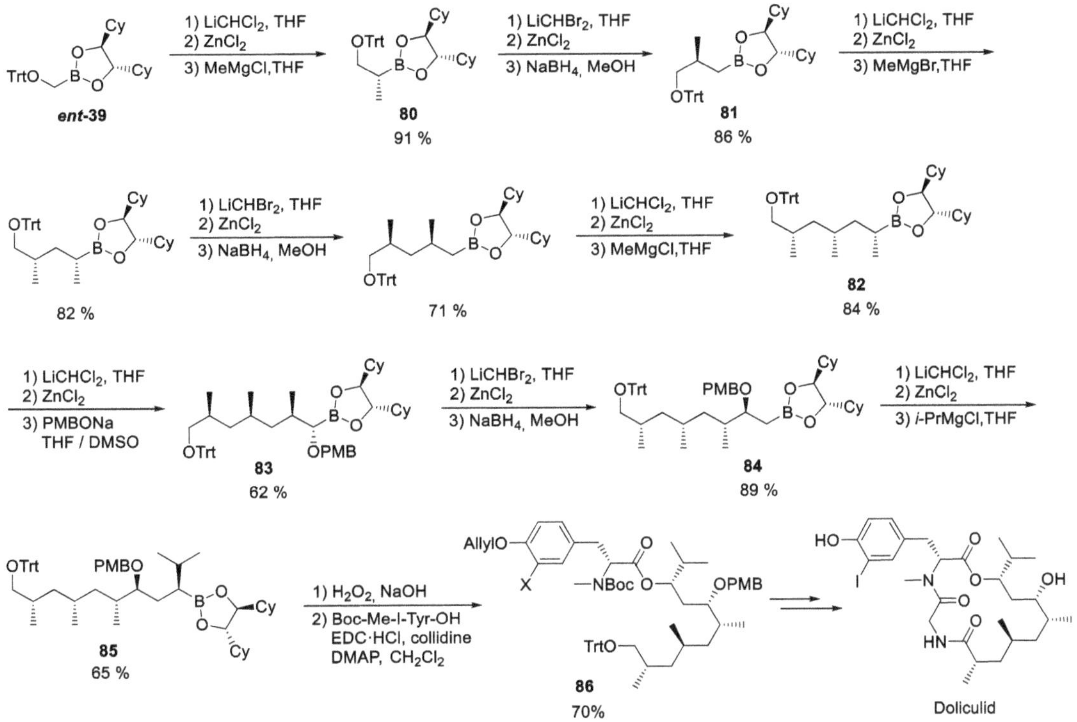

Scheme 20. Synthesis of doliculide according to Kazmaier et al. [44].

The final oxidation of **85** led to the desired protected polyketide precursor which was coupled with *O*-allylated halogenated tyrosine to **86**. Further standard operations gave rise to doliculide. Boronic ester **84** was reacted in an analogous way also with other Grignard reagents (methyl, allyl, progargyl), which allowed the construction of derivatives that could be further modified, e.g., by thiol-ene-click chemistry or [3+2]-cycloadditions [165].

4. Syntheses of Marine Natural Products Using the Lithiation–Borylation Protocol

The lithiation–borylation homologation strategy is based on Hoppe's chiral deprotonated carbamates [50–55] or Beak' aryl esters [56] and has been used by Aggarwal and others in various ways for natural product syntheses [59,166], including a range of marine natural products.

4.1. Solandelactone E and F

Soledanolactones, a group of marine oxylipids, were first isolated from *Solanderia secunda* by Shin and coworkers [167]. As a striking structural feature, they contain an 8-membered lactone ring linked to a *trans*-configured cyclopropane. In soledanolactone E, this unit is linked to a double unsaturated fatty acid residue via an unsaturated *anti*-1,4-ene-diol, while in soledanolactone F this subunit has a *cis* configuration.

In 2010, Aggarwal and co-workers reported on an elegant method for the stereoselective synthesis of such unsaturated *anti*-1,4-diols based on the reaction of chiral lithium carbamates with β-silylvinylboranes [168]. Sparteine-complexed lithiated carbamates react with alkylboranes under inversion, while retention can be observed in the absence of sparteine or other sterically demanding diamine ligands. A 1,2-Shift of the vinyl residue generates chiral allylboranes which can be subjected to allylborations with aldehydes in a highly enantioselective fashion. Due to the steric demand of the bicyclononane scaffold on the boron, the allylic substituent preferentially occupies an axial position in the Zimmermann–Traxler transition state, which ultimately leads to the *anti*-configured product. This reaction sequence was used in the synthesis of soledanolactone A (Scheme 21) [169].

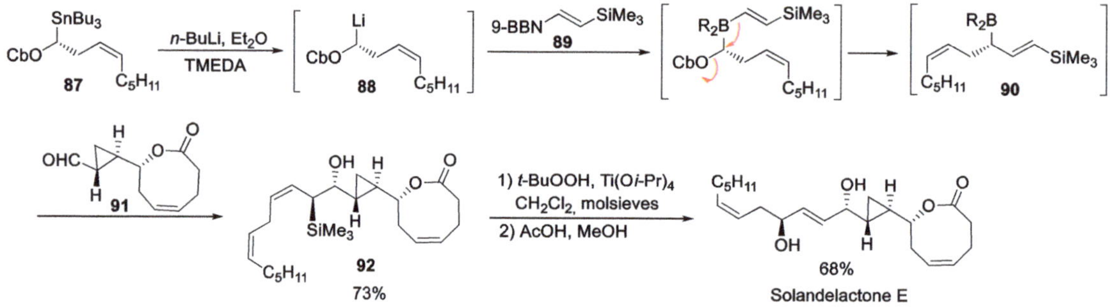

Scheme 21. Synthesis of soledanolactone E according to Aggarwal et al. [169].

For this purpose, the chiral tin reagent **87** was transmetalated with *n*-BuLi (e.r. 10:1) giving rise to an "diamine free" lithiated carbamate **88** which was reacted with the silylated vinyl borane **89** to provide allylborane **90**. The addition of aldehyde **91** to the in situ formed **90** provided the desired allylsilane **92** initially in a rather low yield (15%). The problem resulted from the poor stirrability of the viscous reaction mixture. By adding TMEDA in the transmetalation step, this problem was solved and the yield could be increased to 73%. The diastereomers (i.e., 10:1) could be separated at this stage, whereby the lithium-boron exchange took place under complete retention even in the presence of TMEDA. Sharpless epoxidation of **92** allowed the selective oxidation of the homoallyl alcohol in the presence of the other two double bonds [170]. Acid-catalyzed ring-opening-elimination of the α-silylated epoxide yielded diastereomerically pure soledanolactone E.

Robinson and Aggarwal also developed a slightly modified route that leads to *syn*-2-ene-1,4-diols, such as soledanolactone F [171]. In principle, if the (*E*)-configured allyl silane is preferentially formed in the allylation step, this should provide the *syn*-1,4-ene-diol under the same oxidation/elimination conditions. This could be achieved by using β-silylvinyl-boronic acid ethylene glycol ester. However, boronic esters enter into a 1,2-alkyl shift much more slowly than alkyboranes, and allylboration is usually also slower, but can often be accelerated by adding Lewis acids. For example, no vinyl migration was observed when homoallylcarbamate **87** was reacted with vinyl boronic ester **94**, but it occurred when Beak's TIB ester **93** was used (Scheme 22) [56]. The reaction of the allylborane formed with **91** in the presence of $MgBr_2$ yielded the desired (*E*)-allyl silane **95** in reasonable yield and selectivity. Epoxidation with *m*CPBA and acidic elimination in this case yielded soledanolactone F but only in moderate yield and selectivity.

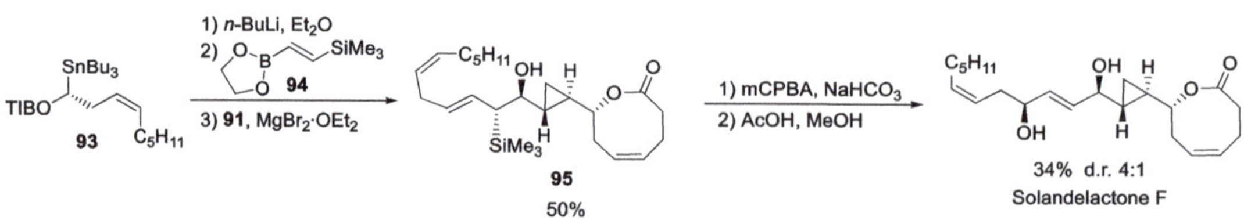

Scheme 22. Synthesis of soledanolactone F according to Robinson and Aggarwal [171].

4.2. *Erogorgiaene*

Erogorgiaene is a marine diterpene natural product isolated from the Pacific horn coral *Pseudopterogorgia elisabethae* that shows promising activity against *Mycobacterium tuberculosis* H37Rov [172]. By applying the lithiation/borylation strategy in combination with protodeborations, the synthesis of four stereoisomers of the erogorgia was achieved. The starting point was the chiral benzyl carbamate **96**, which is easily accessible from *p*-methylacetophenone by Noyori reduction [173]. Reaction with *s*-BuLi and addition of boronic ester **97** yielded tertiary boronic ester **98**, which then protodeborates with TBAF [174] with retention of the configuration (Scheme 23) [175]. Treatment with polyphosphoric acid (PPA) yielded ketone **99**, which was likewise reduced with either the (*S*,*S*) or (*R*,*R*)-Noyori catalyst to obtain the corresponding *trans* and *cis* alcohols enantiomerically pure, in order to subsequently convert them into the desired carbamates **100** and **101**. Such benzylic carbamates can be converted into the corresponding boronates either under retention or inversion, depending on whether alkylborans or boronic esters are used [63]. Model reactions have shown that alkyl dimethylboranes yield the best selectivities with such carbamates, with sterically demanding and seconded alkyl groups migrating preferentially. Therefore, for the introduction of the unsaturated side chain, the chiral boronic pinacol esters **102**, which were accessible via the sparteine route, were converted with MeMgBr into the corresponding dimethylboranes **103**, which were reacted directly with the carbamates **100** and **101**. Final protodeborations with TBAF yielded the desired erogorgiaene and its diastereomers with *d.r.* $\geq$ 9:1.

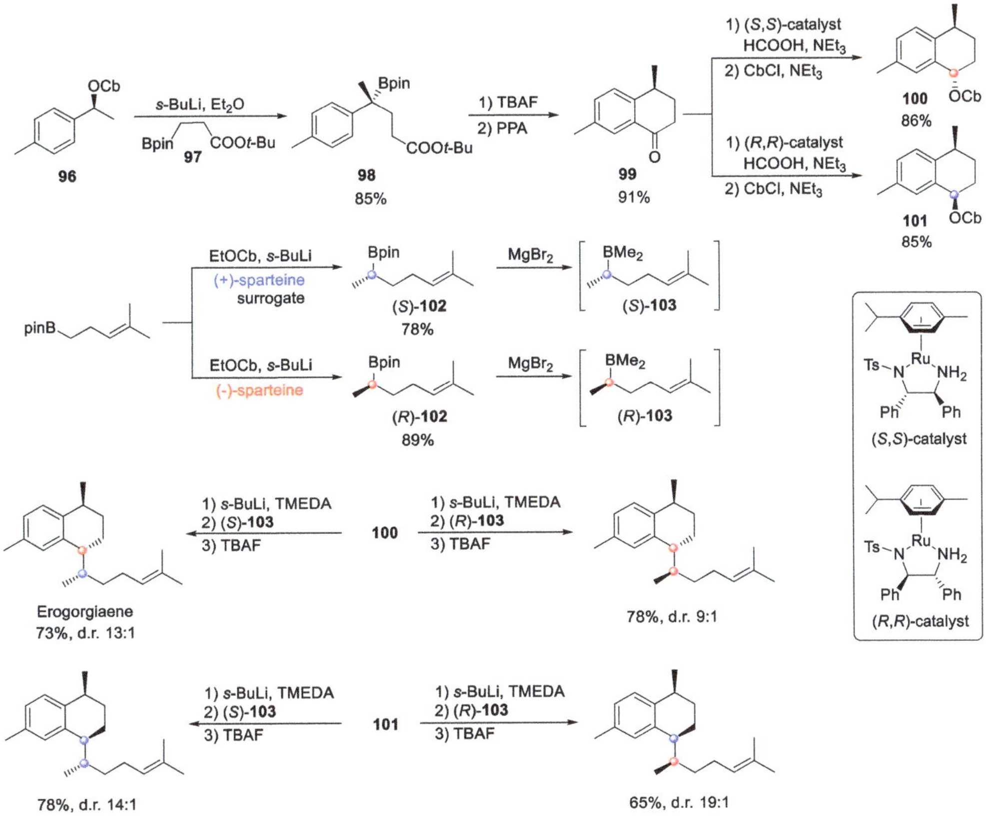

Scheme 23. Synthesis of erogorgiaene and stereoisomers according to Aggarwal et al. [175].

4.3. Sporochnol A

Sporochnol A, isolated from the Caribbean marine alga *Sporochnus bolleanus*, has been shown to exhibit significant feeding deterrence towards herbivorous fish [176]. It can easily be obtained similar to Erogorgiaene from chiral benzyl carbamate **104** (Scheme 24). Reaction with the unsaturated boronic ester **105** yielded the tertiary boronic ester **106**, which was subjected to a Zweifel-olefination [177–179]. The final step was the cleavage of the methyl ether [180]. In a similar way, a number of sesquiterpenes of the Bisabolane family have been obtained [181].

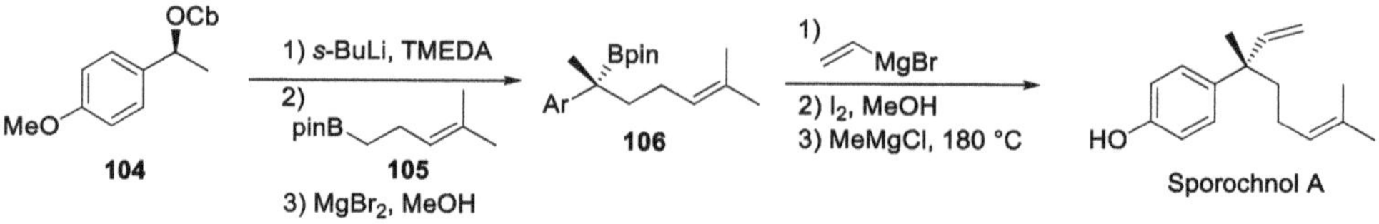

Scheme 24. Synthesis of sporochnol A according to Aggarwal et al. [180].

4.4. Aplysin

Marine mollusks of the *Aplysia* species are known to feed almost exclusively on *Laurencia* algae and store their metabolites with anti-feeding properties to protect themselves from predators [182]. A wide range of sesquiterpenoid natural products have been isolated from these organisms over the last 60 years. Typical representatives are e.g., aplysin and debromoaplysine [183], which are easily accessible via Aggarwal's lithiation-borylation route (Scheme 25) [184].

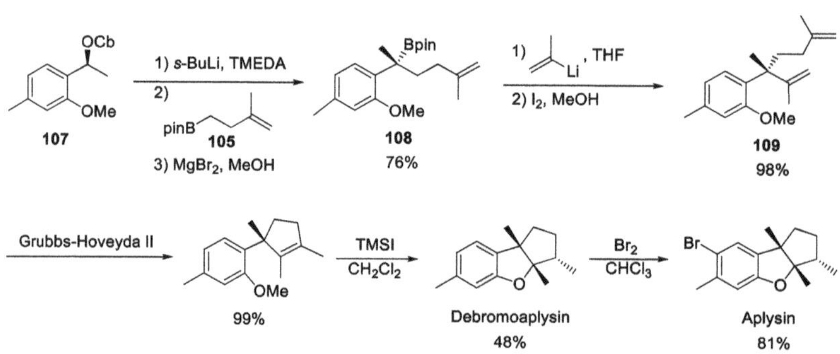

Scheme 25. Synthesis of debromoaplysin and aplysin according to Aggarwal et al. [184].

Again, the key steps were the reaction of a lithiated secondary benzylic carbamate **107** to obtain a tertiary boronic ester **108**, followed by propenylation in which the quaternary stereocenter of **109** was constructed with perfect enantioselectivity. The subsequent ring-closing metathesis, followed by deprotection and in situ cyclization, gave rise to debromoaplysin with good diastereoselectivity. Subsequent bromination provided access to aplysin.

4.5. Filiformin

Filiformin is a sesquiterpene natural compound, isolated from the red seaweed *Laurencia filiformis*, that contains quaternary stereogenic centers [185]. In the synthesis, both a chiral lithiated secondary benzylic and a primary carbamate **111** were used. The latter was generated by transmetalation of the chiral tin compound **110**, which allowed a "diamine-free" reaction (Scheme 26).

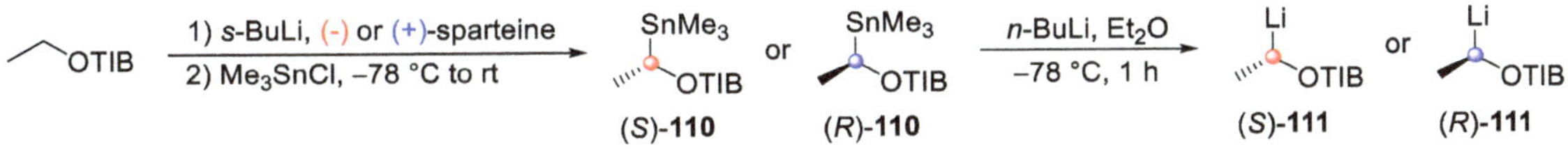

Scheme 26. Generation of "diamine-free" chiral lithiated primary carbamates **111**.

The starting point of the synthesis was the chiral carbamate *ent*-**107**, which, after lithiation, was reacted with the halogenated unsaturated boronic ester **112** to **113** (Scheme 27) [186]. A second homologation with freshly produced (*S*)-**111** delivered the extended boronic ester **114** with perfect enantio- and diastereoselectivity. The key to the success of this challenging homologation was the use of the diamine-free carbenoid **111** and the addition of allyl bromide to quench the benzylic carbanion formed during the 1,2 rearrangement. An intramolecular Zweifel-type olefination yielded methylene cyclopentane **115** in excellent yield. The cleavage of the aromatic methyl ether, acid-catalyzed cyclization and bromination completed the synthesis of the natural product.

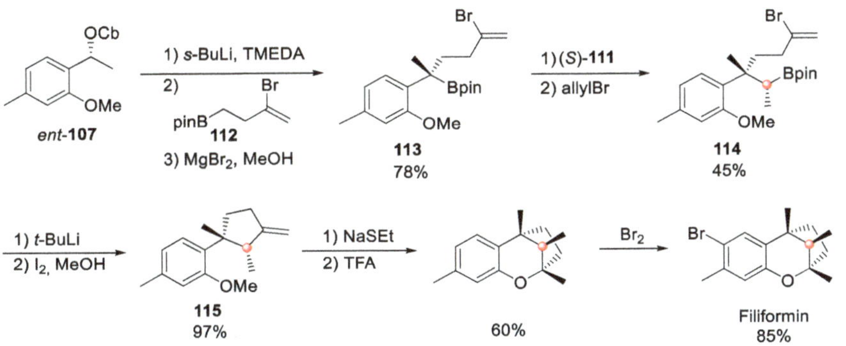

Scheme 27. Synthesis of filiformin according to Aggarwal et al. [186].

4.6. Kalkitoxin

(+)-Kalkitoxin is a neurotoxic lipopeptide isolated from the marine cyanobacterium *Lyngbya majuscula* [187]. The compound showed strong neurotoxicity [188] by blocking the voltage-sensitive Na^+ channel [189]. In this case, only freshly generated lithiated benzoate esters (*S*)-**111** and (*R*)-**111** (Scheme 26), were used to build up the three stereogenic centers of the central polymethylated ω-aminocarboxylic acid [190]. For the introduction of the CH_2 units, $LiCH_2Cl$ (**116**) was freshly prepared using the standard Matteson protocol [38,39].

The synthesis of kalkitoxin started with achiral *p*-methoxybenzyl boronic ester **117** [191], which was successively converted twice with (*S*)-**111**, once with **116**, once with (*R*)-**111** and then twice more with **116** to form the elongated boronic ester **118** (Scheme 28) [192,193]. To introduce the terminal amino group, lithiated *O*-methylhydroxylamine was added [194] and the resulting primary amino group was acylated with **119** and subsequently *N*-methylated. Oxidative cleavage of the electron-rich aromatic ring led to carboxylic acid **120**, which was converted into kalkitoxin.

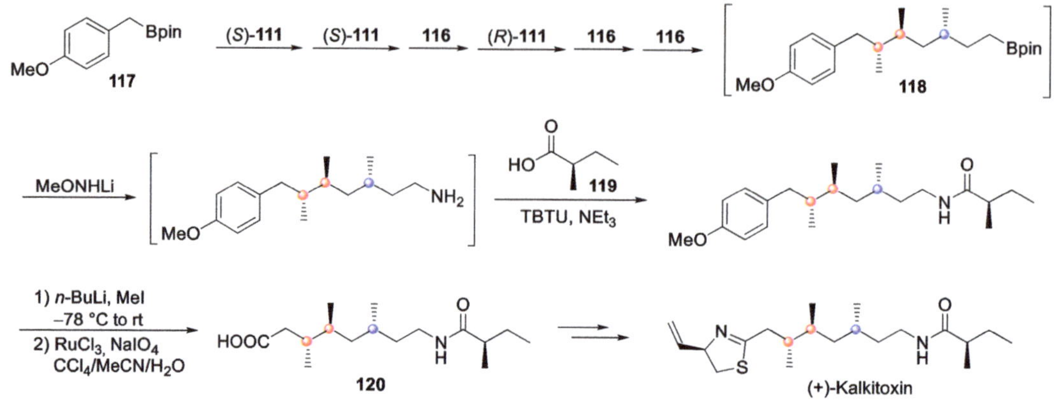

Scheme 28. Synthesis of kalkitoxin according to Aggarwal et al. [192,193].

4.7. Clavosolide A

The clavosolides A–D were isolated from extracts of the sea sponge *Myriastra clavosa*, which was found near the Philippines [195,196]. Crude extracts of *Myriastra clavosa* showed promising cytotoxic and antiproliferative effects in antitumor screenings. However, a detailed investigation of the biological properties was not possible due to the limited quantities available. However, the substance class is not only interesting for synthetic chemists because of its biological activities, but also because of its complex structure. Clavosolide A is a symmetrical dimeric macrolide with highly substituted cyclopropyl, tetrahydropyranyl and glycosidic ring systems.

As part of their synthesis of clavosolide A, Aggarwal and co-workers wanted to show that their lithiation-borylation method can also be used for such complex structures as **121** and used it as a late-stage coupling to perform the last stereoselective C-C coupling (Scheme 29) [197]. The TIB ester proved to be superior as a coordinating group to the initially used Cb-carbamate, as the latter provided only very moderate and varying yields (23–48%) due to competing deprotonation at the glycoside ring. This problem could be circumvented by using the more acidifying TIB-group, which increased the yield in the reaction of **121** with cyclopropane boronic ester **122** to 73%. Direct oxidation of the generated boronic ester yielded the alcohol **123**, which could be converted into clavosolide A in three further standard reactions.

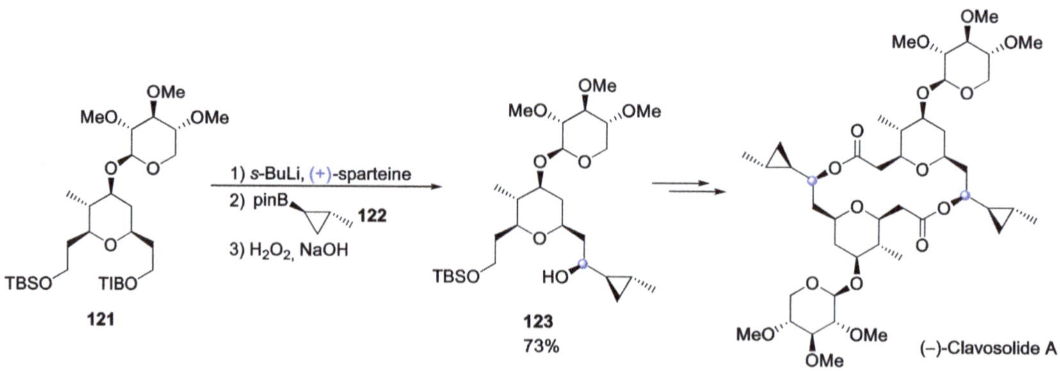

Scheme 29. Synthesis of clavosolide A according to Aggarwal et al. [197].

4.8. Baulamycin A and B

Analysis of extracts of *Streptomyces tempisquensis*, marine bacteria found in the coastal region of Costa Rica led to the isolation of the novel antibiotics baulamycins A and B. These two polyketides are active against the superbug methicillin-resistant *Staphylococcus aureus* (MRSA) and *Bacillus anthracis* [198] as well as several other important bacterial pathogens. Liquid culture studies demonstrated the capacity of these natural products to penetrate bacterial barriers and inhibit the growth of both Gram-positive and Gram-negative species. However, extensive biological studies could not be carried out due to the small amount of material available, and only the smallest amounts of isolated natural products were available for NMR spectroscopic structure determination.

The substitution pattern of the polyketide part is predestined for the application of the assembly line protocol, especially since it allows arbitrary inversion of individual stereocenters. Aggarwal and colleagues were thus able to correct the originally postulated structure by synthesizing various stereoisomers [199]. Their synthesis was based on the linking of two fragments at the central hydroxyl group based on the lithiation-borylation strategy (Scheme 30). The right half of the molecule was converted from boronic ester **124** via assembly-line synthesis into the boronic ester **125**, which was then subjected to a Zweifel olefination. Using a lithiated enol ether in this step yielded **126** as masked ketone. Deprotonation of **126** in the presence of (−)-sparteine followed by a regioselective homologation of the primary boronic ester of **127** resulted in the corresponding 1,3-bis(boric acid ester), which, after oxidation, gave rise to the desired diol in a highly stereoselective fashion. Acid hydrolysis of the protective groups led to the natural products.

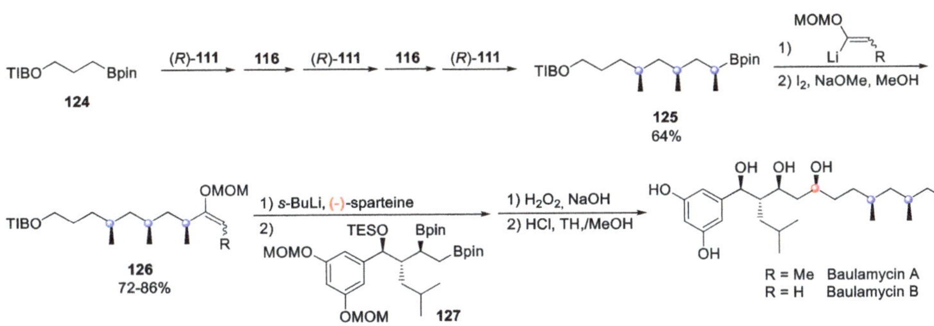

Scheme 30. Syntheses of baulamycin A and B according to Aggarwal et al. [199].

4.9. Bastimolide B

Bastimolide B is a 24-membered polyhydroxylated macrolide isolated from marine cyanobacteria *Okeania hirsute* [200] and, like bastimolide A, has high antimalarial activity, also against multidrug-resistant strains of *Plasmodium falciparum* [201]. Structurally striking is the dense arrangement of hydroxylated stereogenic centers with a 1,5 relationship along a hydrocarbon chain (Figure 4). These 1,5-polyols represent a particularly challenging subject for synthesis, as the distant position of the stereocenters makes their stereoselective generation difficult [202]. To build up such structural motifs, Aggarwal and coworkers have extended their synthetic approach for 1,4-diols to the stereoselective assembly of 1,5 diols [203]. Retrosynthetically, bastimolide B can be split into two main fragments. One is the lactone ring (left half) and the other is the 1,5-polyhydroxylated side chain (right half). The carboxyl terminus of the lactone should be accessible from a terminal alkene via hydroboration/Suzuki coupling. This resulted in the main fragments **128** and **129** that had to be synthesized.

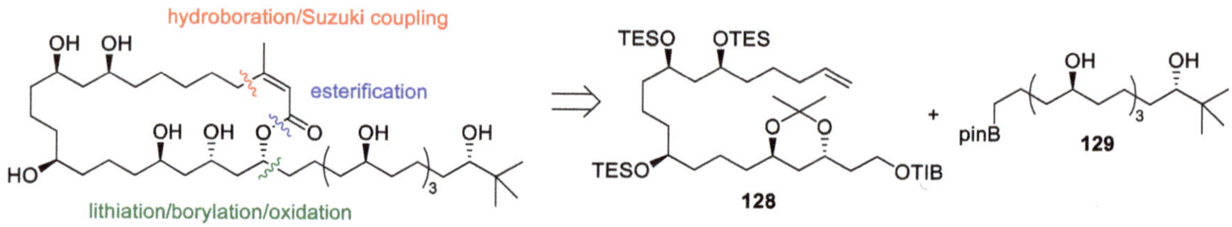

Figure 4. Retrosynthesis of bastimolide B.

The synthesis of fragment **128** started with bisboronic ester **130**, which was obtained from the corresponding homoallylic TIB ester by enantioselective Pt-catalyzed diboration (Scheme 31) [204,205]. Homologation of the primary boron ester with **131**, which was generated in situ from a stable sulfoxide [206,207], and subsequent oxidation yielded 1,3-diol **132**. Repeated enantioselective Pt-catalyzed diboration/homologation/oxidation and final silyl protection yielded the desired building block **128**.

The synthesis of fragment **129** started with the neopentyl TIP ester **133** (Scheme 32). Deprotonation with *s*-BuLi in the presence of (−)-sparteine and subsequent reaction with allyl boronate **134** yielded the desired product **135** with 96% ee, but only in 17% yield, probably due to the steric demand of the sparteine-lithium-carbenoid complex. Therefore, "diamine-free" conditions were used, in which the lithium carbenoid was first transmetalated to the corresponding tin compound and then regenerated on demand "sparteine-free". Under these conditions, the yield of **135** could be increased to 94% (NMR). The crude product was subjected to iridium-catalyzed hydroboration [208–210], and subsequent reaction with magnesium carbenoid **131** yielded the diastereomerically pure 1,5-bisboronic ester. After repeating this sequence twice, the tetraboronic ester was obtained on a gram scale. Oxidation and silyl protection of the tetrol formed yielded the desired fragment **129** after final hydroboration.

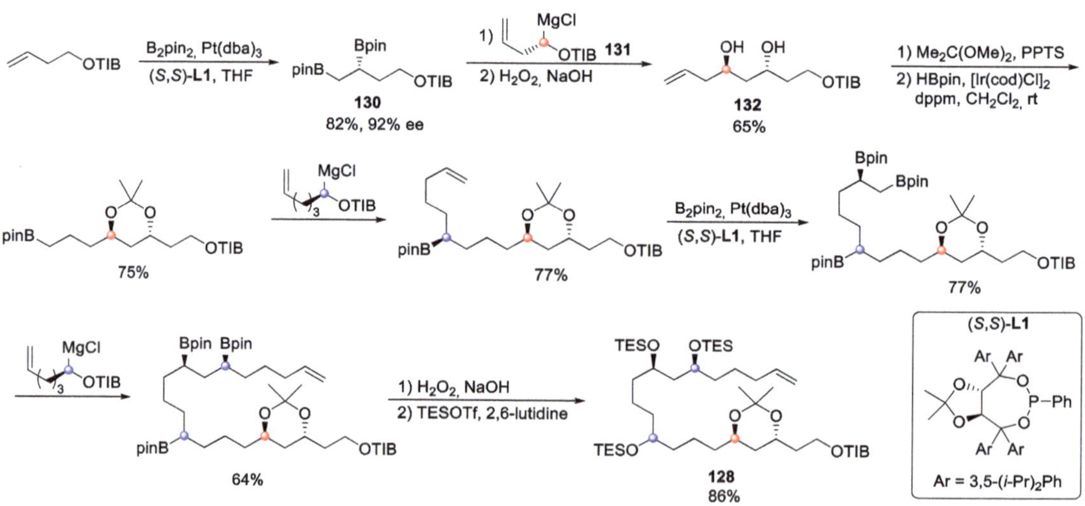

Scheme 31. Syntheses of bastimolide fragment **128**.

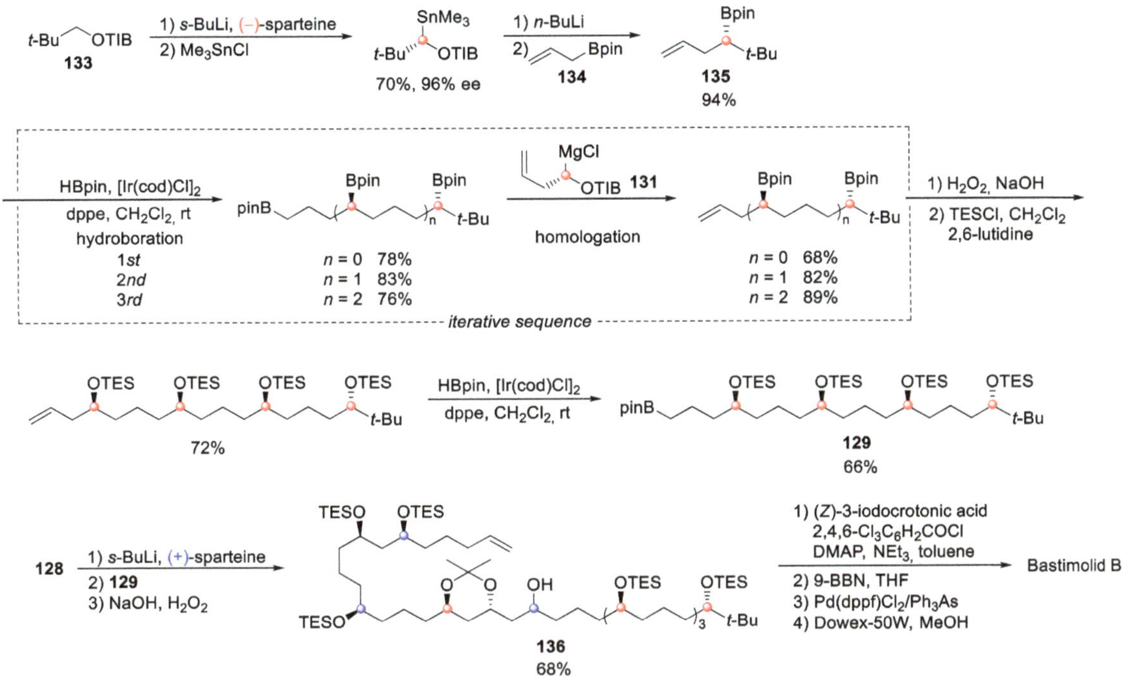

Scheme 32. Syntheses of bastimolide B according to Aggarwal et al. [203].

To connect the two fragments, a slight excess (1.5 equiv.) of **128** was deprotonated in the presence of (+)-sparteine before **129** was added, which led to linear precursor **136** in excellent stereoselectivity after oxidation. Esterification of the secondary alcohol with (Z)-3-iodocrotonic acid, hydroboration of the terminal alkene, and intramolecular Suzuki coupling [211–213] provided the desired macrolactone, which was deprotected under acidic conditions to bastimolide B.

4.10. Rakicidin F

The rakicidines are a family of cyclic depsipeptides isolated from *Streptomyces* sp. and which partially inhibit the invasion of tumor cells [214]. Rakicidin F was extracted from the fermentation broth of the actinomycete strain *Streptomyces* sp. GKU 220, which was isolated from a sea sponge collected in the Andaman Sea near Thailand [215]. Rakicidin F showed moderate growth-inhibiting activity against *B. subtilis* and *E. coli* but no anti-invasive activity, at least at non-cytotoxic concentrations.

The assembly line strategy was well suited for the construction of the tetramethylated β-hydroxy acid. The benzoate ester **137** required could be produced in three steps from the commercially available (S)-Roche ester [216]. Deprotonation in the presence of (+)-sparteine and reaction with $PhMe_2SiBpin$ provided diastereomerically pure boronic ester **138** [166], which was then fed into the cascade of lithiation-borylation reactions to form **139** (Scheme 33). The olefination of **139** to **140** completed the synthesis of the lipophilic side chain, with a yield of 49% over six steps. The subsequent hydrogenation of the double bond initially caused problems, as Pd/C unexpectedly led to the formation of diastereomers, probably due to the migration of the double bond before hydrogenation. However, this problem could be solved by using PtO_2. The subsequent Tamao–Fleming oxidation under Woerpel conditions [217] with simultaneous TES deprotection yielded diol **141** in 92%

over two steps. Oxidation, followed by allylation, resulted in fragment **142**, which was incorporated into the peptide. Final cyclization gave access to rakicidin F.

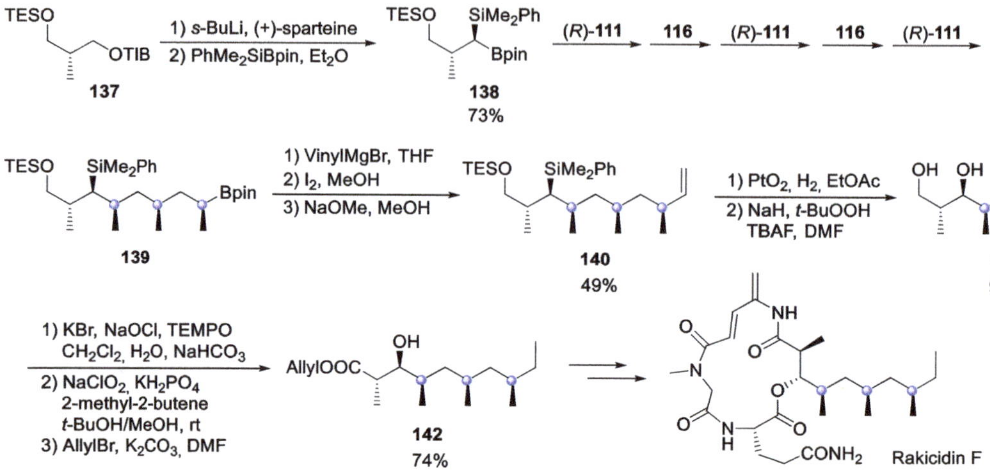

Scheme 33. Syntheses of rakicidin F according to Aggarwal et al. [216].

5. Conclusions

The Matteson homologation, a successive extension of chiral boronic esters, is perfectly suited for the synthesis of complex molecular structures containing many stereogenic centers. The "classical version" allows the introduction of different functional groups in 1,2-*anti*-configuration, but is often limited to this relative configuration, whereby the absolute configuration is determined by the appropriate choice of the chiral auxiliary. The great advantage of the "classical version" results from the multiple use of the chiral auxiliary, since the successive construction of a growing alkyl chain allows the generation of several stereogenic centers controlled by only one auxiliary. In contrast, in Aggarwal's lithiation-borylation strategy, new chiral auxiliary reagents must be used for each reaction step, which on the other hand allows the individual introduction of arbitrary configurations of stereogenic centers. Each method has its individual advantages and disadvantages. Depending on requirements, both synthesis protocols are ideally suited for the synthesis of marine natural products.

Funding: This research was funded by Saarland University and by a grant of the Deutsche Forschungsgemeinschaft (Ka880/13-1 and Bruker Neo 500–447298507) to U.K.

Institutional Review Board Statement: Not applicable.

Informed Consent Statement: Not applicable.

Data Availability Statement: The original contributions presented in this study are included in the article.

Conflicts of Interest: The author declares no competing financial interests.

References

1. Chintoju, N.; Konduru, P.; Kathula, R.L.; Remella, R. Importance of Natural Products in the Modern History. *Res. Rev. J. Hosp. Clin. Pharm.* **2015**, *1*, 5–10.
2. Hamburger, M.; Hostettmann, K. Bioactivity in Plants: The link between Phytochemistry and Medicine. *Phytochemistry* **1991**, *30*, 3864–3874. [CrossRef]

3. Newman, D.J.; Cragg, G.M. Natural Products as Sources of New Drugs over the Last 25 Years. *J. Nat. Prod.* **2007**, *70*, 461–477. [CrossRef] [PubMed]
4. Harvey, A.L. Natural Products in Drug Discovery. *Drug Discov. Today* **2008**, *13*, 894–901. [CrossRef] [PubMed]
5. Mayer, A.M.S.; Glaser, K.B.; Cuevas, C.; Jacobs, R.S.; Kem, W.; Little, R.D.; Mcintosh, J.M.; Newman, D.J.; Potts, B.C.; Shuster, D.E. The Odyssey of Marine Pharmaceuticals: A Current Pipeline Perspective. *Trends Pharmacol. Sci.* **2010**, *31*, 255–265. [CrossRef]
6. Haque, N.; Parveen, S.; Tang, T.; Wei, J.; Huang, Z. Marine Natural Products in Clinical Use. *Mar. Drugs* **2022**, *20*, 528. [CrossRef]
7. Mayer, A.M.S.; Mayer, V.A.; Swanson-Mungerson, M.; Pierce, M.L.; Rodríguez, A.D.; Nakamura, F.; Taglialatela-Scafati, O. Marine Pharmacology in 2019–2021: Marine Compounds with Antibacterial, Antidiabetic, Antifungal, Anti-Inflammatory, Antiprotozoal, Antituberculosis and Antiviral Activities; Affecting the Immune and Nervous Systems, and Other Miscellaneous Mechanisms of Action. *Mar. Drugs* **2024**, *22*, 309. [CrossRef] [PubMed]
8. Tripathi, A.; Puddick, J.; Prinsep, M.R.; Lee, P.P.F.; Tan, L.T. Lagunamides A and B: Cytotoxic and Antimalarial Cyclodepsipeptides from the Marine Cyanobacterium *Lyngbya majuscula*. *J. Nat. Prod.* **2010**, *73*, 1810–1814. [CrossRef] [PubMed]
9. Luesch, H.; Yoshida, W.Y.; Moore, R.E.; Paul, V.J.; Corbett, T.H. Total Structure Determination of Apratoxin A, a Potent Novel Cytotoxin from the Marine Cyanobacterium *Lyngbya majuscule*. *J. Am. Chem. Soc.* **2001**, *123*, 5418–5423. [CrossRef]
10. Zampella, A.; D'Auria, M.V.; Gomez Paloma, L.; Casapullo, A.; Minale, L.; Debitus, C.; Henin, Y. Callipeltin A, an Anti-HIV Cyclic Depsipeptide from the New Caledonian Lithistida Sponge *Callipelta* sp. *J. Am. Chem. Soc.* **1996**, *118*, 6202–6209. [CrossRef]
11. Fuwa, H. Structure Determination, Correction, and Disproof of Marine Macrolide Natural Products by Chemical Synthesis. *Org. Chem. Front.* **2021**, *8*, 3990–4023. [CrossRef]
12. Nájera, C.; Sansano, J.M. Catalytic Asymmetric Synthesis of α-Amino Acids. *Chem. Rev.* **2007**, *107*, 4584–4671. [CrossRef]
13. Perdih, A.; Sollner Dolenc, M. Recent Advances in the Synthesis of Unnatural α-Amino Acids. *Curr. Org. Chem.* **2007**, *11*, 801–832. [CrossRef]
14. Troyano, F.J.A.; Merkens, K.; Anwar, K.; Gómez-Suárez, A. Radical-based Synthesis and Modification of Amino Acids. *Angew. Chem. Int. Ed.* **2021**, *60*, 1098–1115. [CrossRef] [PubMed]
15. Paterson, I.; Lam, N.Y.S. Challenges and Discoveries in the Total Synthesis of Complex Polyketide Natural Products. *J. Antibiot.* **2018**, *71*, 215–233. [CrossRef] [PubMed]
16. Stockdale, T.P.; Lam, N.Y.S.; Anketell, M.J.; Paterson, I. The Stereocontrolled Total Synthesis of Polyketide Natural Products: A Thirty-Year Journey. *Bull. Chem. Soc. Jpn.* **2021**, *94*, 713–731. [CrossRef]
17. Matteson, D.S.; Ray, R. Directed Chiral Synthesis with Pinanediol Boronic Esters. *J. Am. Chem. Soc.* **1980**, *102*, 7590–7591. [CrossRef]
18. Matteson, D.S.; Collins, D.S.L.; Aggarwal, V.K.; Ciganek, E. in The Matteson Reaction. *Org. React.* **2021**, *105*, 427–860. [CrossRef]
19. Matteson, D.S.; Mah, R.W.H. Neighboring Boron in Nucleophilic Displacement. *J. Am. Chem. Soc.* **1963**, *85*, 2599–2603. [CrossRef]
20. Matteson, D.S.; Majumdar, D. α-Chloro boronic esters from homologation of boronic esters. *J. Am. Chem. Soc.* **1980**, *102*, 7588–7590. [CrossRef]
21. Matteson, D.S.; Majumdar, D. Homologation of Boronic Esters to α-Chloro Boronic Esters. *Organometallics* **1983**, *2*, 1529–1535. [CrossRef]
22. Matteson, D.S.; Peterson, M.L. Synthesis of L-(+)-Ribose via (S)-Pinanediol (αS)-α-Bromo Boronic Esters. *J. Org. Chem.* **1987**, *52*, 5116–5121. [CrossRef]
23. Matteson, D.S.; Sadhu, K.M.; Peterson, M.L. 99% Chirally Selective Syntheses via Pinanediol Boronic Esters: Insect Pheromones, Diols, and an Amino Alcohol. *J. Am. Chem. Soc.* **1986**, *108*, 810–819. [CrossRef]
24. Matteson, D.S.; Michnick, T.J. Stereoselective Reaction of an Enolate with Chiral α-Halo Boronic Acid Esters. *Organometallics* **1990**, *9*, 3171–3177. [CrossRef]
25. Matteson, D.S. Boronic Esters in Asymmetric Synthesis. *J. Org. Chem.* **2013**, *78*, 10009–10023. [CrossRef] [PubMed]
26. Ray, R.; Matteson, D.S. Osmium tetroxide catalyzed hydroxylation of hindered olefins. *Tetrahedron Lett.* **1980**, *21*, 449–450. [CrossRef]
27. Matteson, D.S.; Kandil, A.A. (*S*,*S*)-Diisopropylethanediol (diped)—A new chiral director for the α-chloro boronic ester synthesis. *Tetrahedron Lett.* **1986**, *27*, 3831–3834. [CrossRef]
28. Matteson, D.S.; Beedle, E.C.; Kandil, A.A. Preparation of (3*S*,4*S*)-2,5-dimethyl-3,4-hexanediol [(*S*)-DIPED] from (*R*,*R*)-tartaric acid via trimethylsilyl chloride catalyzed acetylation of a hindered 1,4-diol. *J. Org. Chem.* **1987**, *52*, 5034–5036. [CrossRef]
29. Hoffmann, R.W.; Ditrich, K.; Köster, G.; Stürmer, R. Stereoselective synthesis of alcohols, XXXI: Stereoselective C–C bond formation using chiral (*Z*)-pentenylboronates. *Chem. Ber.* **1989**, *122*, 1783–1789. [CrossRef]
30. Hiscox, W.C.; Matteson, D.S. An Efficient Preparation of (R*,R*)-1,2-Dicyclohexylethane-1,2-diol, a Superior Chiral Director for Synthesis with Boronic Esters. *J. Org. Chem.* **1996**, *61*, 8315–8316. [CrossRef] [PubMed]
31. Corey, E.J.; Barnes-Seeman, D.; Lee, T.W. The mechanistic basis for diastereoselectivity in the Matteson rearrangement. *Tetrahedron Asymmetry* **1997**, *8*, 3711–3713. [CrossRef]

32. Midland, M.M. Ab Initio Investigation of the Transition State for Asymmetric Synthesis with Boronic Esters. *J. Org. Chem.* **1998**, *63*, 914–915. [CrossRef]
33. Tripathy, P.B.; Matteson, D.S. Asymmetric Synthesis of the Four Stereoisomers of 4-Methyl-3-heptanol via Boronic Esters: Sequential Double Stereodifferentiation Leads to Very High Purity. *Synthesis* **1990**, *1990*, 200–206. [CrossRef]
34. Rangaishenvi, M.V.; Singaram, B.; Brown, H.C. Chiral Synthesis via Organoboranes. 30. Facile Synthesis, by the Matteson Asymmetric Homologation Procedure, of α-Methyl Boronic Acids Not Available from Asymmetric Hydroboration and Their Conversion into the Corresponding Aldehydes, Ketones, Carboxylic Acids, and Amines of High Enantiomeric Purity. *J. Org. Chem.* **1991**, *56*, 3286–3294. [CrossRef]
35. Matteson, D.S.; Man, H.-W.; Ho, O.C. Asymmetric Synthesis of Stegobinone via Boronic Ester Chemistry. *J. Am. Chem. Soc.* **1996**, *118*, 4560–4566. [CrossRef]
36. Villieras, J.; Bacquet, C.; Masure, D.; Normant, J.F. Les carbénoïdes lithiens dibromés et leur intérêt synthétique. *J. Organomet. Chem.* **1973**, *50*, C7–C11. [CrossRef]
37. Matteson, D.S.; Man, H.W. Enantioselective capture and retroracemization of (1-bromoalkyl)boronic esters by an *n*-propanoyloxazolidinone enolate and iodide-ion. *J. Org. Chem.* **1994**, *59*, 5734–5741. [CrossRef]
38. Sadhu, K.M.; Matteson, D.S. (Chloromethyl) lithium: Efficient generation and capture by boronic esters and a simple preparation of diisopropyl (chloromethyl) boronate. *Organometallics* **1985**, *4*, 1687–1689. [CrossRef]
39. Brown, H.C.; Singh, S.M.; Rangaishenvi, M.V. Organoboranes. 46. New Procedures for the Homologation of Boronic Esters: A Critical Examination of the Available Procedures to Achieve Convenient Homologation of Boronic Esters. *J. Org. Chem.* **1986**, *51*, 3150–3155. [CrossRef]
40. Michnick, T.J.; Matteson, D.S. (Bromomethyl) lithium: Efficient in situ reactions. *Synlett* **1991**, *1991*, 631–632. [CrossRef]
41. Gorovoy, A.S.; Gozhina, O.; Svendsen, J.-S.; Tetz, G.V.; Domorad, A.; Tetz, V.V.; Lejon, T. Syntheses and anti-tubercular activity of β-substituted and α,β-disubstituted peptidyl β-aminoboronates and boronic acids. *J. Pept. Sci.* **2013**, *19*, 613–618. [CrossRef] [PubMed]
42. Gorovoy, A.S.; Gozhina, O.; Svendsen, J.-S.; Domorad, A.A.; Tetz, G.V.; Tetz, V.V.; Lejon, T. Boron-Containing Peptidomimetics—A Novel Class of Selective Anti-tubercular Drugs. *Chem. Biol. Drug Des.* **2013**, *81*, 408–413. [CrossRef] [PubMed]
43. Matteson, D.S.; Soundararajan, R.; Ho, O.C.; Gatzweiler, W. (Alkoxyalkyl)boronic Ester Intermediates for Asymmetric Synthesis. *Organometallics* **1996**, *15*, 152–163. [CrossRef]
44. Tost, M.; Andler, O.; Kazmaier, U. A Matteson Homologation-Based Synthesis of Doliculide and Derivatives. *Eur. J. Org. Chem.* **2021**, *2021*, 6459–6471. [CrossRef]
45. Matteson, D.S.; Kandil, A.A.; Soundararajan, R. Synthesis of Asymmetrically Deuterated Glycerol and Dibenzylglyceraldehyde via Boronic Esters. *J. Am. Chem. Soc.* **1990**, *112*, 3964–3969. [CrossRef]
46. Matteson, D.S. Asymmetric synthesis with boronic esters. *Acc. Chem. Res.* **1988**, *21*, 294–300. [CrossRef]
47. Matteson, D.S. Boronic Esters in Stereodirected Synthesis. *Tetrahedron* **1989**, *45*, 1859–1885. [CrossRef]
48. Matteson, D.S.; Wan, H.-W. Hydrolysis of Substituted 1,3,2-Dioxaborolanes and an Asymmetric Synthesis of a Differently Protected Syn,syn-3-Methyl-2,4-hexanediol. *J. Org. Chem.* **1996**, *61*, 6047–6051. [CrossRef]
49. Matteson, D.S.; Kandil, A.A. Conversion of α-halo boronic esters to inverted α-(methylsulfonyl)oxy boronic esters. *J. Org. Chem.* **1987**, *52*, 5121–5124. [CrossRef]
50. Stymiest, J.L.; Dutheuil, G.; Mahmood, A.; Aggarwal, V.K. Lithiated Carbamates: Chiral Carbenoids for Iterative Homologation of Boranes and Boronic Esters. *Angew. Chem. Int. Ed.* **2007**, *46*, 7491–7494. [CrossRef]
51. Hoppe, D.; Hintze, F.; Tebben, P.; Paetow, M.; Ahrens, H.; Schwerdtfeger, J.; Sommerfeld, P.; Haller, J.; Guarnieri, W.; Kolczewski, S.; et al. Enantioselective synthesis via sparteine-induced asymmetric deprotonation. *Pure App. Chem.* **1994**, *66*, 1479–1486. [CrossRef]
52. Hoppe, D.; Hense, T. Enantioselective Synthesis with Lithium/(−)-Sparteine Carbanion Pairs. *Angew. Chem. Int. Ed. Engl.* **1997**, *36*, 2282–2316. [CrossRef]
53. Hoppe, D.; Hintze, F.; Tebben, P. Chiral Lithium-1-oxyalkanides by Asymmetric Deprotonation; Enantioselective Synthesis of 2-Hydroxyalkanoic Acids and Secondary Alkanols. *Angew. Chem. Int. Ed.* **1990**, *29*, 1422–1424. [CrossRef]
54. Beckmann, E.; Desai, V.; Hoppe, D. Stereospecific Reaction of α-Carbamoyloxy-2-alkenylboronates and α-Carbamoyloxy-alkylboronates with Grignard Reagents—Synthesis of Highly Enantioenriched Secondary Alcohols. *Synlett* **2004**, 2275–2280. [CrossRef]
55. Beckmann, E.; Hoppe, D. Synthesis of an Enantioenriched α-Carbamoyloxy-crotylboronate and Its Homoaldol Reaction with Aldehydes. *Synthesis* **2005**, *2005*, 217–222. [CrossRef]
56. Beak, P.; Baillargeon, M.; Carter, L.G. Lithiation of Ethyl 2,4,6-Triisopropylbenzoate Adjacent to Oxygen: The a-Lithioalkyl Alcohol Synthon. *J. Org. Chem.* **1978**, *43*, 4255–4256. [CrossRef]
57. Dearden, M.J.; Firkin, C.R.; Hermet, J.-P.R.; O'Brien, P. A Readily-Accessible (+)-Sparteine Surrogate. *J. Am. Chem. Soc.* **2002**, *124*, 11870–11871. [CrossRef] [PubMed]

58. Firth, J.D.; Canipa, S.J.; Ferris, L.; O'Brien, P. Gram-Scale Synthesis of the (−)-Sparteine Surrogate and (−)-Sparteine. *Angew. Chem. Int. Ed.* **2018**, *57*, 223–226. [CrossRef]
59. Leonori, D.; Aggarwal, V.K. Lithiation−Borylation Methodology and Its Application in Synthesis. *Acc. Chem. Res.* **2014**, *47*, 3174–3183. [CrossRef]
60. Linne, Y.; Schönwald, A.; Weißbach, S.; Kalesse, M. Desymmetrization of C2-Symmetric Bis(Boronic Esters) by Zweifel Olefinations. *Chem. Eur. J.* **2020**, *26*, 7998–8002. [CrossRef] [PubMed]
61. Hoppe, D.; Carstens, A.; Krämer, T. Generation of a Configurationally Stable Chiral Benzyllithium Derivative, and the Capricious Stereochemistry of Its Electrophilic Substitution. *Angew. Chem. Int. Ed.* **1990**, *29*, 1424–1425. [CrossRef]
62. Derwing, C.; Hoppe, D. Synthesis of Enantioenriched Tertiary Benzylic Alcohols via Stereospecific Lithiation of Secondary Benzyl Carbamates—Design of Dialkylcarbamates, Cleavable under Basic, Mild Conditions. *Synthesis* **1996**, *1996*, 149–154. [CrossRef]
63. Scott, H.K.; Aggarwal, V.K. Highly Enantioselective Synthesis of Tertiary Boronic Esters and their Stereospecific Conversion to other Functional Groups and Quaternary Stereocentres. *Chem. Eur. J.* **2011**, *17*, 13124–13132. [CrossRef]
64. Stymiest, J.L.; Bagutski, V.; French, R.M.; Aggarwal, V.K. Enantiodivergent conversion of chiral secondary alcohols into tertiary alcohols. *Nature* **2008**, *456*, 778–782. [CrossRef] [PubMed]
65. Bagutski, V.; French, R.M.; Aggarwal, V.K. Full Chirality Transfer in the Conversion of Secondary Alcohols into Tertiary Boronic Esters and Alcohols Using Lithiation–Borylation Reactions. *Angew. Chem. Int. Ed.* **2010**, *49*, 5142–5145. [CrossRef] [PubMed]
66. Linne, Y.; Bonandi, E.; Tabet, C.; Geldsetzer, J.; Kalesse, M. The Total Synthesis of Chondrochloren A. *Angew. Chem. Int. Ed.* **2021**, *60*, 6938–6942. [CrossRef]
67. Linne, E.; Kalesse, M. Stereoselective Construction of β-chiral Homoallyl Functionalities by Substrate- and Reagent-Controlled Iterative 1,2-Metallate Rearrangements. *Org. Lett.* **2023**, *25*, 8210–8214. [CrossRef]
68. Linne, Y.; Birkner, M.; Flormann, J.; Lücke, D.; Becker, J.A.; Kalesse, M. Sparteine-Free, Highly Stereoselective Construction of Complex Allylic Alcohols Using 1,2-Metallate Rearrangements. *J. Am. Chem. Soc. Au* **2023**, *3*, 1695–1710. [CrossRef]
69. Blakemore, P.R.; Burge, M.S. Iterative Stereospecific Reagent-Controlled Homologation of Pinacol Boronates by Enantioenrichedalpha-Chloroalkyllithium Reagents. *J. Am. Chem. Soc.* **2007**, *129*, 3068–3069. [CrossRef] [PubMed]
70. Blakemore, P.R.; Burge, M.S.; Stephton, M.A. Competing reaction pathways from α-halo-α-protioalkyl aryl sulfoxides initiated by organometallic reagents. *Tetrahedron Lett.* **2007**, *48*, 3999–4002. [CrossRef]
71. Drago, C.; Caggiano, L.; Jackson, R.F.W. Vanadium-Catalyzed Sulfur Oxidation/Kinetic Resolution in the Synthesis of Enantiomerically Pure Alkyl Aryl Sulfoxides. *Angew. Chem. Int. Ed.* **2005**, *44*, 7221–7223. [CrossRef] [PubMed]
72. Cogan, D.A.; Liu, G.; Kim, K.; Backes, B.J.; Ellman, J.A. Catalytic Asymmetric Oxidation of tert-Butyl Disulfide. Synthesis of tert-Butanesulfinamides, tert-Butyl Sulfoxides, and tert-Butanesulfinimines. *J. Am. Chem. Soc.* **1998**, *120*, 8011–8019. [CrossRef]
73. Bolm, C.; Bienewald, F. Asymmetric Sulfide Oxidation with Vanadium Catalysts and H_2O_2. *Angew. Chem. Int. Ed. Engl.* **1995**, *34*, 2640–2642. [CrossRef]
74. Satoh, T.; Oohara, T.; Ueda, Y.; Yamakawa, K. The practical procedure for a preparation of 1-chloroalkyl p-tolyl sulfoxides in high optically active form: A very short synthesis of optically active disparlure. *Tetrahedron Lett.* **1988**, *29*, 313–316. [CrossRef]
75. Hoyt, A.L.; Blakemore, P.R. On the nature of the chainextending species in organolithium initiated stereospecific reagentcontrolled homologation reactions using α-chloroalkyl aryl sulfoxides. *Tetrahedron Lett.* **2015**, *56*, 2980–2982. [CrossRef]
76. Emerson, C.R.; Zakharov, L.N.; Blakemore, P.R. Investigation of Functionalized α-Chloroalkyllithiums for a Stereospecific Reagent-Controlled Homologation Approach to the Analgesic Alkaloid (−)-Epibatidine. *Chem. Eur. J.* **2013**, *19*, 16342–16356. [CrossRef]
77. Sun, X.; Blakemore, P.R. Programmed Synthesis of a Contiguous Stereotriad Motif by Triple Stereospecific Reagent-Controlled Homologation. *Org. Lett.* **2013**, *15*, 4500–4503. [CrossRef] [PubMed]
78. Emerson, C.R.; Zakharov, L.N.; Blakemore, P.R. Iterative Stereospecific Reagent-Controlled Homologation Using a Functionalized α-Chloroalkyllithium: Synthesis of Cyclic Targets Related to Epibatidine. *Org. Lett.* **2011**, *13*, 1318–1321. [CrossRef] [PubMed]
79. Blakemore, P.R.; Marsden, S.P.; Vater, H.D. Reagent-Controlled Asymmetric Homologation of Boronic Esters by Enantioenriched Main-Group Chiral Carbenoids. *Org. Lett.* **2006**, *8*, 773–776. [CrossRef]
80. Jadhav, P.K.; Man, H.-W. Enantiotopic Differentiation of pro-R or pro-S Chlorides in (Dichloromethyl)borates by Chiral Lewis Acids: Enantioselective Synthesis of (α-Chloroalkyl)boronates. *J. Am. Chem. Soc.* **1997**, *119*, 846–847. [CrossRef]
81. Smith, K.; Saleh, B.A.; Alshammari, M.B.; El-Hiti, G.A.; Elliott, M.C. Studies on a catalytic version of the Matteson asymmetric homologation reaction. *Org. Biomol. Chem.* **2021**, *19*, 4279–4284. [CrossRef]
82. Sharma, H.A.; Essman, J.Z.; Jacobsen, E.N. Enantioselective Catalytic 1,2-Boronate Rearrangements. *Science* **2021**, *374*, 752–757. [CrossRef] [PubMed]
83. Essman, J.Z.; Sharma, H.A.; Jacobsen, E.N. Development of Enantioselective Lithium-Isothiourea-Boronate–Catalyzed Matteson Homologations. *Synlett* **2023**, *34*, 2061. [CrossRef] [PubMed]

84. Angle, S.R.; Sharma, H.A.; Choi, C.K.; Carlson, K.E.; Hou, Y.; Nwachukwu, J.C.; Kim, S.H.; Katzenellenbogen, B.S.; Nettles, K.W.; Katzenellenbogen, J.A.; et al. Iterative Catalyst-Controlled Diastereoselective Matteson Homologations Enable the Selective Synthesis of Benzestrol Isomers. *J. Am. Chem. Soc.* **2024**, *146*, 30771–30777. [CrossRef] [PubMed]
85. Janetzko, J.; Batey, R.A. Organoboron-Based Allylation Approach to the Total Synthesis of the Medium-Ring Dilactone (+)-Antimycin A1b. *J. Org. Chem.* **2014**, *79*, 7415–7424. [CrossRef] [PubMed]
86. Lebarbier, C.; Carreaux, F.; Carboni, B. Synthesis of as boronic acid Analoque of L-ornithine. *Synthesis* **1996**, 1371–1374. [CrossRef]
87. Andler, O.; Kazmaier, U. Stereoselective Synthesis of the Side Chain of Meliponamycin A. *Org. Lett.* **2022**, *24*, 2541–2545. [CrossRef]
88. Kohr, M.; Papenkordt, N.; Jung, M.; Kazmaier, U. Total synthesis and biological evaluation of the histone deacetylase inhibitor WF-3161. *Org. Biomol. Chem.* **2023**, *21*, 4382–4387. [CrossRef]
89. Kempf, M.; Andler, O.; Kazmaier, U. Total synthesis of salviaquinesin A using the homologation approach of Matteson. *Helv. Chim. Acta* **2023**, e202300136. [CrossRef]
90. Andler, O.; Kazmaier, U. Matteson Homologation-based total synthesis of meliponamycin A. *Org. Lett.* **2024**, *26*, 148–152. [CrossRef]
91. Yue, G.; Yang, L.; Yuan, C.; Du, B.; Liu, B. Total syntheses of lindenane-type sesquiterpenoids: (±)-chloranthalactones A, B, F, (±)-9-hydroxy heterogorgiolide, and (±)-shizukanolide E. *Tetrahedron* **2012**, *68*, 9624–9637. [CrossRef]
92. Struth, F.R.; Hirschhäuser, C. A Modular Approach to the Asymmetric Synthesis of Cytisine. *Eur. J. Org. Chem.* **2016**, *2016*, 958–964. [CrossRef]
93. Matteson, D.S.; Singh, R.P.; Schafman, B.; Yang, J.-J. Asymmetric Synthesis of Serricornin via Boronic Esters. *J. Org. Chem.* **1998**, *63*, 4466–4469. [CrossRef]
94. Matteson, D.S.; Sadhu, K.M. Boronic ester homologation with 99% chiral selectivity and its use in syntheses of the insect pheromones (3S,4S)-4-methyl-3-heptanol and exo-brevicomin. *J. Am. Chem. Soc.* **1983**, *105*, 2077–2078. [CrossRef]
95. Matteson, D.S.; Man, H.-W. High-Precision Asymmetric Synthesis of Stegobiol and Stegobinone over Boronic Acid Esters. *J. Org. Chem.* **1993**, *58*, 6545–6547. [CrossRef]
96. Anderbrant, O.; Matteson, D.S.; Unelius, C.R.; Pharazyn, P.S.; Santangelo, E.M.; Schlyter, F.; Birgersson, G. Pheromone of the elm bark beetle *Scolytus laevis* (Coleoptera: Scolytidae): Stereoisomers of 4-methyl-3-heptanol reduce interspecific competition. *Chemoecology* **2010**, *20*, 179–187. [CrossRef]
97. Moore, R.E.; Pettus, J.A., Jr.; Doty, M.S. Dictyopterene A. An odoriferous constituent from algae of the genus dictyopteris. *Tetrahedron Lett.* **1968**, *9*, 4787–4790. [CrossRef]
98. Hohn, E.; Paleček, J.; Pietruszka, J. Synthesis of Dictyopterene A. *Synlett* **2008**, 971–974. [CrossRef]
99. Jang, J.-H.; Kanoh, K.; Adachi, K.; Shizuri, Y. Awajanomycin, a Cytotoxic γ-Lactone-δ-lactam Metabolite from Marine-Derived *Acremonium* sp. *AWA16-1*, *J. Nat. Prod.* **2006**, *69*, 1358–1360. [CrossRef]
100. Wohlfahrt, M.; Harms, K.; Koert, U. Total Synthesis of (+)-Awajanomycin. *Eur. J. Org. Chem.* **2012**, 2260–2265. [CrossRef]
101. Chen, L.L.; Pousada, M.; Haines, T.H.J. The flagellar membrane of *Ochromonas danica*. Lipid composition. *J. Biol. Chem.* **1976**, *251*, 1835–1842. [CrossRef] [PubMed]
102. Landry, M.L.; Hu, D.X.; McKenna, G.M.; Burns, N.Z. Catalytic Enantioselective Dihalogenation and the Selective Synthesis of (−)-Deschloromytilipin A and (−)-Danicalipin A. *J. Am. Chem. Soc.* **2016**, *138*, 5150–5158. [CrossRef] [PubMed]
103. Chen, J.L.-Y.; Scott, H.K.; Hesse, M.J.; Willis, C.L.; Aggarwal, V.K. Highly diastereo- and enantioselective allylboration of aldehydes using α-substituted allyl/crotyl pinacol boronic esters via in situ generated borinic esters. *J. Am. Chem. Soc.* **2013**, *135*, 5316–5319. [CrossRef] [PubMed]
104. Chen, J.L.-Y.; Aggarwal, V.K. Highly Diastereoselective and Enantiospecific Allylation of Ketones and Imines Using Borinic Esters: Contiguous Quaternary Stereogenic Centers. *Angew. Chem. Int. Ed.* **2014**, *53*, 10992–10996. [CrossRef]
105. De Silva, E.D.; Williams, D.E.; Andersen, R.J.; Klix, H.; Holmes, C.F.B.; Allen, T.M. Motuporin, a potent protein phosphatase inhibitor isolated from the Papua New Guinea sponge *Theonella swinhoei* Gray. *Tetrahedron Lett.* **1992**, *33*, 1561–1564. [CrossRef]
106. Honkanen, R.A.; Dukelow, M.; Zwiller, J.; Moore, R.A.; Khatra, B.S.; Boynton, A. L Cyanobacterial nodularin is a potent inhibitor of type 1 and type 2A protein phosphatases. *Mol. Pharmacol.* **1991**, *40*, 577–583. [PubMed]
107. Honkanen, R.A.; Zwiller, J.; Moore, R.A.; Dailey, S.L.; Khatra, B.S.; Dukelow, M.; Boynton, A.L. Characterization of microcystin-LR, a potent inhibitor of type 1 and type 2A protein phosphatases. *J. Biol. Chem.* **1990**, *265*, 19401–19404. [CrossRef] [PubMed]
108. Matteson, D.S.; Sadhu, K.M. Synthesis of 1-Amino-2-phenylethane-I-boronic Acid Derivatives. *Organometallics* **1984**, *3*, 614–618. [CrossRef]
109. Matteson, D.S.; Jesthi, P.K.; Sadhu, K.M. Synthesis and Properties of Pinanediol a-Amido Boronic Esters. *Organometallics* **1984**, *3*, 1284–1288. [CrossRef]
110. Matteson, D.S.; Beedle, E.C. A direct chiral synthesis of amino acids from boronic esters. *Tetrahedron Lett.* **1987**, *28*, 4499–4502. [CrossRef]

111. Matteson, D.S.; Majumdar, D. Iodomethaneboronic esters and aminomethaneboronic esters. *J. Organomet. Chem.* **1979**, *170*, 259–264. [CrossRef]
112. Matteson, D.S.; Lu, J. Asymmetric synthesis of 1-acyl-3,4-disubstituted pyrrolidine-2-boronic acid derivatives. *Tetrahedron Asymmetry* **1998**, *9*, 2423–2436. [CrossRef]
113. Matteson, D.S.; Singh, R.P.; Sutton, C.H.; Verheyden, J.D.; Lu, J. An Exploratory Study of Silylated Amino Boronic Ester Chemistry. *Heteroatom Chem.* **1997**, *8*, 487–494. [CrossRef]
114. Bauer, S.M.; Armstrong, R.W. Total Synthesis of Motuporin (Nodularin-V). *J. Am. Chem. Soc.* **1999**, *121*, 6355–6366. [CrossRef]
115. Matteson, D.S.; Beedle, E.C. A chiral synthesis of (2S, 3S)-phenylalanine-3-2H via boronic esters. *J. Label Compd. Radiopharm.* **1988**, *25*, 675–683. [CrossRef]
116. Dess, D.B.; Martin, J.C. Readily Accessible 12-I-5 Oxidant for the Conversion of Primary and Secondary Alcohols to Aldehydes and Ketones. *J. Org. Chem.* **1983**, *48*, 4155–4156. [CrossRef]
117. Tanaka, T.; Oikawa, Y.; Hamada, T.; Yonemitsu, O. Total synthesis of tylonolide, the aglycone of the 16-membered ring macrolide tylosin, from D-glucose. Selective application of MPM and DMPM protecting groups for hydroxy functions. *Tetrahedron Lett.* **1986**, *27*, 3651–3654. [CrossRef]
118. Bal, B.S.; Childers, W.E.; Pinnick, H.W. Oxidation of α, β-unsaturated aldehydes. *Tetrahedron* **1981**, *37*, 2091–2096. [CrossRef]
119. D'Auria, M.V.; Zampella, A.; Paloma, L.G.; Minale, L.; Debitus, C.; Roussakis, C.; Le Bert, V. Callipeltins B and C.; Bioactive Peptides from a Marine Lithistida Sponge *Callipelta* sp. *Tetrahedron* **1996**, *52*, 9589–9596. [CrossRef]
120. Zampella, A.; Randazzo, A.; Borbone, N.; Luciani, S.; Trevisi, L.; Debitus, C.; D'Auria, M.V. Isolation of callipeltins A–C and of two new open-chain derivatives of callipeltin A from the marine sponge *Latrunculia* sp. A revision of the stereostructure of callipeltins. *Tetrahedron Lett.* **2002**, *43*, 6163–6166. [CrossRef]
121. Sepe, V.; D'Orsi, R.; Borbone, N.; D'Auria, M.V.; Bifulco, G.; Monti, M.C.; Catania, A.; Zampella, A. Callipeltins F–I: New antifungal peptides from the marine sponge *Latrunculia* sp. *Tetrahedron* **2006**, *62*, 833–840. [CrossRef]
122. Stierhof, M.; Hansen, K.Ø.; Sharma, M.; Feussner, K.; Subko, K.; Díaz-Rullo, F.F.; Isaksson, J.; Pérez-Victoria, I.; Clarke, D.; Hansen, E.; et al. New cytotoxic callipeltins from the Solomon Island marine sponge *Asteropus* sp. *Tetrahedron* **2016**, *72*, 6929–6934. [CrossRef]
123. Horn, A.; Kazmaier, U. Synthesis of the cyclic heptapeptide nucleus of Callipeltin A. *Org. Chem. Front.* **2022**, *9*, 5213–5218. [CrossRef]
124. Horn, A.; Kazmaier, U. Stereoselective synthesis of the side chain of Callipeltin A. *Org. Lett.* **2022**, *24*, 7072–7076. [CrossRef]
125. Horn, A.; Papadopoulos, E.; Kinsinger, T.; Greve, J.; Bickel, E.; Pachoula, S.; Kazmaier, U. Stereoselective synthesis of α-azido esters and α-amino acid derivatives via Matteson homologation of boron esters. *Z. Anorg. Allg. Chem.* **2024**, *650*, e202400113. [CrossRef]
126. Bickel, E.; Kazmaier, U. Simple syntheses of bottromycin derivatives via Ugi reactions and Matteson homologations. *Org. Biomol. Chem.* **2024**, *22*, 8811–8816. [CrossRef]
127. Cheng, X.C.; Kihara, T.; Kusakbe, H.; Magea, J.; Kobayashi, Y.; Fang, R.P.; Ni, Z.F.; Shen, Y.C.; Ko, K.; Yamaguchi, I.; et al. A new antibiotic, tautomycin. *J. Antibiot.* **1987**, *40*, 907–909. [CrossRef]
128. Maurer, K.W.; Armstrong, R.W. Synthesis of the C1-C21 Fragment of the Serine/Threonine Phosphatase Inhibitor Tautomycin. *J. Org. Chem.* **1996**, *61*, 3106–3116. [CrossRef] [PubMed]
129. Takai, K.; Niit, K.; Utimoton, K. Simple and Selective Method for RCHO to (*E*)-RCH=CHX Conversion by Means of a CHX3–$CrCl_2$ System. *J. Am. Chem. Soc.* **1986**, *108*, 7408–7410. [CrossRef]
130. Kishi, Y. Applications of Ni (II)/Cr (II)-mediated coupling reactions to natural products syntheses. *Pure Appl. Chem.* **1992**, *64*, 343–350. [CrossRef]
131. Takai, K.; Tagashira, M.; Kuroda, T.; Oshima, K.; Utimoto, K.; Nozaki, H. Reactions of alkenylchromium reagents prepared from alkenyl trifluoromethanesulfonates (triflates) with chromium(II) chloride under nickel catalysis. *J. Am. Chem. Soc.* **1986**, *108*, 6048–6050. [CrossRef]
132. Priester, R.; Kazmaier, U. A Straightforward Synthesis of Emericellamide A using Matteson's Homologation Approach. *Synlett* **2023**, *34*, 2159–2164. [CrossRef]
133. Nakao, Y.; Age, W.Y.; Takada, Y.; Kimura, J.; Yang, L.; Mooberry, S.L.; Scheuer, P.J. Kulokekahilide-2, a Cytotoxic Depsipeptide from a Cephalaspidean Mollusk *Philinopsis speciosa*. *J. Nat. Prod.* **2004**, *67*, 1332–1340. [CrossRef]
134. Takada, Y.; Mori, E.; Umehara, M.; Nakao, Y.; Kimura, J. Reinvestigation of the stereochemistry of kulokekahilide-2. *Tetrahedron Lett.* **2007**, *48*, 7653–7656. [CrossRef]
135. Takada, Y.; Umehara, M.; Nakao, Y.; Kimura, J. Revised absolute stereochemistry of natural kulokekahilide-2. *Tetrahedron Lett.* **2008**, *49*, 1163–1165. [CrossRef]
136. Sueyoshi, K.; Kaneda, M.; Sumimoto, S.; Oishi, S.; Fujii, N.; Suenaga, K.; Teruya, T. Odoamide, a cytotoxic cyclodepsipeptide from the marine cyanobacterium *Okeania* sp. *Tetrahedron* **2016**, *72*, 5472–5478. [CrossRef]

137. Suenaga, K.; Mutou, T.; Shibata, T.; Itoh, T.; Kigoshi, H.; Yamada, K. Isolation and stereostructure of aurilide, a novel cyclodepsipeptide from the Japanese sea hare *Dolabella auricularia*. *Tetrahedron Lett.* **1996**, *37*, 6771–6774. [CrossRef]
138. Suenaga, K.; Mutou, T.; Shibata, T.; Itoh, T.; Fujita, T.; Takada, N.; Hayamizu, K.; Takagi, M.; Irifune, T.; Kigoshi, H.; et al. Aurilide, a cytotoxic depsipeptide from the sea hare *Dolabella auricularia*: Isolation, structure determination, synthesis, and biological activity. *Tetrahedron* **2004**, *60*, 8509–8527. [CrossRef]
139. Han, B.; Gross, H.; Goeger, D.E.; Mooberry, S.L.; Gerwick, W.H. Aurilides B and C, Cancer Cell Toxins from a Papua New Guinea Collection of the Marine Cyanobacterium *Lyngbya majuscule*. *J. Nat. Prod.* **2006**, *69*, 572–575. [CrossRef] [PubMed]
140. Huang, X.; Huang, W.; Li, L.; Sun, X.; Song, S.; Xu, Q.; Zhang, L.; Wei, B.; Deng, X. Structure Determinants of Lagunamide A for Anticancer Activity and Its Molecular Mechanism of Mitochondrial Apoptosis. *Mol. Pharm.* **2016**, *13*, 3756–3763. [CrossRef] [PubMed]
141. Hu, Y.; Mostert, D.; Orgler, C.; Andler, O.; Zischka, H.; Kazmaier, U.; Vollmar, A.M.; Braig, S.; Sieber, S.A.; Zahler, S. Lagunamide A causes potent antiproliferative and pro-apoptotic effects in cancer cells by targeting EYA3. *ChemBioChem* **2024**, e202400024. [CrossRef]
142. Suenaga, K.; Kajiwara, S.; Kuribayashi, S.; Handa, T.; Kigoshi, H. Synthesis and cytotoxicity of aurilide analogs. *Bioorg. Med. Chem. Lett.* **2008**, *18*, 3902–3905. [CrossRef]
143. Andler, O.; Kazmaier, U. A Straightforward Synthesis of Polyketides via Ester Dienolate Matteson Homologation. *Chem. Eur. J.* **2021**, *27*, 949–953. [CrossRef] [PubMed]
144. Gutiérrez, M.; Suyama, T.L.; Engene, N.; Wingerd, J.S.; Matainaho, T.; Gerwick, W.H. Apratoxin D, a Potent Cytotoxic Cyclodepsipeptide from Papua New Guinea Collections of the Marine Cyanobacteria *Lyngbya majuscula* and *Lyngbya sordida*. *J. Nat. Prod.* **2008**, *71*, 1099–1103. [CrossRef]
145. Matthew, S.; Schupp, P.J.; Luesch, H. Apratoxin E, a Cytotoxic Peptolide from a Guamanian Collection of the Marine Cyanobacterium *Lyngbya bouillonii*. *J. Nat. Prod.* **2008**, *71*, 1113–1116, Erratum in *J. Nat. Prod.* **2018**, *81*, 217–217. [CrossRef]
146. Thornburg, C.C.; Cowley, E.S.; Sikorska, J.; Shaala, L.A.; Ishmael, J.E.; Youssef, D.T.A.; McPhail, K.L. Apratoxin H and Apratoxin A Sulfoxide from the Red Sea Cyanobacterium *Moorea producens*. *J. Nat. Prod.* **2013**, *76*, 1781–1788. [CrossRef]
147. Tarsis, E.M.; Rastelli, E.J.; Wengryniuk, S.E.; Coltart, D.M. The apratoxin marine natural products: Isolation, structure determination, and asymmetric total synthesis. *Tetrahedron* **2015**, *71*, 5029–5044. [CrossRef]
148. Liu, Y.; Law, B.K.; Luesch, H. Apratoxin A Reversibly Inhibits the Secretory Pathway by Preventing Cotranslational Translocation. *Mol. Pharmacol.* **2009**, *76*, 91–104. [CrossRef] [PubMed]
149. Luesch, H.; Chanda, S.K.; Raya, R.M.; DeJesus, P.D.; Orth, A.P.; Walker, J.R.; Izpisúa Belmonte, J.C.; Schultz, P.G. A functional genomics approach to the mode of action of apratoxin A. *Nat. Chem. Biol.* **2006**, *2*, 158–167. [CrossRef]
150. Wan, X.; Serrill, J.D.; Humphreys, I.R.; Tan, M.; McPhail, K.L.; Ganley, I.G.; Ishmael, J.E. ATG5 Promotes Death Signaling in Response to the Cyclic Depsipeptides Coibamide A and Apratoxin A. *Mar. Drugs* **2018**, *16*, 77. [CrossRef] [PubMed]
151. Chen, Q.; Liu, Y.; Luesch, H. Systematic Chemical Mutagenesis Identifies a Potent Novel Apratoxin A/E Hybrid with Improved in Vivo Antitumor Activity. *ACS Med. Chem. Lett.* **2011**, *2*, 861–865. [CrossRef]
152. Andler, O.; Kazmaier, U. Total synthesis of apratoxin A and B using Matteson's homologation approach. *Org. Biomol. Chem.* **2021**, *19*, 4866–4870. [CrossRef] [PubMed]
153. Ishiwata, H.; Nemoto, T.; Ojika, M.; Yamada, K. Isolation and Stereostructure of Doliculide, a Cytotoxic Cyclodepsipeptide from the Japanese Sea Hare *Dolabella auricularia*. *J. Org. Chem.* **1994**, *59*, 4710–4711. [CrossRef]
154. Harrigan, G.G.; Luesch, H.; Yoshida, W.Y.; Moore, R.E.; Nagle, D.G.; Paul, V.J.; Mooberry, S.L.; Corbett, T.H.; Valeriote, F.A. Symplostatin 1: A Dolastatin 10 Analogue from the Marine Cyanobacterium *Symploca hydnoides*. *J. Nat. Prod.* **1998**, *61*, 1075–1077. [CrossRef] [PubMed]
155. Bai, R.; Covell, D.G.; Liu, C.; Ghosh, A.K.; Hamel, E. (−)-Doliculide, a New Macrocyclic Depsipeptide Enhancer of Actin Assembly. *J. Biol. Chem.* **2002**, *277*, 32165–32171. [CrossRef] [PubMed]
156. Franklin-Tong, V.E.; Gourlay, C.W. A Role for Actin in Regulating Apoptosis/Programmed Cell Death: Evidence Spanning Yeast, Plants and Animals. *Biochem. J.* **2008**, *413*, 389–404. [CrossRef] [PubMed]
157. Pollard, T.D.; Cooper, J.A. Actin, a Central Player in Cell Shape and Movement. *Science* **2009**, *326*, 1208–1212. [CrossRef]
158. Matcha, K.; Madduri, A.V.R.; Roy, S.; Ziegler, S.; Waldmann, H.; Hirsch, A.K.H.; Minnaard, A.J. Total Synthesis of (−)-Doliculide, Structure–Activity Relationship Studies and Its Binding to F-Actin. *ChemBioChem* **2012**, *13*, 2537–2548. [CrossRef] [PubMed]
159. Foerster, F.; Braig, S.; Chen, T.; Altmann, K.-H.; Vollmar, A.M. Pharmacological Characterization of Actin-Binding (−)-Doliculide. *Bioorg. Med. Chem.* **2014**, *22*, 5117–5122. [CrossRef]
160. Sumiya, E.; Shimogawa, H.; Sasaki, H.; Tsutsumi, M.; Yoshita, K.; Ojika, M.; Suenaga, K.; Uesugi, M. Cell-Morphology Profiling of a Natural Product Library Identifies Bisebromoamide and Miuraenamide A as Actin Filament Stabilizers. *ACS Chem. Biol.* **2011**, *6*, 425–431. [CrossRef] [PubMed]

161. Moser, C.; Rüdiger, D.; Förster, F.; von Blume, J.; Yu, P.; Küster, B.; Kazmaier, U.; Vollmar, A.M.; Zahler, S. Persistent inhibition of pore-based cell migration by sub-toxic doses of miuraenamide, an actin filament stabilizer. *Sci. Rep.* **2017**, *7*, 16407. [CrossRef] [PubMed]
162. Wang, S.; Meixner, M.; Yu, L.; Karmann, L.; Kazmaier, U.; Vollmar, A.M.; Antes, I.; Zahler, S. Turning the Actin Nucleating Compound Miuraenamide into Nucleation Inhibitors. *ACS Omega* **2021**, *6*, 22165–22172. [CrossRef] [PubMed]
163. Foerster, F.; Chen, T.; Altmann, K.-H.; Vollmar, A.M. Actin-Binding Doliculide Causes Premature Senescence in P53 Wild Type Cells. *Bioorg. Med. Chem.* **2016**, *24*, 123–129. [CrossRef] [PubMed]
164. Ho, O.C.; Soundararajan, R.; Lu, J.; Matteson, D.S.; Wang, Z.; Chen, X.; Wei, M.; Willett, R.D. ((Trityloxy)methyl)boronic Esters. *Organometallics* **1995**, *14*, 2855–2860. [CrossRef]
165. Tost, M.; Kazmaier, U. Synthesis and Late-Stage Modification of (−)-Doliculide Derivatives Using Matteson's Homologation Approach. *Mar. Drugs* **2024**, *22*, 165. [CrossRef] [PubMed]
166. Millán, A.; Martinez, P.D.G.; Aggarwal, V.K. Stereocontrolled Synthesis of Polypropionate Fragments based on a Building Block Assembly Strategy using Lithiation-Borylation Methodologies. *Chem. Eur. J.* **2018**, *24*, 730–735. [CrossRef] [PubMed]
167. Seo, Y.; Cho, K.W.; Rho, J.-R.; Shin, J. Solandelactones A-I, Lactonized Cyclopropyl Oxylipins Isolated from the Hydroid Solanderia secunda. *Tetrahedron* **1996**, *52*, 10583–10596. [CrossRef]
168. Binanzer, M.; Fang, G.Y.; Aggarwal, V.K. Asymmetric Synthesis of Allylsilanes by the Borylation of Lithiated Carbamates: Formal Total Synthesis of (−)-Decarestrictine D. *Angew. Chem. Int. Ed.* **2010**, *49*, 4264–4268. [CrossRef] [PubMed]
169. Robinson, A.; Aggarwal, V.K. Asymmetric Total Synthesis of Solandelactone E: Stereocontrolled Synthesis of the 2-ene-1,4-diol Core Through a Lithiation–Borylation—Allylation Sequence. *Angew. Chem. Int. Ed.* **2010**, *49*, 6673–6675. [CrossRef]
170. Landais, Y.; Parra-Rapado, L. Epoxidation and cyclopropanation of 2-silyl-3-alkenols. A study of 1,2-asymmetric induction. *Tetrahedron Lett.* **1996**, *37*, 1205–1208. [CrossRef]
171. Robinson, A.; Aggarwal, V.K. Stereocontrolled asymmetric synthesis of syn-E-1,4-diol-2-enes using allyl boronates and its application in the total synthesis of solandelactone F. *Org. Biomol. Chem.* **2012**, *10*, 1795–1801. [CrossRef] [PubMed]
172. Rodriguez, A.D.; Ramirez, C. Serrulatane Diterpenes with Antimycobacterial Activity Isolated from the West Indian Sea Whip *Pseudopterogorgia elisabethae*. *J. Nat. Prod.* **2001**, *64*, 100–102. [CrossRef] [PubMed]
173. Fujii, A.; Hashiguchi, S.; Uematsu, N.; Ikariya, T.; Noyori, R. Ruthenium(II)-Catalyzed Asymmetric Transfer Hydrogenation of Ketones Using a Formic Acid−Triethylamine Mixture. *J. Am. Chem. Soc.* **1996**, *118*, 2521–2522. [CrossRef]
174. Nave, S.; Sonawane, R.P.; Elford, T.G.; Aggarwal, V.K.J. Protodeboronation of Tertiary Boronic Esters: Asymmetric Synthesis of Tertiary Alkyl Stereogenic Centers. *J. Am. Chem. Soc.* **2010**, *132*, 17096–17098. [CrossRef]
175. Elford, T.G.; Nave, S.; Sonawane, R.P.; Aggarwal, V.K. Total Synthesis of (+)-Erogorgiaene Using Lithiation–Borylation Methodology, and Stereoselective Synthesis of Each of Its Diastereoisomers. *J. Am. Chem. Soc.* **2011**, *133*, 16798–16801. [CrossRef]
176. Shen, Y.-C.; Tsai, P.I.; Fenical, W.; Hay, M.E. Secondary metabolite chemistry of the caribbean marine alga *Sporochnus bolleanus*: A basis for herbivore chemical defence. *Phytochemistry* **1993**, *52*, 71. [CrossRef]
177. Zweifel, G.; Arzoumanian, H.; Whitney, C.C. A Convenient Stereoselective Synthesis of Substituted Alkenes via Hydroboration-Iodination of Alkynes. *J. Am. Chem. Soc.* **1967**, *89*, 3652–3653. [CrossRef]
178. Zweifel, G.; Polston, N.L.; Whitney, C.C. A stereoselective synthesis of conjugated dienes from alkynes via the hydroboration-iodination reaction. *J. Am. Chem. Soc.* **1968**, *90*, 6243–6245. [CrossRef]
179. Evans, D.A.; Crawford, T.C.; Thomas, R.C.; Walker, J.A. Studies directed toward the synthesis of prostaglandins. Useful boron-mediated olefin syntheses. *J. Org. Chem.* **1976**, *41*, 3947–3953. [CrossRef]
180. Sonawane, R.P.; Jheengut, V.; Rabalakos, C.; Larouche-Gauthier, R.; Scott, H.K.; Aggarwal, V.K. Enantioselective Construction of Quaternary Stereogenic Centers from Tertiary Boronic Esters: Methodology and Applications. *Angew. Chem. Int. Ed.* **2011**, *50*, 3760–3763. [CrossRef]
181. Aggarwal, V.K.; Ball, L.T.; Carobene, S.; Connelly, R.L.; Hesse, M.J.; Partridge, B.M.; Roth, P.; Thomas, S.P.; Webster, M.P. Application of the lithiation–borylation reaction to the rapid and enantioselective synthesis of the bisabolane family of sesquiterpenes. *Chem. Commun.* **2012**, *48*, 9230–9232. [CrossRef] [PubMed]
182. Jongaramruong, J.; Blackman, A.J.; Skelton, B.W.; White, A.H. Chemical relationships between the sea hare *Aplysia parvula* and the red seaweed *Laurencia filiformis* from Tasmania. *Aust. J. Chem.* **2002**, *55*, 275–280. [CrossRef]
183. Yamamura, S.; Hirata, Y. Structures of aplysin and aplysinol, naturally occurring bromo compounds. *Tetrahedron* **1963**, *19*, 1485–1496. [CrossRef]
184. Fletcher, C.J.; Blair, D.J.; Wheelhouse, K.M.P.; Aggarwal, V.K. The total synthesis of (−)-aplysin via a lithiation–borylation–propenylation sequence. *Tetrahedron* **2012**, *68*, 7598–7604. [CrossRef]
185. Kazlauskas, R.; Murphy, P.T.; Quinn, R.J.; Wells, R.J. New laurene derivatives from *Laurencia filiformis*. *Aust. J. Chem.* **1976**, *29*, 2533–2539. [CrossRef]
186. Blair, D.J.; Fletcher, C.J.; Wheelhouse, K.M.P.; Aggarwal, V.K. Stereocontrolled Synthesis of Adjacent Acyclic Quaternary-Tertiary Motifs: Application to a Concise Total Synthesis of (−)-Filiformin. *Angew. Chem. Int. Ed.* **2014**, *53*, 5552–5555. [CrossRef]

187. Wu, M.; Okino, T.; Nogle, L.M.; Marquez, B.L.; Williamson, R.T.; Sitachitta, N.; Berman, F.W.; Murray, T.F.; McGough, K.; Jacobs, R.; et al. Structure, Synthesis, and Biological Properties of Kalkitoxin, a Novel Neurotoxin from the Marine Cyanobacterium Lyngbya majuscule. *J. Am. Chem. Soc.* **2000**, *122*, 12041–12042. [CrossRef]
188. Berman, F.W.; Gerwick, W.H.; Murray, T.F. Antillatoxin and kalkitoxin, ichthyotoxins from the tropical cyanobacterium Lyngbya majuscula, induce distinct temporal patterns of NMDA receptor-mediated neurotoxicity. *Toxicon* **1999**, *37*, 1645–1648. [CrossRef] [PubMed]
189. Manger, R.L.; Leja, L.S.; Lee, S.Y.; Hungerford, J.M.; Hokama, Y.; Dickey, R.W.; Granade, H.R.; Lewis, R.; Yasumoto, T.; Wekell, M.M. Detection of sodium channel toxins: Directed cytotoxicity assays of purified ciguatoxins, brevetoxins, saxitoxins, and seafood extracts. *J. AOAC Int.* **1995**, *78*, 521–527. [CrossRef]
190. Burns, M.; Essafi, S.; Bame, J.R.; Bull, S.P.; Webster, M.P.; Balieu, S.; Dale, J.W.; Butts, C.P.; Harvey, J.N.; Aggarwal, V.K. Assembly-line synthesis of organic molecules with tailored shapes. *Nature* **2014**, *513*, 183–188. [CrossRef] [PubMed]
191. Balieu, S.; Hallett, G.E.; Burns, M.; Bootwicha, T.; Studley, J.; Aggarwal, V.K. Toward Ideality: The Synthesis of (+)-Kalkitoxin and (+)-Hydroxyphthioceranic Acid by Assembly-Line Synthesis. *J. Am. Chem. Soc.* **2015**, *137*, 4398–4403. [CrossRef] [PubMed]
192. Bootwicha, T.; Feilner, J.M.; Myers, E.L.; Aggarwal, V.K. Iterative assembly line synthesis of polypropionates with full stereocontrol. *Nat. Chem.* **2017**, *9*, 896–902. [CrossRef] [PubMed]
193. Yeung, K.; Mykura, R.C.; Aggarwal, V.K. Lithiation–borylation methodology in the total synthesis of natural products. *Nat. Synth.* **2022**, *1*, 117–126. [CrossRef]
194. Mlynarski, S.N.; Karns, A.S.; Morken, J.P. Direct Stereospecific Amination of Alkyl and Aryl Pinacol Boronates. *J. Am. Chem. Soc.* **2012**, *134*, 16449–16451. [CrossRef]
195. Rao, R.M.; Faulkner, D.J. Clavosolides A and B, Dimeric Macrolides from the Philippines Sponge *Myriastra clavosa*. *J. Nat. Prod.* **2002**, *65*, 386–388. [CrossRef]
196. Erickson, K.L.; Gustafson, K.R.; Pannell, L.K.; Beutler, J.A.; Boyd, M. New Dimeric Macrolide Glycosides from the Marine Sponge *Myriastra clavosa*. *J. Nat. Prod.* **2002**, *65*, 1303–1306. [CrossRef] [PubMed]
197. Millán, A.; Smith, J.R.; Chen, J.L.-Y.; Aggarwal, V.K. Tandem Allylboration–Prins Reaction for the Rapid Construction of Substituted Tetrahydropyrans: Application to the Total Synthesis of (−)-Clavosolide A. *Angew. Chem. Int. Ed.* **2016**, *55*, 2498–2502. [CrossRef] [PubMed]
198. Tripathi, A.; Schofield, M.M.; Chlipala, G.E.; Schultz, P.J.; Yim, I.; Newmister, S.A.; Nusca, T.D.; Scaglione, J.B.; Hanna, P.C.; Tamayo-Castillo, G.; et al. Baulamycins A and B, broad-spectrum antibiotics identified as inhibitors of siderophore biosynthesis in *Staphylococcus aureus* and *Bacillus anthracis*. *J. Am. Chem. Soc.* **2014**, *136*, 1579–1586. [CrossRef]
199. Wu, J.; Lorenzo, P.; Zhong, S.; Ali, M.; Butts, C.P.; Myers, E.L.; Aggarwal, V.K. Synergy of synthesis, computation and NMR reveals correct baulamycin structures. *Nature* **2017**, *547*, 436–440. [CrossRef]
200. Shao, C.-L.; Mou, X.-F.; Cao, F.; Spadafora, C.; Glukhov, E.; Gerwick, L.; Wang, C.-Y.; Gerwick, W.H. Bastimolide B, an Antimalarial 24-Membered Marine Macrolide Possessing a tert-Butyl Group. *J. Nat. Prod.* **2018**, *81*, 211–215. [CrossRef]
201. Shao, C.-L.; Linington, R.G.; Balunas, M.J.; Centeno, A.; Boudreau, P.; Zhang, C.; Engene, N.; Spadafora, C.; Mutka, T.S.; Kyle, D.E.; et al. Bastimolide A, a Potent Antimalarial Polyhydroxy Macrolide from the Marine Cyanobacterium *Okeania hirsute*. *J. Org. Chem.* **2015**, *80*, 7849–7855. [CrossRef] [PubMed]
202. Friestad, G.K.; Sreenilayam, G. 1,5-Polyols: Challenging Motifs for Configurational Assignment and Synthesis. *Pure Appl. Chem.* **2011**, *83*, 461–478. [CrossRef]
203. Fiorito, D.; Keskin, S.; Bateman, J.M.; George, M.; Noble, A.; Aggarwal, V.K. Stereocontrolled Total Synthesis of Bastimolide B Using Iterative Homologation of Boronic Esters. *J. Am. Chem. Soc.* **2022**, *144*, 7995–8001. [CrossRef] [PubMed]
204. Kliman, L.T.; Mlynarski, S.N.; Ferris, G.E.; Morken, J.P. Catalytic Enantioselective 1,2-Diboration of 1,3-Dienes: Versatile Reagents for Stereoselective Allylation. *Angew. Chem. Int. Ed.* **2012**, *51*, 521–524. [CrossRef] [PubMed]
205. Coombs, J.R.; Haeffner, F.; Kliman, L.T.; Morken, J.P. Scope and Mechanism of the Pt-Catalyzed Enantioselective Diboration of Monosubstituted Alkenes. *J. Am. Chem. Soc.* **2013**, *135*, 11222–11231. [CrossRef] [PubMed]
206. Casoni, G.; Kucukdisli, M.; Fordham, J.M.; Burns, M.; Myers, E.L.; Aggarwal, V.K. α-Sulfinyl Benzoates as Precursors to Li and Mg Carbenoids for the Stereoselective Iterative Homologation of Boronic Esters. *J. Am. Chem. Soc.* **2017**, *139*, 11877–11886. [CrossRef] [PubMed]
207. Blair, D.J.; Chitti, S.; Trobe, M.; Kostyra, D.M.; Haley, H.M.S.; Hansen, R.L.; Ballmer, S.G.; Woods, T.J.; Wang, W.; Mubayi, V.; et al. Automated Iterative Csp^3–C Bond Formation. *Nature* **2022**, *604*, 92–97. [CrossRef]
208. Crudden, M.C.; Hleba, Y.B.; Chen, A.C. Regio- and Enantiocontrol in the Room-Temperature Hydroboration of Vinyl Arenes with Pinacol Borane. *J. Am. Chem. Soc.* **2004**, *126*, 9200–9201. [CrossRef] [PubMed]
209. Yamamoto, Y.; Fujikawa, R.; Umemoto, T.; Miyaura, N. Iridium-Catalyzed Hydroboration of Alkenes with Pinacolborane. *Tetrahedron* **2004**, *60*, 10695–10700. [CrossRef]
210. Fiorito, D.; Mazet, C. Ir-Catalyzed Selective Hydroboration of 2-Substituted 1,3-Dienes: A General Method to Access Homoallylic Boronates. *ACS Catal.* **2018**, *8*, 9382–9387. [CrossRef]

211. Chemler, S.R.; Trauner, D.; Danishefsky, S.J. The B-Alkyl Suzuki-Miyaura Cross-Coupling Reaction: Development, Mechanistic Study, and Applications in Natural Product Synthesis. *Angew. Chem. Int. Ed.* **2001**, *40*, 4544–4568. [CrossRef]
212. Kallan, N.C.; Halcomb, R.L. Synthesis of the Ring System of Phomactin D Using a Suzuki Macrocyclization. *Org. Lett.* **2000**, *2*, 2687–2690. [CrossRef] [PubMed]
213. Chemler, S.R.; Danishefsky, S.J. Transannular Macrocyclization via Intramolecular B-Alkyl Suzuk.i Reaction. *Org. Lett.* **2000**, *2*, 2695–2698. [CrossRef]
214. Igarashi, Y.; Shimasaki, R.; Miyanaga, S.; Oku, N.; Onaka, H.; Sakurai, H.; Saiki, I.; Kitani, S.; Nihira, T.; Wimonsiravude, W.; et al. Rakicidin D, ein Inhibitor der Tumorzellinvasion aus marinen *Streptomyces* sp. *J. Antibiot.* **2010**, *63*, 563–565. [CrossRef] [PubMed]
215. Kitani, S.; Ueguchi, T.; Igarashi, Y.; Leetanasaksakul, K.; Thamchaipenet, A.; Nihira, T. Rakicidin F, a new antibacterial cyclic depsipeptide derived from a marine sponge-derived *Streptomyces* sp. *J. Antibiot.* **2018**, *71*, 139–141. [CrossRef] [PubMed]
216. Bold, C.P.; Yeung, K.; Pape, F.; Kaiser, D.; Aggarwal, V.K. Application of Lithiation–Borylation to the Total Synthesis of (−)-Rakicidin F. *Organic Lett.* **2022**, *24*, 9398–9402. [CrossRef] [PubMed]
217. Smitrovich, J.H.; Woerpel, K.A. Oxidation of Sterically Hindered Alkoxysilanes and Phenylsilanes under Basic Conditions. *J. Org. Chem.* **1996**, *61*, 6044–6046. [CrossRef]

marine drugs

MDPI

Review

Marine Natural Products in Preclinical Cancer Studies: Ten Years of Advanced Total Synthesis

Ester Colarusso [1], Assunta Giordano [2], Maria Giovanna Chini [3], Giuseppe Bifulco [1,*] and Gianluigi Lauro [1,*]

[1] Department of Pharmacy, University of Salerno, Via Giovanni Paolo II 132, 84084 Fisciano, SA, Italy; ecolarusso@unisa.it
[2] Institute of Biomolecular Chemistry (ICB), Consiglio Nazionale Delle Ricerche (CNR), Via Campi Flegrei 34, 80078 Pozzuoli, NA, Italy; assunta.giordano@cnr.it
[3] Department of Biosciences and Territory, University of Molise, Contrada Fonte Lappone, 86090 Pesche, IS, Italy; mariagiovanna.chini@unimol.it
* Correspondence: bifulco@unisa.it (G.B.); glauro@unisa.it (G.L.)

Abstract

Marine ecosystems represent an exceptional reservoir of structurally diverse metabolites with remarkable pharmacological potential. Over the past decades, the exploration of marine organisms has led to the discovery of an ever-expanding number of bioactive compounds. Many of these metabolites display highly original chemical scaffolds that are not typically found in terrestrial organisms, offering new opportunities for drug discovery. Among the most promising applications is their development as anticancer agents, given their ability to interfere with key cellular processes. This review highlights marine natural products currently under investigation in preclinical studies as potential anticancer lead compounds. The molecules are classified into major structural families: aromatic and heterocyclic alkaloids, terpenes and their derivatives, macrolide frameworks, and diverse peptide-based scaffolds, alongside other complex classes (polyketides, thiazole lipids, alkylamino alcohols, and pyrrolocarbazole derivatives). A particular emphasis has been placed on the role of total synthesis over the last decade. Advances in synthetic methodology have not only enabled the production of these complex metabolites in sufficient quantities but have also facilitated the development of novel chemotherapeutic agents. To overcome the challenges of limited natural availability, the advanced synthetic approaches are crucial for harnessing the full therapeutic potential of marine-derived compounds.

Keywords: marine-derived compounds; anticancer activities; total synthesis

1. Introduction

More than 80% of all plant and animal species on Earth can be found in the oceans, along with an astounding variety of microbes. This exceptionally high level of biodiversity and chemodiversity, often substantially different from terrestrial ones, is explained by considering different factors; among these, the temperatures, which can vary greatly (from 35.0 °C to 1.5 °C), are of pivotal importance [1,2].

The marine environment has recently yielded a large number of bioactive compounds (e.g., peptides, alkaloids, macrocyclic lactones), offering a novel source of medications to treat serious illnesses such as inflammation and cancer [3]. Some marine-derived drugs have already been released into the market, while preclinical or early clinical development is underway for many other medicinal compounds from marine sources.

Despite growing interest, several challenges remain. Exploring deep-sea ecosystems requires specialised equipment and technology, making the process both expensive and logistically demanding. Consequently, most research still focuses on marine organisms found in shallow waters, leaving vast areas of marine biodiversity largely unexplored. Furthermore, the overharvesting of marine species for scientific purposes can compromise the integrity of fragile ecosystems and harm sensitive species, thereby raising significant ethical and environmental concerns.

Many marine organisms are also complex to cultivate or sustain in laboratory settings, which limits the ability to reproduce their bioactive compounds.

Lastly, international regulations and biodiversity agreements (such as the Nagoya Protocol) can further restrict access to marine genetic resources. Given the importance of these species and the difficulty in isolating them from the sea, approved products are commonly produced through synthetic processes.

The first FDA-approved drug derived from a marine source was Cytarabine (Ara-C, Figure 1), approved in 1969 [4]. It was initially isolated from the marine sponge *Cryptotethya crypta* and is an analogue of cytidine that combines a cytosine base with an arabinose sugar [5]. Its discovery marked the beginning of drug development from marine environments. Cytarabine is primarily used to treat various forms of leukaemia, including acute myelocytic leukaemia, lymphocytic leukaemia, meningeal leukaemia, and the blast crisis phase of chronic myelogenous leukaemia [6–9]. Even today, it remains a key chemotherapeutic agent in clinical practice. Its success laid the foundation for the continued exploration of the oceans as a valuable source of new pharmaceuticals.

Since then, numerous compounds derived from marine sources have been approved. Trabectedin (Figure 1), an alkaloid originally derived from the sea squirt *Ecteinascidia turbinate* [10], was the first marine-derived anticancer drug approved in the EU (2007) and later by the FDA (2015) for soft tissue sarcoma and ovarian cancer [11].

Dolastatin 10 (Figure 1) is an anticancer peptide derived from the sea hare *Dolabella auricularia* [12] and is currently in phase I clinical trials. It strongly inhibits the growth of human prostate cancer DU-145 cells in culture at very low concentrations (IC_{50} = 0.5 nM), causing cell cycle arrest in the G2/M phase and depolymerization of α-tubulin [13]. In animal studies, treatment with 5 μg every four days prevented tumour invasion in mice. Dolastatin 10 is therefore a promising marine-derived compound for prostate cancer therapy, acting through tubulin depolymerization rather than apoptosis induction [13].

Moreover, numerous Antibody Drug Conjugates inspired by marine peptides were approved by EMA and FDA for different treatments (e.g., polatuzumab vedotin (Polivy), enfortumab vedotin (Padcev), etc.) [14].

While Cytarabine, Trabectedin, and Dolastatin 10 are either approved drugs or currently in clinical trials, this review focuses specifically on marine-derived compounds that are in preclinical studies as anticancer agents. Emphasis is placed on their unique chemical structures and on the total synthesis approaches that have been optimised over the last decade, highlighting their promising therapeutic potential and the opportunities they offer for future drug development. These compounds of marine origin are of great importance for drug development; however, their limited availability from natural sources restricts their use. Therefore, chemical synthesis is necessary to ensure an adequate supply. These marine-derived compounds are classified in different classes: aromatic and heterocyclic alkaloids (Table 1 and Figure 2); terpenes and derivatives (Table 2 and Figure 3); macrolydes (Table 3 and Figure 4); linear, cyclic and depsipeptides (Table 4 and Figure 5) and other classes (e.g., polyketide, thiazole lipid, alkylamino alcohol, pyrrolocarbazole derivatives) (Table 5 and Figure 6).

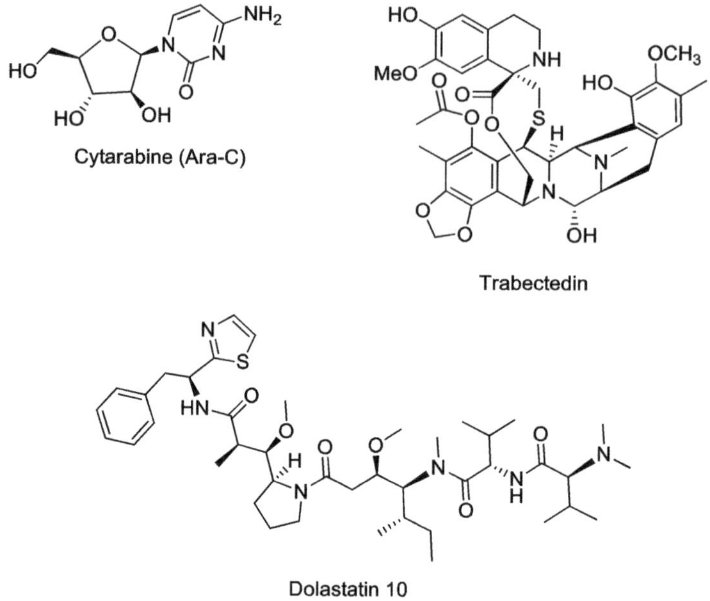

Figure 1. Structure of Cytarabine (Ara-C), Trabectedin, and Dolastatin 10.

2. Marine Natural Products in Preclinical Cancer Research

2.1. Aromatic and Heterocyclic Alkaloids

Ascididemin (Figure 2) is the first marine-derived pyridoacridine alkaloid, isolated in 1988 [15]. Originally obtained from the ascidian *Didemnum* sp., it has strong anticancer properties. Ascididemin inhibits topoisomerase II [16], an enzyme essential for DNA replication and repair, by intercalating into DNA, leading to DNA damage, cell death, and suppression of cancer cell growth. Ascididemin has been shown to exhibit cytotoxic effects against a variety of cancer cell types (HL-60, MCF7, HCT-116, and A549) with IC_{50} values ranging from nanomolar to micromolar [16,17]. Additionally, Vollmar's group demonstrated that ascididemin causes leukaemia Jurkat T cells to undergo apoptosis through a signalling cascade that necessitates the activation of the initiator caspase-2 upstream of mitochondria. Ultimately, in the same work, its cytotoxicity was demonstrated even against cancer cells that were resistant to many drugs [18].

In 1985, Faulkner and coworkers reported the first isolation of the lamellarin class marine alkaloids, lamellarins A, B, C, and D, from the prosobranch mollusk, *Lamellaria* sp. Since then, more than 50 lamellarins have been isolated from several marine organisms [19]. Among these aromatic and heterocyclic alkaloids, lamellarin D (Figure 2) is a potent anticancer compound. By inhibiting topoisomerase I, it exhibited mitochondrial pro-apoptotic activity, with in vitro cytotoxicity against various tumour cell lines (IC_{50} < 1 μM), including drug-resistant models [20]. In vivo, it demonstrated anticancer activity by slowing the growth of tumours in murine xenograft models. Among the series of natural compounds, lamellarin D is one of the most powerful [21], and it seems to be more well-tolerated than similar substances like ascididemin; nevertheless, comprehensive information on pharmacokinetics and systemic toxicity is still scarce [22].

In Antarctica, the sponge *Kirkpatrickia variolosa* is the source of the unique marine natural substance variolin B (Figure 2) [2]. Given its demonstrated pro-apoptotic properties, variolin B was a novel and highly effective natural cytotoxic agent [23]. Nevertheless, the poor stability of variolin B in solution restricts its application. This drawback of the original molecule has been addressed by the creation of a deoxyvariolin B (Figure 2) analogue that is far more stable and soluble. The biological activity of this deoxy analogue was comparable to that of variolin B, with a modest increase in potency that is probably due to its increased solubility and stability [24].

Both variolin B and deoxy variolin [25], show potent cytotoxic effects on a variety of tumour cell lines (IC_{50} in the 50–100 nM range). Due to their cytotoxic activities, Simone et al. [26] determined the molecular target of these substances. Their studies revealed that cyclin-dependent kinases (CDKs) are the main targets of these compounds, and consistent with their cell cycle-blocking properties, they preferentially inhibit the phosphorylation of histone H1 mediated by CDK1 and CDK2, but also inhibit CDK4 and CDK7.

Then, Meijer and colleagues [27] additional investigations supported this CDK inhibition profile and demonstrated that variolin B inhibits CDK9 even more potently than CDK1 or CDK2 (IC_{50} = 26 nM). Thus, its peculiar heterocyclic structure became a new scaffold for creating novel CDK inhibitors, and deoxy-variolin B was selected for preclinical development by PharmaMar due to its improved physicochemical properties over variolin B, including better solubility and stability [24,28]. Structural analogues (≥16 compounds) with modifications at positions C5 and C7 were synthesised; some of these analogues displayed antiproliferative activity comparable to or greater than variolin B across several cancer cell lines (colon, breast, melanoma, ovary, lung, pancreas, etc.) [28].

There are several methods to synthesise variolin B and deoxy variolin B. The first process is an 8-step procedure that begins with 4-chloro-2-methylthiopyrimidine and yields a 17% overall yield [24]. In 2008, Baeza et al. [29] introduced a new method based on selective Pd-catalysed C–N, C–C, and C–O bond formations on a trihalo-substituted pyridopyrrolopyrimidine intermediate to build the variolin B framework. In 2010, the same group published a new, more efficient route for synthesising variolins and potential analogues through a selective palladium-mediated functionalization of the pyrido [3′,2′:4,5]pyrrolo[1,2-*c*]pyrimidine core to rapidly install key substituents [30]. However, we will not go into greater detail about these works in this review since this topic was not further investigated in published papers in the last 10 years.

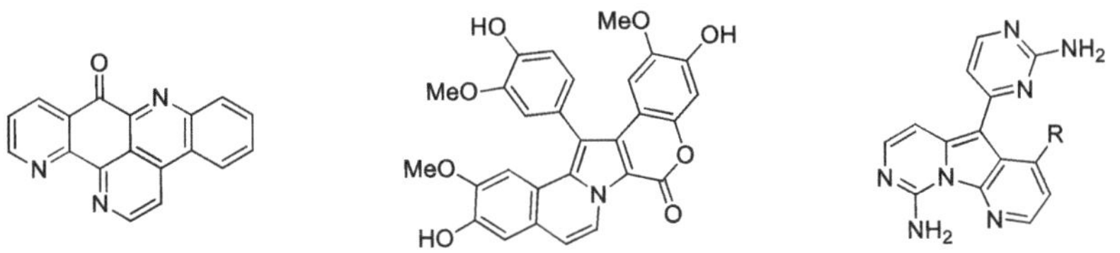

Ascididemin

Lamellarin D

R= OH, Variolin B
R= H, Deoxyvariolin B

Figure 2. Structure of ascididemin, lamellarin D, variolin B and deoxyvariolin B.

Table 1. Marine-derived aromatic and heterocyclic alkaloids with anticancer activities: chemical classification, source and involvement in cancer.

Compound (Isolation)	Class	Source	Cancer Type
Ascididemin (1988)	Aromatic alkaloid	*Didemnum* sp. (sponge)	Leukaemia
Lamellarin D (1985)	Pyrrole alkaloid	*Lamellaria* sp. (mollusc/corals)	Leukaemia, colon cancer
Variolins (1994)	Heterocyclic alkaloid	*Kirkpatrickia variolosa* (sponge)	Leukaemia, brain tumours

Lamellarin D Total Syntheses

The first total synthesis of lamellarin D was accomplished by Iwao and co-workers in 1997 [31]. Over the years, numerous total syntheses of lamellarin D have been performed [32–36]. In 2015, Chittchang [37] and coworkers published a common general approach to lamellarin D and azalamellarin D (Scheme 1). Starting from 4-(benzyloxy)-3-methoxybenzaldehyde (**1**), the bromination with pyridinium tribromide gave compound **2**, which reacted with ethyl 2-nitroacetate, in the presence of $Et_2NH{\cdot}HCl$, in toluene at reflux, to give compound **3**. This underwent a crucial Michael reaction with benzyl dihydroisoquinoline **7**, producing the 2-carboethoxypyrrole intermediate **4**. The pyrrole carboxylic acid (compound **5**) was unexpectedly obtained by the attempted amination of the pyrrole ester using $NaNH_2$, in dioxane at 100 °C. The resulting acid was then cyclized to form a lactone via microwave-assisted intramolecular C–O bond formation in the presence of copper(I) thiophene-2-carboxylate (CuTC). Subsequently, a global DDQ-mediated oxidation was performed, followed by a TFA-mediated acidolysis in thioanisole, which efficiently removed all -OBn-type protecting groups in a single step, affording the lamellarin D in excellent yield.

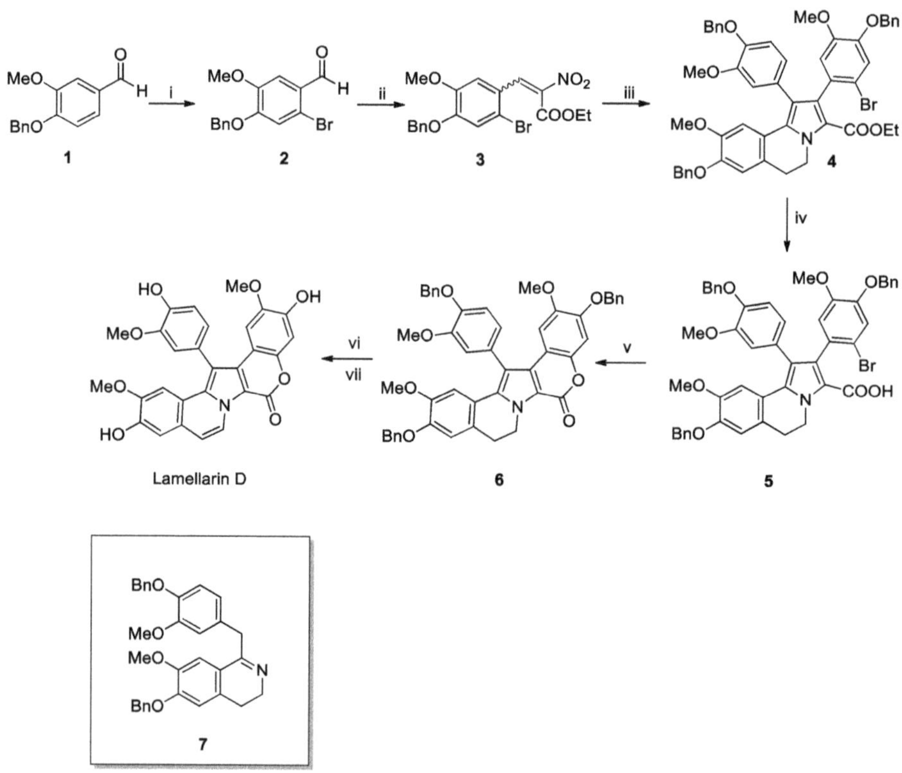

Scheme 1. Synthesis of lamellarin D reported by Chittchang's group in 2015 [37]. Reagents and conditions: (i) $PyHBr_3$, MeOH, r.t., 3 h; (ii) ethyl 2-nitroacetate, $Et_2NH{\cdot}HCl$, toluene, reflux, Ar (g), 3 days; (iii) **7**, $NaHCO_3$, MeCN, reflux, O/N; (iv) $NaNH_2$, anh. 1,4-dioxane, 100 °C, 18 h; (v) CuTC, DMF, MW (200 W, 150 °C), 45 min; (vi) DDQ, CH_2Cl_2, r.t., 4 h; (vii) TFA, thioanisole, r.t., 6 h.

Yang and coworkers reported two different methodologies for synthesizing the lamellarin core [38]. In 2016, they reacted 4-chloro-3-nitrocoumarin (**8**) and 1-methylisoquinoline (**9**) in basic conditions to give 4-(isoquinolin-1-ylmethyl)-3-nitro-2*H*-chromen-2-one (**10**), which was converted to **11** by visible-light-mediated cyclisation reaction. Unfortunately, this procedure failed when applied to 1-benzylisoquinoline; therefore, they opted for a direct coupling of **8** and **13**, catalysed by $Yb(OTf)_3$ Lewis acid in xylene under reflux, to give the lamellarin core **15**. This optimised methodology was then utilised in the preparation of lamellarin D trimethyl ether (**16**), by coupling 4-chloro-6,7-dimethoxy-3-nitrocoumarin (**12**) with commercially available papaverine (**14**) to give lamellarin D trimethyl ether (**16**) in 8% overall yield in three steps (Scheme 2). Subsequent exhaustive demethylation of **17** using boron tribromide afforded the natural product lamellarin H.

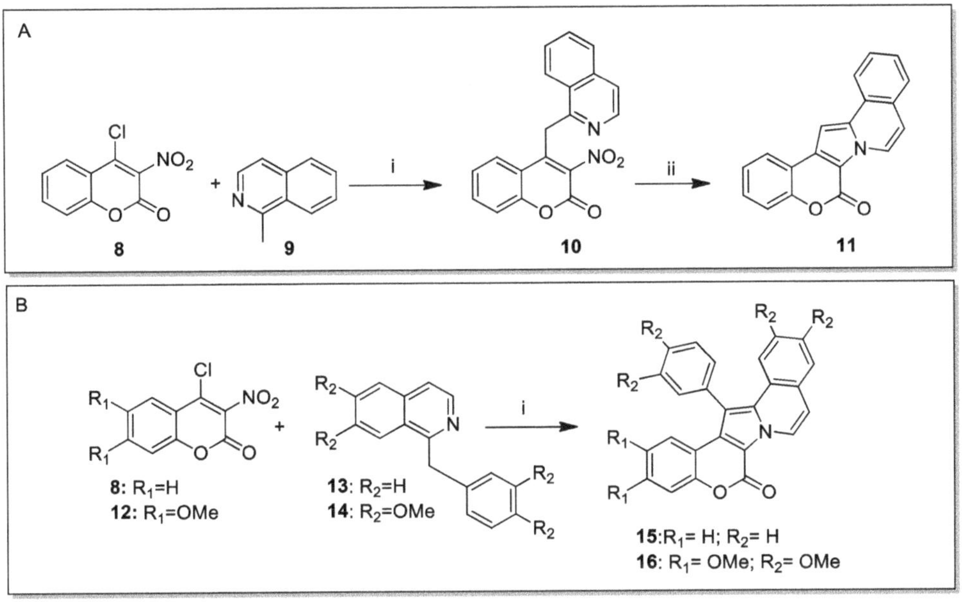

Scheme 2. (**A**) Synthesis of compound **11** [38]. Reagents and conditions: (i) K_2CO_3, DCE, reflux, 12 h; (ii) visible light, acetonitrile, 12 h; (**B**) Synthesis of lamellarian core [38]. Reagents and conditions: (i) cat $Yb(OTf)_3$, xylene, 130 °C, 2 days.

In a subsequent work, the same group described the synthesis of lamellarin D (Scheme 3) along with that of lamellarin H [39]. The Grob coupling reaction between 3-nitrocoumarin **17** and 1-methylisoquinoline **18** was employed for the synthesis of the key intermediate **19** by using $NaHCO_3$ and xylene in a sealed tube at 120 °C for 18 h. The building block was subsequently brominated and then coupled with [4-(benzyloxy)-3-methoxyphenyl]boronic acid to give the intermediate **20**. Finally, the debenzylation mediated by $Pd(OH)_2$ and AcOEt afforded the lamellarin D product. Moreover, in the same work, the authors demonstrated how to obtain intermediate **20** through a direct coupling between 3-nitrocoumarin **17** and benzylisoquinoline **21** under similar coupling conditions, by using $NaHCO_3$ and xylene in a sealed tube, this time at 130 °C for 24 h. This work represents the shortest route reported to date to obtain the lamellarin D.

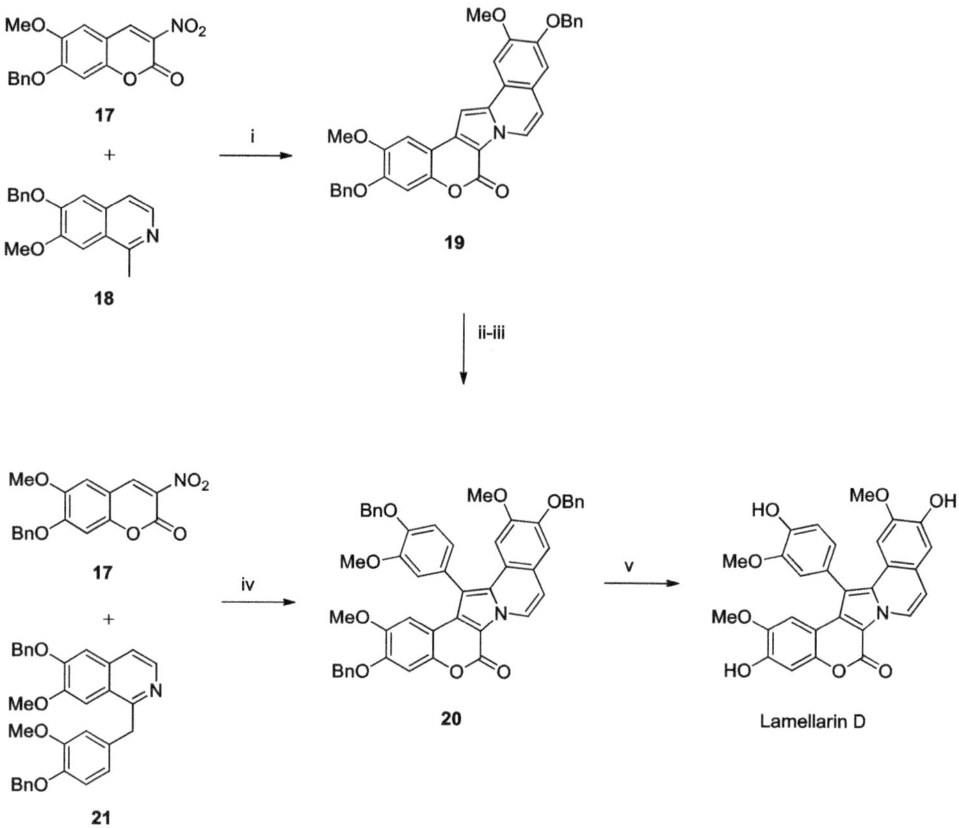

Scheme 3. Synthesis of lamellarin D reported by Yang's group in 2017 [39]. Reagents and conditions: (i) $NaHCO_3$, xylene, sealed tube, 120 °C, 18 h; (ii) NBS, THF, 0 °C-r.t., overnight; (iii) (4-(benzyloxy)-3-methoxyphenyl)boronic acid, CSF, Ag_2O, $Pd(PPh_3)_4$, DME, reflux, 24 h; (iv) $NaHCO_3$, xylene sealed tube, 130 °C, 24 h; (v) H_2, $Pd(OH)_2/C$, AcOEt, r.t., 8 h.

In 2017, Chandrasekhar's group synthesised lamellarin D (Scheme 4) [40]. The procedure began with compound **22**. By using the $[RuCl_2(p\text{-cymene})]_2$ and $AgSbF_6$, in the presence of $Cu(OAc)_2{\cdot}H_2O$ as the oxidant, in PEG-400, the diarylpyrrole-5-carboxylate **24** was obtained. Afterwards, the obtained pyrrole **24**, once brominated, was coupled by a Suzuki–Miyaura reaction, giving the tetrasubstituted pyrrole **26**, which was subjected to a Pomeranz–Fritsch reaction to create the lactone ring, affording the desired lamellarins H and D, with an overall yield of 29% and 37%, respectively.

Almost simultaneously, Ackermann's group published a synthesis of lamellarin D and H [41] using the same procedure described by Chandrasekhar's group (Scheme 4). In this case, Ackermann's group took advantage of the recent advancements in the application of Ru(II) catalysts for C–H/N–H activation. The central pyrrol ring of the alkaloids was obtained by a Ru-catalysed (3 + 2) oxidative annulation between enamide **23** with alkyne **22**. The optimisation of reaction conditions resulted in a gram-scale synthesis of intermediate **24** (Scheme 4).

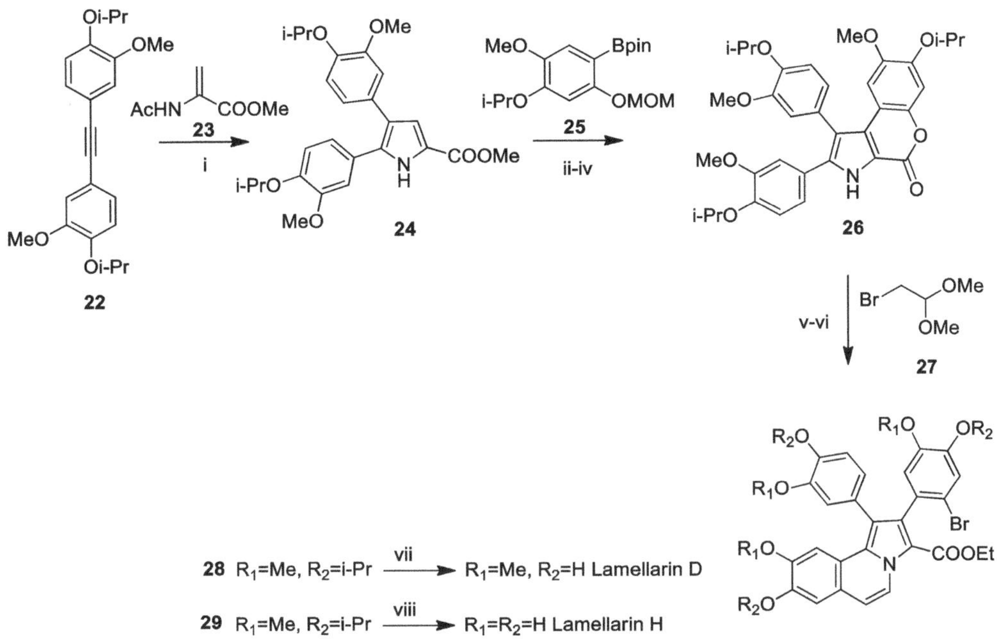

Scheme 4. Synthesis of lamellarin D reported by Chandrasekhar's group in 2017 [40]. Reagents and conditions: (i) $[RuCl_2(p\text{-cymene})]_2$, $Cu(OAc)_2{\cdot}H_2O$ PEG-400, 110 °C, 24 h; (ii) NBS, DMF, 0 °C to r.t., 12 h; (iii) **25**, $Pd_2(dba)_3$, dppf, DME/H_2O, 110 °C, 36 h; (iv) pTsOH, MeOH, 16 h, 110 °C; (v) **27**, Cs_2CO_3, DMF, 110 °C, 24 h; (vi) TfOH, CH_2Cl_2, 0 to 24 °C, 1.5 h; (vii) BCl_3, CH_2Cl_2, –78 to 24 °C, 3.5 h; (viii) BBr_3, CH_2Cl_2, –78 to 24 °C, 17 h.

In 2019 Shirley et al. published [42] a chemical synthesis procedure (Scheme 5) starting from compound **30** that was cyclized to obtain the pyrrole ring by using an excess of NH_4OAc in acetic acid at 110 °C for 30 min. The debenzylation of intermediate **31** involves the subsequent processes, which include lactonisation with K_2CO_3 in ethanol to obtain compound **32**. Compound **33** was then produced by alkylating the pyrrole with bromoacetaldehyde acetate, which, by eliminating the acetal intermediate in situ using catalytic TfOH, gave compound **34**. The last synthesis steps involved CH-arylation of molecule **34** with previously synthesised 4-bromo-1-isopropoxy-2-methoxybenzene, followed by the selective deprotection of the isopropoxy groups using BCl_3, yielding lamellarin D.

This approach was very innovative because bicyclic ring pyrrolo-benzofurans are obtained in a single system from a 1,4-dicarbonyl intermediate. Moreover, it was the first time that the C-H arylation on a late pyrrole was applied in the total synthesis of a lamellarin. The direct arylation reaction catalysed by Pd(II) was performed without the need for pre-activation of the pyrrole (e.g., bromuration followed by coupling), overcoming the limitations of the classical strategies based on halogenation and Suzuki/Stille coupling.

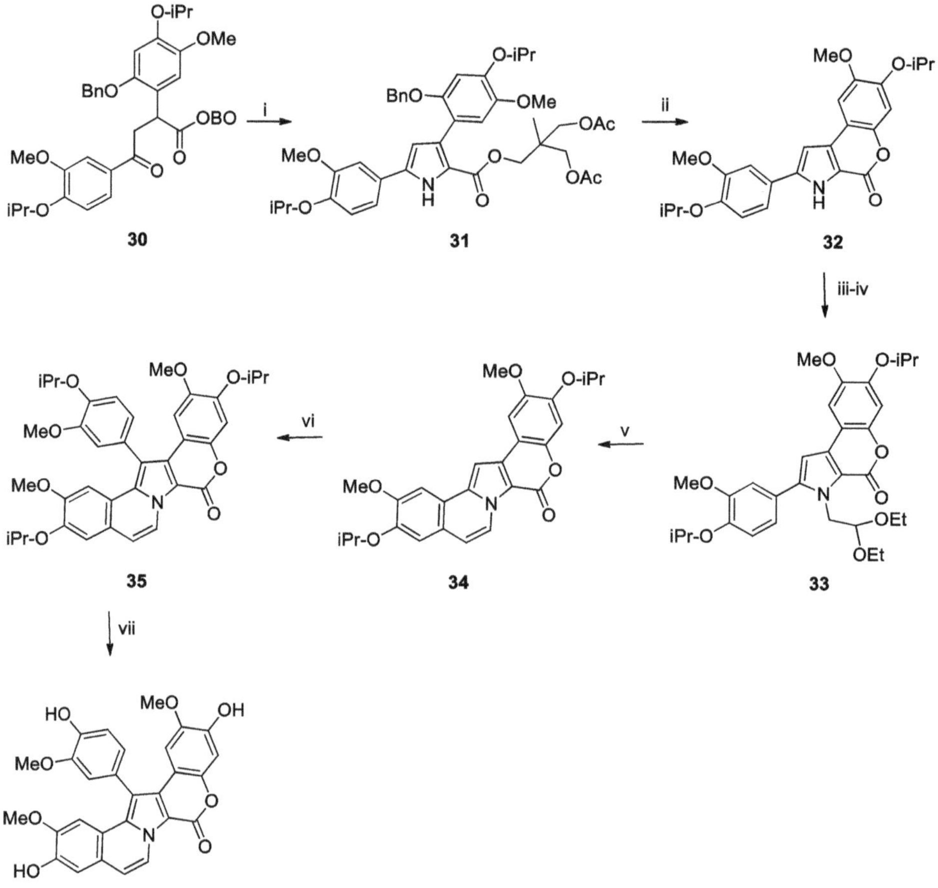

Lamellarin D

Scheme 5. Synthesis of lamellarin D reported by Shirley et al. in 2019 [42]. Reagents and conditions: (i) NH_4OAc, AcOH, 110 °C, 30 min; (ii) H_2, Pd/C, EtOH, rt, 6.5 h; (iii) K_2CO_3, EtOH, 90 °C, 2 h; (iv) $BrCH_2CH(OEt)_2$, Cs_2CO_3, DMF, 110 °C, 24 h; (v) TfOH, DCM, −10 °C to −5 °C, 24 h; (vi) $Pd(PPh_3)_2Cl_2$ (5 mol%), KOAc, 4-bromo-1-isopropoxy-2-methoxybenzene, DMA, 150 °C, 22 h; (vii) BCl_3, DCM, −78 °C to rt, 3.5 h. OBO= oxabicyclo [2.2.2]octyl orthoester.

2.2. *Terpenes and Derivatives*

Among terpenes and their derivatives, sarcodictyins are a family of cembranoid diterpenes isolated from soft corals of the genus *Sarcodictyon* [43]. Sarcodictyin B has also demonstrated some antimitotic activity [44]; however, sarcodictyin A (Figure 3 and Table 2) remains the reference compound for preclinical studies. It demonstrated antitumor activity [45] in preclinical models. Its mechanism of action is similar to that of paclitaxel (Taxol), acting by stabilising microtubules and thereby preventing cell division (mitosis). Sarcodictyin A was studied in vitro and in animal models for the treatment of various cancers, including breast cancer, ovarian cancer, and solid drug-resistant tumours [46,47].

Eleutherobin (Figure 3 and Table 2) is another naturally occurring terpene that stabilises microtubules. Initially identified from the rare soft coral *Eleutherobia* sp. in 1997 in Western Australia [48], it contains a central nine-membered unsaturated heterocyclic ring, showing an antitumor potency ten times greater than those of Taxol and Docetaxel [44,48].

Eleutherobin demonstrated potent cytotoxic activity against multiple tumour cell lines [49], and it showed nearly 100-fold greater potency against lung, ovarian, kidney, and breast cancer cells, as evaluated in a screening made by The National Cancer Institute (NCI) against 60 cancer cell lines. Finally, the NCI analysis revealed that its tumour selectivity pattern substantially matches that of paclitaxel [48]. Due to its antitumor properties, significant efforts were made toward the total synthesis of this marine natural compound.

In 2011, Su et al. [50] isolated ircinolin A, 15-acetylirciformonin B, and 10-acetylirciform onin B from the marine sponge *Ircinia* sp. Ircinolin A is the first metabolite generated from C_{21} terpenoid identified in *Ircinia*. In that same paper [50], two novel C_{22} furanoterpenoid metabolites were identified: 15-acetylirciformonin B and 10-acetylirciformonin B. The cytotoxicity of each of these substances was evaluated against several cancer cell lines, including the leukaemia line K562, the colon cancer cell line DLD-1, and the liver cancer cell lines HepG2 and Hep3B. In these screening tests, 15-acetylirciformonin B was the most effective of all. IC_{50} values were 0.03 μM (DLD-1), 0.5 μM (HepG2), 1.1 μM (Hep3B), and approximately 5.4 μM (K562). No complete synthesis of ircinolin A, 15-acetylirciformonin B, or 10-acetylirciformonin B has been documented as of the most recent literature.

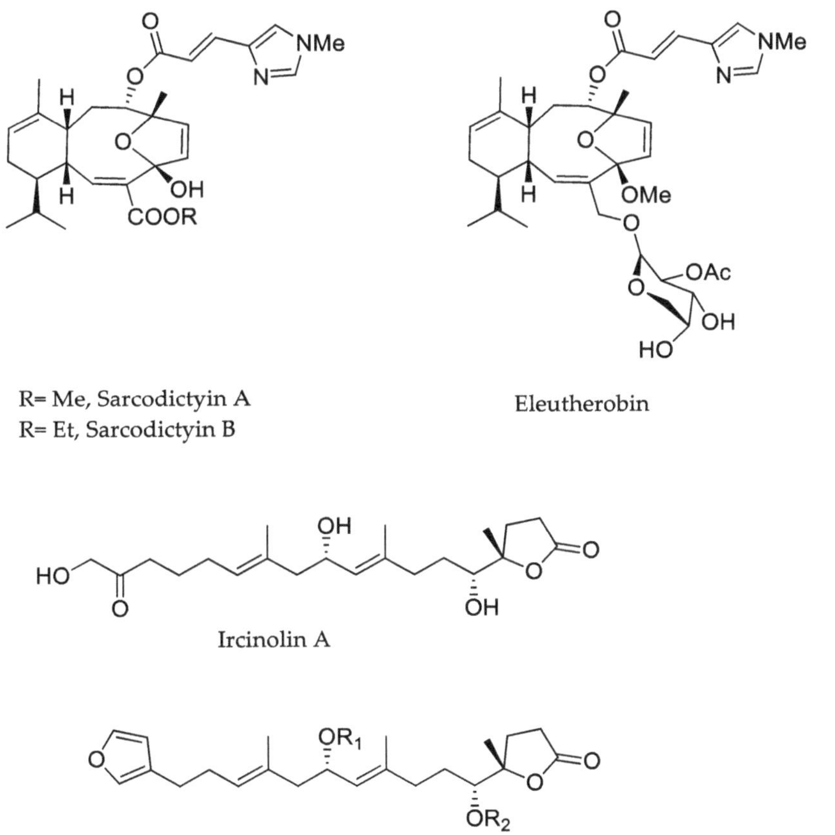

R_1=H, R_2=Ac 15-acetylirciformonin B
R_1=Ac, R_2=H 10-acetylirciformonin B

Figure 3. Structure of sarcodictyins, eleutherobin, 15-acetylirciformonin B and 10-acetylirciformonin B.

Table 2. Marine-derived terpenes and derivatives with anticancer activities: chemical classification, source, and involvement in cancer.

Compound (Isolation)	**Class**	**Source**	**Cancer Type**
Sarcodictyins (1987s)	Diterpene	*Sarcodictyon roseum* (sponge)	Ovarian, breast cancer, solid tumours
Eleutherobin 1997	Diterpene glycoside	*Eleutherobia* sp./*Erythropodium* (sponge)	Leukaemia, breast cancer
Ircinolin A 2011	Norsesterterpenoid	*Sponge Ircinia* sp. (sponge)	Leukaemia, colon cancer, hepatocellular carcinoma
15-acetylirciformonin B 2011	Furanosesterterpenoids	*Sponge Ircinia* sp. (sponge)	Leukaemia, colon cancer, hepatocellular carcinoma
10-Acetylirciformonin B 2011	Furanosesterterpenoids	*Sponge Ircinia* sp. (sponge)	Leukaemia, colon cancer, hepatocellular carcinoma

Recent Synthesis of Sarcodictyins and Eleutherobin

K.C. Nicolaou and colleagues were the first to complete a total synthesis of sarcodictyins A and B [51]. They developed two distinct approaches to access both compounds, starting from (+)-carvone, completing the synthesis in 29 linear steps. Since then, no new total syntheses of sarcodictyins have been published until 2025.

Very recently, the Britton group published a new synthesis of sarcodictyins and eleutherobin (Schemes 6 and 7) [52]. Their synthesis of sarcodictyins (Scheme 6) began from intermediate **36**, also known as eunicellin. After several trials, the C7–C8 alkene was *si*-face epoxidised with remarkable selectivity using the fructose-derived catalyst (compound **43**), yielding compound **37** as a single diastereomer. Subsequently, bromination at position 3 was achieved using *N*-bromosuccinimide (NBS), which reacted in situ with lithium bis(trimethylsilyl)amide (LiHMDS) in the presence of NEt_3 and TMSCl. In the next step, epoxide ring opening yielded a diol (**39**), in which the hydroxy group at position 7 reacted with the carbonyl at position 4 to form a hemiacetal group, characteristic of compound **40**. This crucial step was achieved by Leonori photochemical halogen atom transfer reaction by using the photocatalyst 4CzIPN, diisopropylethylamine, and a cobalt(III) cocatalyst. The desired alkene **41** was then obtained in good yield using the Leonori photochemical catalyst [53]. Finally, the reaction of compound **41** with (*E*)-3-(1-methyl-1*H*-imidazol-4-yl)acrylic acid produced sarcodictyin B methyl acetal (**42**), which was subsequently converted to sarcodictyin B through hydrolysis of the methyl acetal.

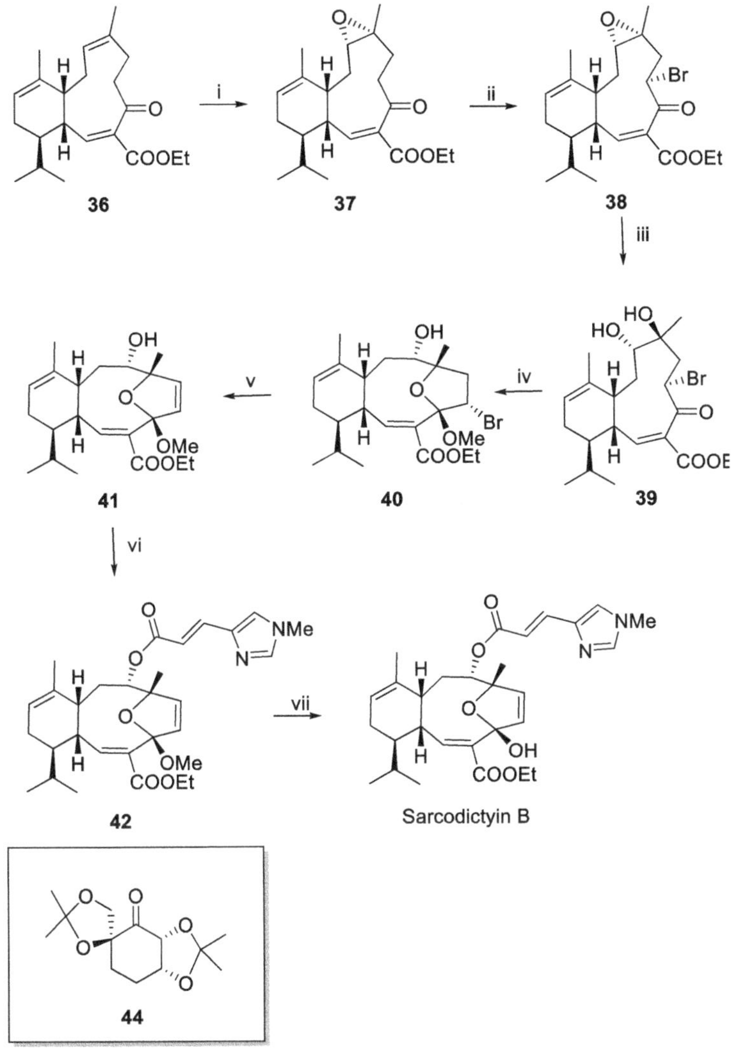

Scheme 6. Synthesis of sarcodictyins reported by Britton's group in 2025 [52]. Reagents and conditions: (i) Compound **44**, oxone, K_2CO_3, $Bu_4N(HSO_4)$, Na_2EDTA, $Na_2B_4O_7{\cdot}H_2O$, MeCN; DMM, H_2O, r.t.; (ii) LiHMDS, NEt_3, TMSCl, NBS, THF, −78° to −10 °C; (iii) TsOH H_2O, $MeCN/H_2O$, 70 °C; (iv) PPTS, MeOH, 50 °C; (v) $Co(dmgH)_2PyCl$, 4CzIPN, DIPEA, MeCN, blu LEDs, r.t.; (vi) (*E*)-3-(1-methyl-1*H*-imidazol-4-yl)acrylic acid, DCC, DMAP, $CDCl_3$, 50 °C; (vii) CSA, CH_2Cl_2, H_2O, r.t.

The groups of Nicolaou and Danishefsky reported the first two total syntheses of eleutherobin [54–56], after which other methods for synthesising have been reported over the years [57,58]. The last work on the synthesis of eleutherobin dates back to Britton's group, in the same work in which the synthesis of sarcodictyins is reported [52]. The synthesis of eleutherobin (Scheme 7) and its analogues was investigated, successfully reducing the number of linear steps to 18 compared to previous syntheses requiring 26–28 steps. Starting from the same intermediate **41,** the ethyl ester at position 15 was first reduced using DIBAL-H in CH_2Cl_2 at −78 °C. This was followed by selective esterification at C8 with (*E*)-3-(1-methyl-1*H*-imidazol-4-yl)acrylic acid to afford intermediate **45.**

Then, a glycosyl iodide (**48**) solution (previously obtained from the TMS-protected sugar and trimethylsilyl iodide) reacted with compound **45** using 2,6-di-tert-butylpyridine as a base in CH_2Cl_2 at room temperature. The resulting glycosylated product (**46**) was peracetylated using acetic anhydride and DMAP (**47**). Finally, deprotection with PPTS in refluxing methanol liberated the 3′- and 5′-hydroxyl groups, affording the fully elaborated eleutherobin.

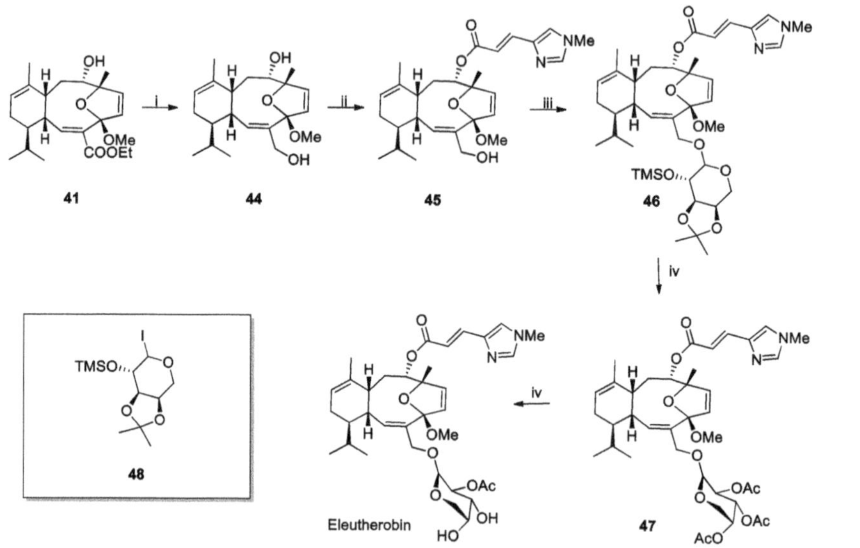

Scheme 7. Synthesis of eleutherobin reported by Britton's group in 2025 [52]. Reagents and conditions: (i) DIBAL-H, CH_2Cl_2, −78 °C; (ii) DCC, DMAP, $CHCl_3$, 3 °C, (*E*)-3-(1-methyl-1*H*-imidazol-4-yl)acrylic acid; (iii) **48**, Ac_2O, pyridine, DMAP, (iv) PPTS, MeOH, reflux.

2.3. Macrolides

Isolated from *Halichondria* sponges, halichondrin B (Figure 4 and Table 3) is a complex polyether macrolide with marine origins [59]. Halichondrin B primarily exerts its activity by inhibiting the formation of microtubules, which are necessary for mitosis and other biological functions [60]. Despite its potency, halichondrin B has a very low natural abundance, making it challenging to extract large amounts from natural sources for in-depth study and therapeutic use. Because of this paucity, chemists worked to fully synthesise halichondrin B and its analogues. Notably, its synthetic analogue eribulin (E7389) was approved by the FDA as an anticancer medication for liposarcoma and breast cancer [61].

Laulimalide (Figure 4 and Table 3) was first discovered from the marine sponge Cacospongia mycofijiensis [62] and is a strong macrolide generated from marine sources with significant anticancer properties. The primary way in which laulimalide acts as an anticancer drug is by stabilising microtubules in a manner similar to paclitaxel [63,64], but at a different binding location on β-tubulin [65]. In light of this, it is effective against cancer cells that are resistant to paclitaxel because it does not compete with it for the binding site. Moreover, laulimalide shows nanomolar IC_{50} values against a broad panel of human cancer cell lines, including breast, colon, lung, and ovarian cancers [63].

(−)-Lasonolide A also belongs to this class of compounds (Figure 4 and Table 3). It was first isolated from the marine sponge *Forcepia* sp. and found in waters close to the Bahamas [66]. (−)-Lasonolide A exhibits nanomolar potency to a number of human cancer cell lines [67]. Zhang et al. [68] revealed the exceptional potency of lasonolide A, inducing a reversible chromosome condensation, acting independently of the mitotic CDK1 pathway and involving histone modifications and topoisomerase activation. In addition, the authors described the (−)-lasonolide A as a promising research tool and a potential anticancer lead, though its exact target and therapeutic window remain to be defined.

Additionally, peloruside A (Figure 4 and Table 3) was discovered in 2000 by Northcote and colleagues [69] from the marine sponge *Mycale hentscheli* and collected in Pelorus Sound, New Zealand. De Brabander's [70] first complete synthesis revealed its absolute configuration; since then, several complete syntheses were reported [71–73] but none in the past decade. Regarding the biological effect, peloruside A is a powerful microtubule stabiliser; it binds to a unique site on the tubulin α,β-heterodimer and, for this reason, it may act synergistically with paclitaxel (needed to be optimised), docetaxel (Taxotere), epothilone A, and discodermolide B [74]. Studies in cultured cells showed enhanced antiproliferative and microtubule-stabilising effects when peloruside A was combined with these agents [74].

Moreover, additional studies revealed that peloruside A is very effective at stopping the growth of lung and P-glycoprotein-overexpressing breast tumours in vivo and, more importantly, was better-tolerated than doxorubicin or paclitaxel.

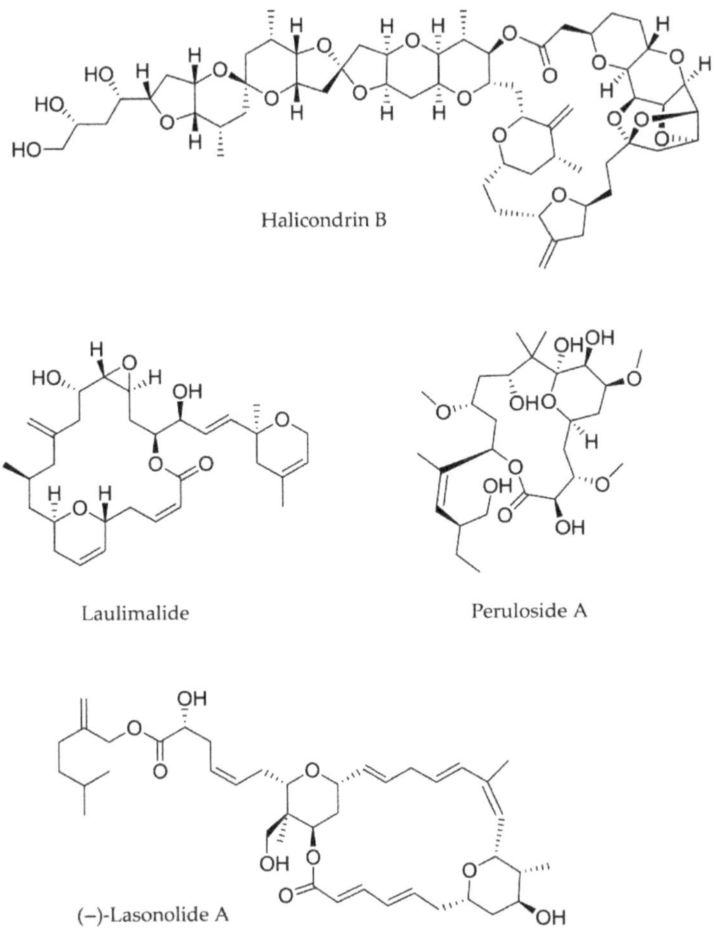

Figure 4. Structure of halichondrin B, laulimalide, peloruside A and lasonolide.

Table 3. Marine-derived macrolide compounds with anticancer activities: chemical classification, source, and involvement in cancer.

Compound (Isolation)	Class	Source	Cancer Type
Halichondrin B (1986)	Macrolide	*Halichondria okadai* (sponge)	Breast, lung
Laulimalide 1988	Macrolide	*Cacospongia mycofijiensis* (sponge)	Lung, ovarian
(−)-Lasonolide A 1994	Macrolide	*Forcepia* sp. *(sponge)*	Lung pancreas
Peloruside A 2003	Macrolide	*Mycale hentscheli* (sponge)	Non-small cell, lung, ovarian

Recent Synthesis of Halichondrin B and (−)-Lasonolide A

With more than 70 stages and sophisticated stereoselective techniques, the first complete synthesis of halichondrin B represents a significant turning point in organic chemistry, since this polyether macrolide features 32 stereocenters. In 1992, Yoon, S. K produced the first total synthesis of Halichondrin B [75]. Many other full syntheses of halichondrin B and other members of the family, such as norhalichondrin B and homohalichondrin B, have been published since then [76–80]. In 2021, Nicolau et al. [81] described a novel, versatile strategy for the synthesis of halichondrin B in 25 linear steps starting from commercially available reagents.

The authors began by synthesising all the key fragments. The synthesis of halichondrin B (Scheme 8) started with the coupling of fragments **49** and **50** (previously synthesised) mediated by NEt_3 and LiCl; then, the use of a high concentration of HF permits the one-pot desilylation, the removal of the acetonide moiety, and the intramolecular cycloetherification to obtain the intermediate **51** as a mixture of its C12 diastereoisomer. Then, the addition of DDQ and light followed by MsCl in the presence of Et_3N gave intermediate **52**. The latter are involved in the nucleophilic attack on the aldehyde group of compound **57**, achieved by using $NiCl_2$, $CrCl_2$, and Et_3N, and by using (*S*)-N-(2-(4-isopropyl-4,5-dihydrooxazol-2-yl)-6-methylphenyl)methanesulfonamide as a catalyst. The intermediate **53** was subjected to hydrolysis and cycloesterification to obtain compound **54**. These steps are very critical and need to be optimised. The best conditions were achieved in KOH and 18-crown-6 in toluene/MeOH at 60 °C, and with the next addition of KOH (1M) in MeOH to afford the desired carboxylic acid. After the coupling between the carboxylic acid and the hydroxy group at position 3 on the pyran ring, the demethylation of the hydroxy group on the hydrofuran ring was achieved in the next step using PTSA. The final stages are represented by the formation of lactol phosphonate **55** (deriving from the reaction with dimethyl (diazomethyl)phosphonate and $SnCl_2$) followed by the coupling with compound **58** in the presence of Et_3N and LiBr. Finally, halichondrin B was obtained by cleaving the TBS and PMB protecting groups and cyclizing with DDQ to generate the cast ring of halichondrin B.

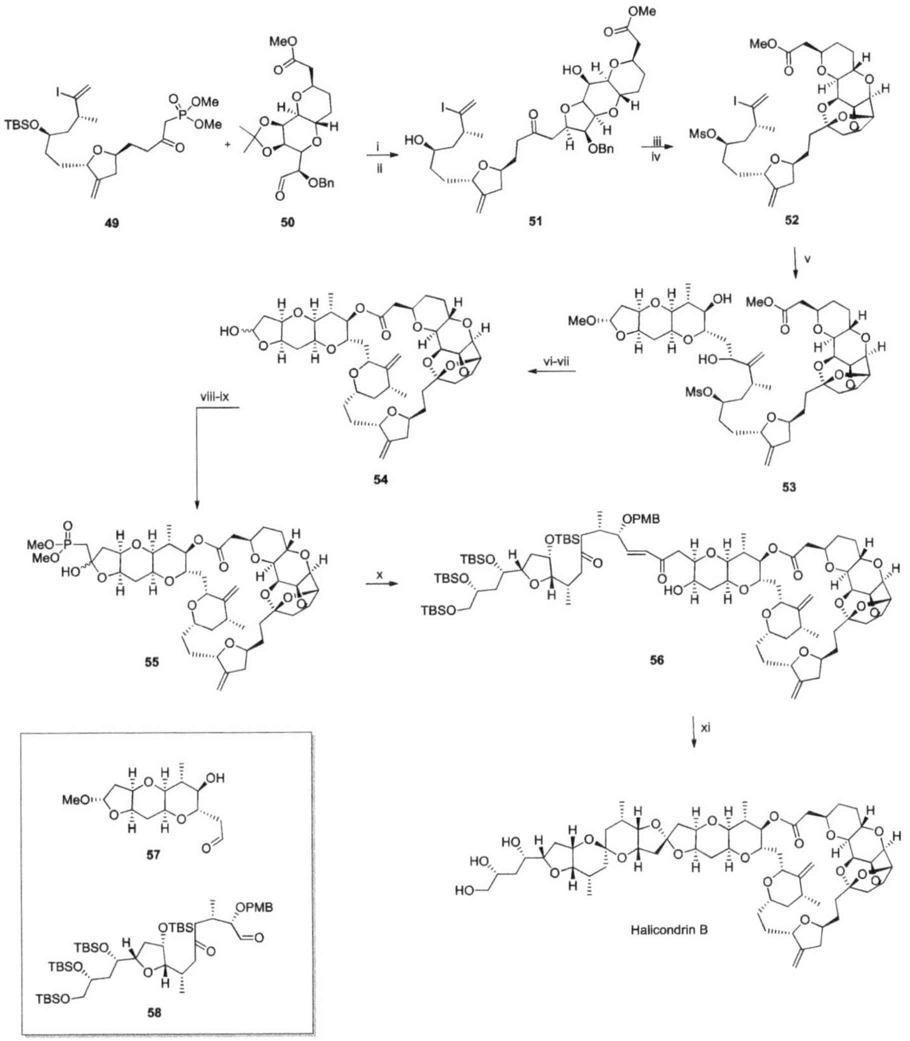

Scheme 8. Synthesis of halicondrin B reported by Nicolau's group in 2021 [81]. Reagent and conditions: (i) Et_3N, LiCl; CH_3CN, 0 °C to 23 °C; (ii) HF·Py (excess), CH_3CN, 23 °C 3 h; (iii) hv, DDQ; (iv) MsCl, Et_3N, DMAP, CH_2Cl_2, O °C, 15 min; (v) **57**, $CrCl_2$, $NiCl_2$, Et_3N, (*S*)-*N*-(2-(4-isopropyl-4,5-dihydrooxazol-2-yl)-6-methylphenyl)methanesulfonamide; (vi) KOH, 18-crown-6, then KOH, MeOH; (vii) MNBA, DMAP, i-Pr_2NEt; (viii) PTSA·H_2O; (ix) dimethyl (diazomethyl)phosphonate, $SnCl_2$; (x) **58**, Et_3N, LiBr, (xi) TBAF/AcOH, DDQ.

(−)-Lasonolide A shows a complex structure as well, and its complete synthesis has been a major achievement in organic chemistry. Asymmetric synthesis, macrolactonization, and convergent methods are employed in the various synthetic pathways that have been documented [82–88].

In 2016, Trost et al. [89] accomplished the last total synthesis of (−)-lasonolide A starting from two key intermediates synthesised by the same group (compounds **64** and **67**, Scheme 9A,B). The coupling between these two compounds was performed and optimised by using Ru-catalysed coupling (Scheme 9C) [90]. Both intermediates **64** and **68** were used for the reaction of acetonide with CSA to obtain both **69** and **70**. Then, the protection of the most accessible alcohols in TMSCl, ImH, 1M HCl, followed by macrolactonization with the Yamaguchi reagent, produced the TBS-protected (−)-lasonolide A.

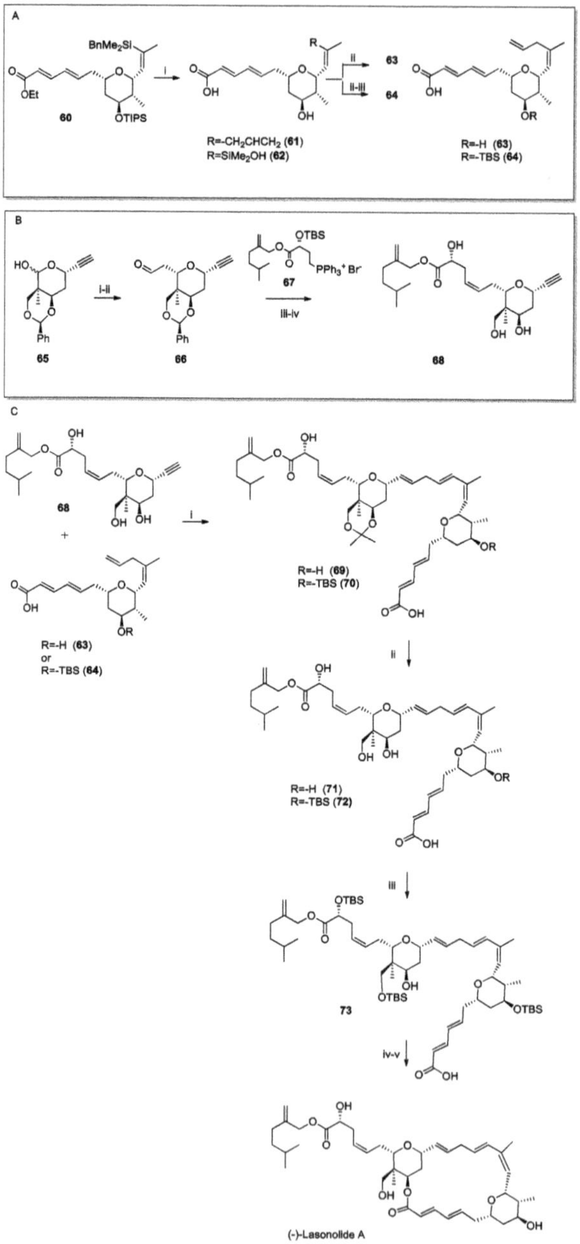

Scheme 9. (**A**) Synthesis of compound **64** [89]. Reagent and conditions: (i) $Pd_2(dba)_3{\cdot}CHCl_3$, allyl acetate, TBAF; (ii) LiOH; (iii) TBSOTf, 2,6-luditine. (**B**) Synthesis of Compound **68** [89]. Reagent and conditions: (i) Tert-butyl 2-(diethoxyphosphoryl)acetate, NaH, THF; (ii) DIBAL-H, CH_2Cl_2; (iii) **67**, KHMDS, THF; (iv) $LiBF_4$, aq. MeCN. (**C**) Synthesis of (−)-Lasonolide A [89]. Reagent and conditions: (i) $[CpRu(MeCN)_3]PF_6$, (ii) CSA; (iii) TBSCl, ImH, 1M HCl; (iv) 2,4,6-trichlorobenzoyl chloride, Et_3N, DMAP; (v) HF·Pyr.

2.4. Peptides: Linear, Cyclic, and Depsipeptides

Dolastatins, diazonamide A, thiocoraline, and vitilevuamide (Figure 5 and Table 4) are among the marine-derived natural peptides that have garnered considerable attention due to their potent anticancer activity. These compounds display unique structural features and mechanisms of action, making them valuable leads for the development of novel chemotherapeutic agents. However, the total syntheses of these molecules were accomplished years ago, and no recent synthetic advancements have been reported, reflecting both the complexity of their structures and the challenges associated with their large-scale production.

Dolastatins (Figure 5 and Table 4) and a few other related substances are antineoplastic pseudopeptides that were extracted from the nudibranch *Dolabella auricularia* [91,92]. Dolastatin 10 and 15 exhibited the most pronounced antiproliferative effect among all the metabolites and are currently being assessed for clinical studies [91]. The stereochemical features and structure of dolastatin-16 were clarified by X-ray crystallography in 2011. Surprisingly, unlike the natural extract, a later complete synthesis produced a molecule that was spectroscopically equivalent to the natural product but lacked nanomolar anticancer action in vitro [93]. It has been suggested that the bioactivity that was previously ascribed to the natural extract might have been caused by certain conformations that were missing from the synthesised molecule or by unknown impurities [93]. As a result, there are still many questions regarding dolastatin 16's actual anticancer potential. Due to the lack of activity seen in its synthetic form, dolastatin 16 never reached the clinical stage, unlike dolastatins 10 and 15, which advanced to phase I–III clinical trials as already reported above.

On the other hand, the ascidians *Diazona angulate* are the source of a complex of the macrocyclic peptides named diazonamides [94]. The anticancer properties of diazonamide A (Figure 5 and Table 4) were assessed among other diazolamides [94]. It binds tubulin and stops the cell cycle during the G2/M phase. In animal models, diazonamide A is a potential chemotherapeutic drug that does not cause severe toxicity [95]. Nicolaou's group accomplished the first complete synthesis of diazonamide A in 2002 [96]. This work is very significant since it combines Pd-boryl annulation for the second ring, Mg^{2+}-assisted macro-aldolization with DAST for the first ring, and asymmetric catalysis mediated by the iminium ion to create a complex macrocycle. Despite having an overall yield of less than 2% and being finished in 20 linear steps, the total synthesis is particularly noteworthy in the field of total synthesis. In order to avoid the macro-aldolizations employed in the first procedure, the second synthesis of diazonamide, carried out by the same group [97], adopts a totally new approach, using SmI_2 for a ring-closing sequence and a unique Pd-mediated oxidation to transform an indoline into an oxindole. Furthermore, MacMillan group total synthesis of diazonamide A [98] (2010) involved an iminium-catalysed stereoselective cascade to construct the furanoindoline core and C(10) quaternary centre. Macrocycle formation depended on Pd-catalysed borylation/annulation and Mg^{2+}-mediated aldolization, completing the synthesis in 20 steps with an overall yield of 1.8%.

The marine bacterium *Micromonospora marina* is the source of the cyclic depsipeptide thiocoraline (Figure 5 and Table 4) [99]. Thiocoraline does not inhibit DNA topoisomerase II or cause DNA strand breaks. Instead, its anticancer activity is linked to inhibition of DNA replication [100]. Primer extension assays showed that thiocoraline blocks DNA elongation by DNA polymerase α at concentrations that also halt cell-cycle progression and colony formation, indicating that the inhibition of DNA polymerase α activity is the primary mechanism [100]. Strong cytotoxicity is demonstrated by thiocoraline against a variety of cancer cell lines, especially colon cancer cell lines and those that are resistant to drugs [101]. Thiocoraline has not yet progressed to clinical trials, despite showing promise in preclinical research. A disulfide bridge connects a symmetrical dimer in its complicated structure. Because of its intricate symmetrical bicyclic depsipeptide structure, which consists of two identical peptide chains connected by a disulfide bridge, synthetic chemists have found it difficult to synthesise thiocoraline in its entirety. In the early 2000s, Boger and colleagues accomplished the first total synthesis [102]. Prior to dimerisation and the creation of disulfide bonds, they assembled each half of the molecule independently using a convergent strategy. This entire synthesis provides access to synthetic analogues that enhance pharmacological properties and enable thorough biological assessments [103].

Vitilevuamide (Figure 5 and Table 4) is a bicyclic peptide that was extracted from marine ascidians and exhibits strong cytotoxicity against a variety of tumour cell lines (LC_{50}: 6–311 nM) and acts as a tubulin polymerisation inhibitor, displaying potency comparable to colchicine [104]. In vitro, vitilevuamide inhibits tubulin assembly ($IC_{50} \approx 2$ μM) and causes G_2/M cell-cycle arrest with 78% of cells becoming tetraploid. It also noncompetitively inhibits vinblastine binding and stabilises colchicine binding, suggesting interaction at a distinct tubulin site. In vivo, it significantly prolonged the survival of mice with P388 leukaemia by 70% at 30 μg/kg, confirming its antimitotic and antitumor activity [104].

Vitilevuamide has not yet been completely synthesised and published in peer-reviewed literature. The majority of the published data focuses on the compound's structural characterisation by NMR and MS/MS, as well as its isolation from the ascidians *Didemnum cuculiferum* and *Polysyncraton lithostrotum*. Its potent in vitro and in vivo tubulin-inhibiting action is one of the biological data; nevertheless, no comprehensive synthesis pathway has been revealed thus far.

Table 4. Marine-derived peptides and depsipeptides with anticancer activities: chemical classification, source, and involvement in cancer.

Compound (Isolation)	Class	Source	Cancer Type
Dolastatin 15 (1987)	Linear peptide	*Dolabella auricularia* (mollusc)	Lymphoma, breast cancer
Diazonamide (1994)	Cyclic peptide	*Diazona angulata* (tunicate)	Colon, pancreatic cancers
Thiocoraline (1999)	Depsipeptide	*Micromonospora marina* (bacterium)	Neuroblastoma, lung cancer
Vitilevuamide (2002)	Cyclic peptide	*Didemnuin cuculiferum* (tunicates)	Lung, breast cancers

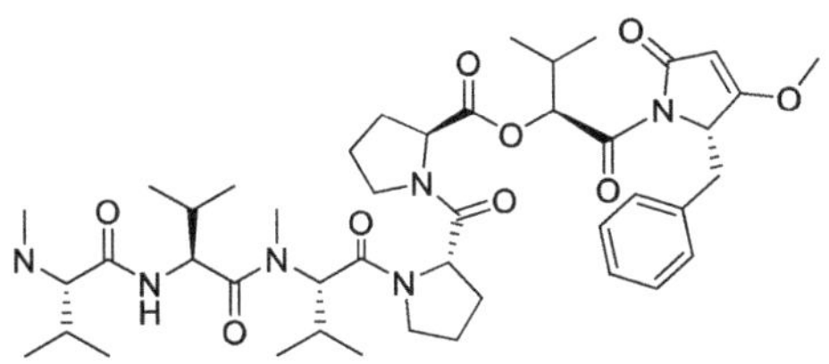

Dolastatin 15

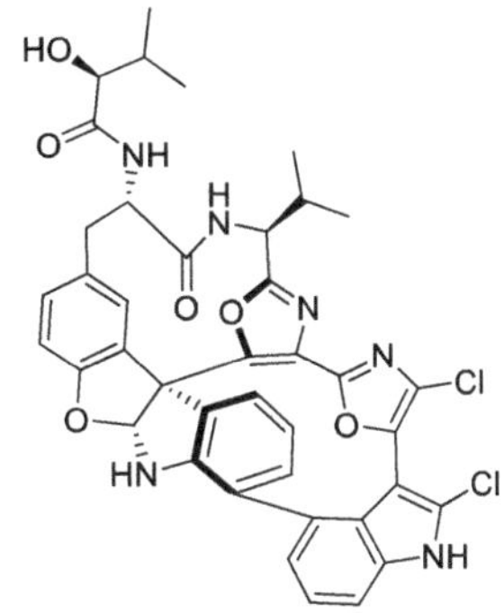

Diazonamide A

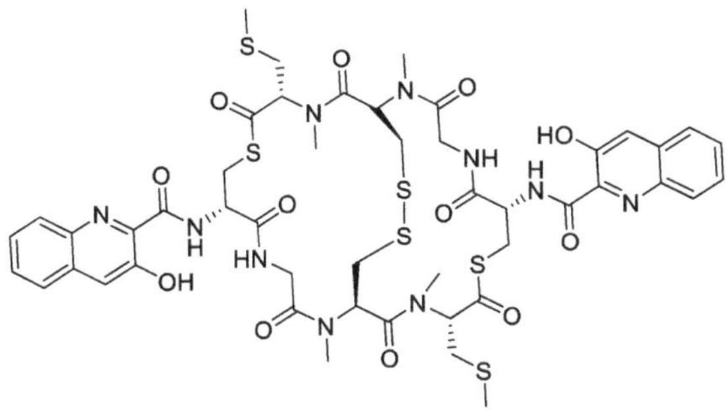

Thiocoraline

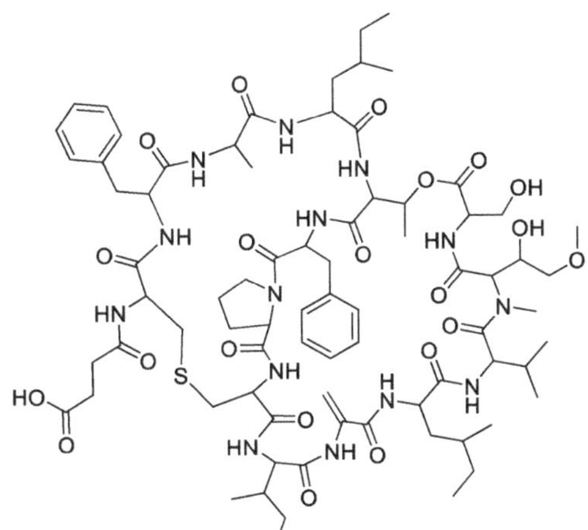

Vitilevuamide

Figure 5. Structure of dolastatins [91], diazonamide [94], thiocoraline [99], and vitilevuamide [104].

2.5. Other Classes

Further marine-derived compounds belong to different chemical classes. In this paragraph, we will describe curacin A, spisulosin 1, and dictyodendrins A–E as the only known members of these classes able to exhibit notable antitumor activity.

A naturally occurring substance with strong anticancer effects, curacin A is a thiazole lipid (Figure 6 and Table 5) and it was extracted from the marine cyanobacterium *Lyngbya majuscula*. Curacin A attaches itself to β-tubulin's colchicine-binding site. Since microtubules are necessary for the creation of mitotic spindles, their formation is inhibited [105]. Consequently, apoptosis results from the arrest of cancer cells in the G2/M phase of the cell cycle.

In vitro, curacin A has shown strong antiproliferative actions against HT-29, MCF-7, and A549 [105]. The clinical development of curacin A is severely hampered by its low water solubility and lack of chemical stability; in light of this, analogues and derivatives have been investigated for increased stability and bioavailability for in vivo applications, although they have been mostly examined in vitro [105].

On the other hand, originally obtained from the arctic surf clam *Spisula polynyma*, spisulosine 1 (Figure 6 and Table 5) is a marine-derived aminodiol molecule that shares structural similarities with sphingosine. When spisulosine 1 was initially isolated from the clam *Spisula polynyma* (syn. *Mactrometris polynyma*), it exhibited a high IC_{50} for cytotoxic activity against both solid tumour cells and leukaemia cell lines [106–108].

Padrón and colleagues further demonstrated that this compound has extraordinary antiproliferative efficacy on a number of cancer cells (HBL-100, HeLa, SW1573, T-47D, and WiDr) and acts as a specific inhibitor of casein kinase 1ε (CK1ε). In human pulmonary artery smooth muscle cells (PASMCs), Bittman and colleagues discovered that spisulosine specifically inhibits sphingosine kinase (SphK1) to cause its ubiquitin-proteasomal degradation, with an IC_{50} of 7.1 ± 0.75 mM, and also considerably suppresses the production of DNA in PASMC. Fusetani and Matsunaga identified dictyodendrins A−E (Figure 6 and Table 5) from the *Dictyodendrilla verongiformis* sponge collected off the coast of southern Japan [109]. These substances are members of a novel class of alkaloids that have at least one sulphate group on the periphery and a distinctive pyrrolo[2,3-c]carbazole moiety. Telomerase inhibition is a prospective target for cancer chemotherapy since the telomerase enzyme is overexpressed in >85% of tumour cells but not in normal cells [110]. Due to their distinct chemical structures and encouraging biological activities, numerous chemists have studied the complete synthesis of dictyodendrins [111–119].

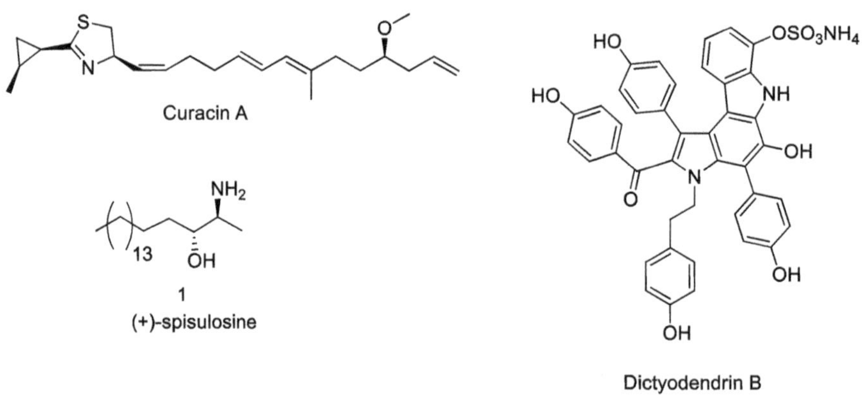

Figure 6. Structure of curacin A, spisulosine, and dictyodendrins.

Table 5. Curacin A, spisulosine, dictyodendrins: chemical classification, source, and involvement in cancer.

Compound (Isolation)	Class	Source	Cancer Type
Curacin A (1994)	Thiazole lipid	*Lyngbya majuscula* (cyanobacterium)	Colon cancer
Spisulosine (ES-285) (2000)	Alkylamino alcohol	*Mactromeris polynyma* (mollusc)	Breast cancer
Dictyodendrins (1993–2012)	Pyrrolocarbazole derivatives	*Dictyodendrilla verongiformis* (sponge)	Melanoma, glioblastoma

Recent Total Synthesis of Spisulosine and Dictyodendrin B

In 2010, Arun K. Shaw and Partha Ghosal [120] achieved the total synthesis of spisulosine. They first prepared (*S*)-Garner's aldehyde in nine steps. To establish the desired 2*S*,3*R* configuration, a key step involved a diastereoselective vinyl Grignard addition to Garner's aldehyde. The long C_{18} alkyl chain was introduced via olefin cross-metathesis, and final hydrogenation afforded (+)-spisulosine (ES 285). Since then, the total synthesis of this natural compound has also been reported by other groups [121,122].

In 2016, Göngiovà group [123] reported the synthesis of (+)-spisulosine (Scheme 10) and its anticancer activity, which shows an IC_{50} value < 1 μM on different cancer cell lines. Regarding the synthesis, the authors started from D-isoascorbic acid (**74**), which was converted into intermediate **75**, as previously reported by Abushanab et al. [124]. Compound **75** was then subjected to benzylation of the free hydroxy group using BnBr and Ag_2O in CH_2Cl_2, followed by reduction of the ester function to yield compound **76**. A one-pot IBX oxidation/Wittig olefination of compound **76** produced a mixture of α,β-unsaturated esters **77**, with the *E* isomer predominating over the *Z* (ratio 88:12). After chromatographic separation, the major *E*-ester was reduced using DIBAL-H, affording the required allylic alcohol. Subsequent reaction with MsCl and Et_3N, followed by treatment with KSCN in MeCN, yielded the corresponding isothiocyanate in two diastereomeric forms (compounds **79** and **80**). This step can be performed under different conditions: microwave irradiation at 70 °C for 1 h yields a 78:22 ratio of the two diastereomers, and similar results are obtained under conventional heating at 90 °C for 1 h. The authors observed that increasing the reaction time and temperature favoured the formation of compound **79**, likely due to the higher stability of this diastereomer compared to the other.

Isothiocyanate **80** was transformed into carbamate **81** over two steps: reaction with MeONa, followed by treatment with mesityl nitrile oxide (MNO). Ozonolysis of compound **81**, followed by a reductive treatment with $NaBH_4$, furnished compound **82**. Following the procedure described by Garegg's group, alcohol **82** was converted into iodide, which underwent catalytic hydrogenation (10% Pd/C) in the presence of Et_3N. To overcome the low yield in this transformation, the carbamate nitrogen was protected with a benzyl group, yielding the desired derivative **83**. Subsequent p-toluenesulfonic acid-mediated acetonide hydrolysis afforded compound **84**. This functionalized intermediate was subjected to oxidative fragmentation with $NaIO_4$ to give the corresponding aldehyde, which was treated with LHMDS and compound **87** in THF, resulting in a poorly separable mixture of olefins **85**. Catalytic hydrogenation saturated the double bond and removed both benzyl ether protecting groups, converting compound **85** into **86**. Finally, base hydrolysis (2 M aqueous NaOH in EtOH, reflux) provided the target compound, (+)-spisulosine.

Regarding the dictyodendrin B, in 2015, Gaunt [125] performed an efficient and innovative approach to synthesise it (Scheme 11), starting from a simple and commercially available indole building block. One of the main strengths of the synthesis is the use of catalytic C–H functionalization reactions and highly selective electrophilic aromatic substitutions, even in complex molecular environments. Another notable aspect is the use of flow chemistry for the late-stage formation of the carbazole ring, which adds both precision and scalability to the process. Overall, the method is modular and streamlined, allowing for the production of over a gram of the protected natural product and paving the way for the creation and testing of various analogues with potentially enhanced biological activity. In more detail, the indole's C7 position is targeted for iridium-catalysed C–H borylation, taking advantage of the directing ability of the indole nitrogen. This borylated intermediate is then directly subjected to a Suzuki–Miyaura coupling with 4-iodoanisole, installing an aryl group at C7 and yielding compound **88**. With the C7 arylation complete, attention turns to the N1 position, which is alkylated using 4-methoxyphenethyl bromide under basic conditions. The resulting product compound **90** is then subjected to a second Suzuki coupling at the C4 position, using a specially prepared nitrophenol-derived boronic ester. This step introduces the final aryl ring. The newly installed nitrophenyl group allows for selective bromination at C6 using N-bromosuccinimide (NBS). Directly in the same pot, the resulting aryl bromide is converted into a methoxy group via copper-catalysed substitution, producing compound **91**. The nitro group is then transformed into an azide through a three-step sequence: reduction, diazotisation, and azidation, yielding compound **92**. This azide is a key precursor for forming the central carbazole ring of dictyodendrin B, applying a continuous-flow process to thermally decompose the azide. This generates a nitrene intermediate that undergoes intramolecular C–H amination, forming the fused carbazole core in compound **93**. At this point, the final stages involve the removal of the tert-butyl ether and sulfonylation of the newly formed hydroxy group, demethylation of the other hydroxy group, and finally, reductive desulfonylation. These transformations culminate in the formation of dictyodendrin B, whose structure matches the natural product in all respects.

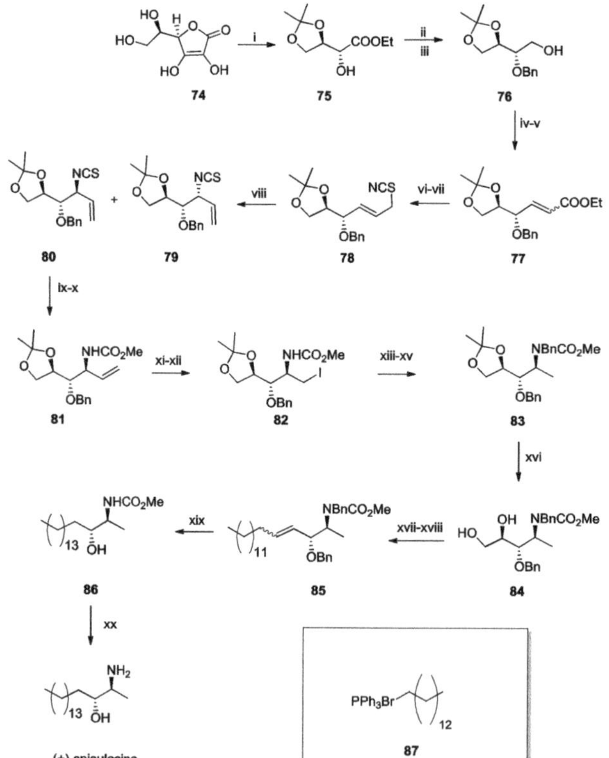

Scheme 10. Synthesis of (+)-spisulosine reported by Göngiovà group [123]. Reagents and conditions: (i) Ref. [124]; (ii) BnBr, Ag_2O, CH_2Cl_2, rt; (iii) $LiAlH_4$, THF, rt; (iv) IBX, MeCN, reflux; (v) $Ph_3P = CHCO_2Et$, CH_2Cl_2, rt; (vi) DIBAl-H, CH_2Cl_2, −50 °C; (vii) MsCl, Et_3N, CH_2Cl_2, 0 °C to r.t.; (viii) KSCN, MeCN, 0 °C to r.t.; (viii) heptane, MW, 70 °C, 1 h or Δ, 90 °C, 1 h; (ix) MeONa, MeOH, 0 °C to r.t.; (x) mesitylnitrile oxide (MNO), MeCN, rt; (xi) O_3, $MeOH/CH_2Cl_2$, −78 °C; (xii) $NaBH_4$, −78 °C to 0 °C; (xiii) Ph_3P, I_2, imidazole, $Et_2O/MeCN$, r.t.; (xiv) H_2, 10% Pd/C, MeOH, Et_3N, r.t.; (xv) BnBr, NaH, TBAI, DMF, 0 °C to r.t.; (xvi) p-TsOH, MeOH, r.t.; (xvii) $NaIO_4$, $MeOH/H_2O$ (1:1), r.t.; (xviii) LHMDS, THF, **87**, r.t.; (xix) H_2, 10% Pd/C/20% $Pd(OH)_2/C$ (1:1), MeOH, 60 °C; (xx) 2M aq NaOH, EtOH, reflux.

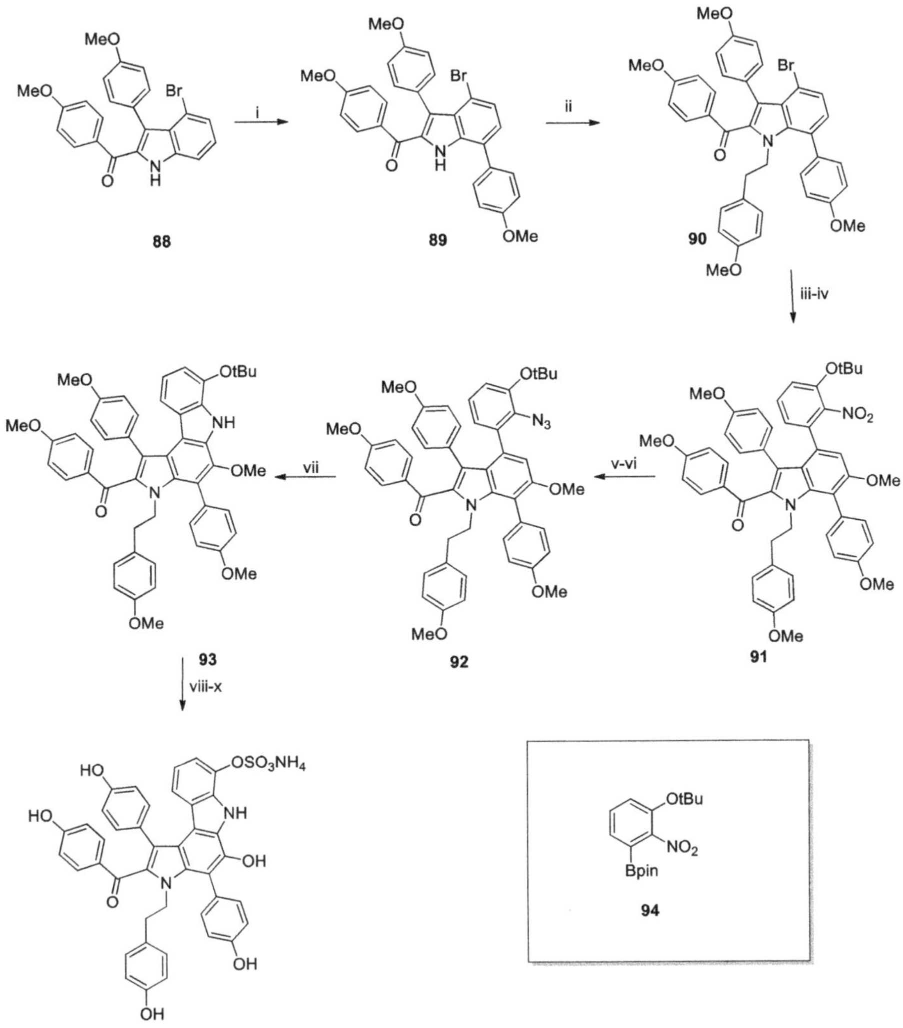

Scheme 11. Synthesis of dictyodendrin B reported by M. J. Gaunt [125]. Reagent and conditions: (i) $(Bpin)_2$, [{IrCl(cod)}leo$_2$], 4,4′-di-tert-butyl-2,2′-dipyridyl, THF, 90 °C, 1.5 h; 4-iodoanisole, [$PdCl_2$(dppf)], KOH, 80 °C, 30 min; (ii) 4-methoxyphenethylbromide, K_2CO_3, DMF, 100 °C, 16 h; (iii) **94**, [$PdCl_2$(dppf)], K_2CO_3, dioxane, 90 °C, 20 h; (iv) NBS, DMF, rt, 24 h, NaOMe, CuI, 80 °C 18.5 h; (v) $Pd(OH)_2$, H_2, MeCN, 24 h; (vi) AcOH, tBuONO, $TMSN_3$, RT, 20 min; (vii) dioxane, 180 °C, 30 min residence time, 0.333 mL min, Vapourtec R2+/R4 system; (viii-x) see Ref. [111].

In 2020, Ohno's group [126] reported the total synthesis of dictyodendrin B (Scheme 12) and the formal synthesis of the other dictyodendrins. Starting from compound **95**, the Boc group was first removed with NaOMe to increase the bromination in NBS in THF. In the next step, the alkylation of the nitrogen of the indole ring was obtained with NaOH, 18-crown-6, and H_2O. Finally, the Suzuki cross-coupling with 4-methoxyphenyl boronic acid, [$Pd(tBu_3P)_2$], K_3PO_4, dioxane/H_2O gave compound **94**. This was selectively brominated, which undergoes Ley–Griffith oxidation. Ullmann coupling with NaOMe was used to introduce a methoxy group at the C5 position, affording compound **97**.

Compound **97** was then subjected to the removal of the OtBu group with BCl_3 at −78 °C, formation of the sulphate group (following Tokuyama's protocol) and removal of the remaining protecting groups (BCl_3 + Zn), to yield dictyodendrin B.

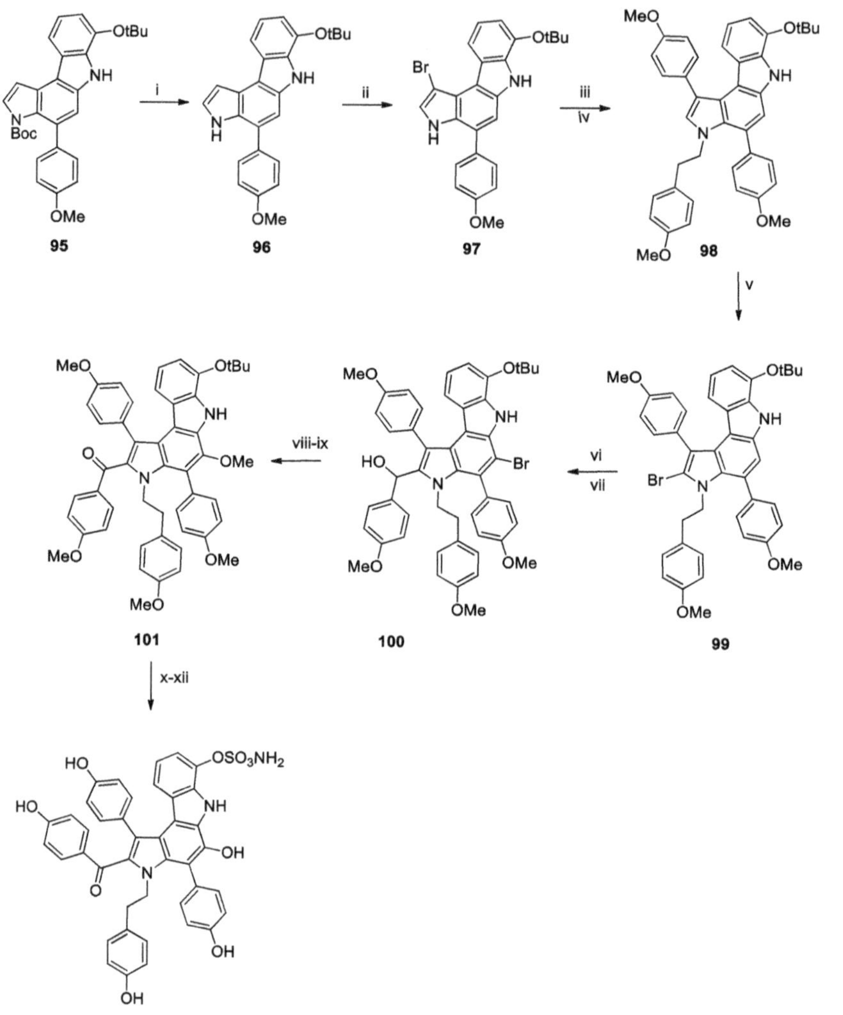

Dictyodendrin B

Scheme 12. Synthesis of dictyodendrin B reported by Ohno's group [126]. Reagent and conditions: (i) NaOMe, THF; (ii) NBS, THF; (iii) 1-(2-bromoethyl)-4-methoxybenzene, NaOH, 18-C-6, H_2O; (iv) (4-methoxyphenyl)boronic acid, $[Pd(tBu_3P)_2]$, K_3PO_4, dioxane/H_2O; (v) NBS, THF; (vi) MeLi, nBuLi, p-anisaldehyde; (vii) NBS, THF; (viii) [TRAP]NMO, CH_2Cl_2; (ix) CuI, NaOMe, DMF; (x) BCl_3, C_6HMe_5, CH_2Cl_2; (xi) $CCl_3CH_2OSO_2Cl$, DABCO, CH_2Cl_2; (xii) BCl_3, nBuNI, CH_2Cl_2; (xiii) Zn dust, HCO_2NH_4, MeOH.

3. Conclusions

Marine organisms, such as sponges, algae, and tunicates, have yielded a variety of secondary metabolites over the past few decades, including peptides, alkaloids, macrocyclic lactones, and terpenes. Some of these compounds have successfully advanced to the pharmaceutical market, while many others are progressing through preclinical and early clinical evaluation, particularly as candidates for cancer therapy. This review highlights the subset of marine natural products that are currently being studied for their anticancer properties, with a particular focus on how total synthesis has contributed to their production. Drug development and widespread use are severely hampered by the structural complexity and paucity of these metabolites from natural sources. Therefore, chemical synthesis and/or semi-synthetic approaches are necessary to ensure long-term access and facilitate structure–activity connection research. Specifically, we focus our attention on the more recent total synthesis, with a particular emphasis on the past decade.

Aromatic and heterocyclic alkaloids, terpenes and their derivatives, macrolides and macrocycles, linear, cyclic, or depsipeptide peptides, and other diverse frameworks such as polyketides, thiazole lipids, alkylamino alcohols, and pyrrolocarbazole derivatives are the main classes into which the compounds discussed here can be broadly divided. This work demonstrates the remarkable potential of marine natural products for cancer medication development and encourages further.

Author Contributions: Conceptualisation, E.C. and A.G.; methodology, E.C., A.G., M.G.C., G.B. and G.L.; writing—original draft preparation, E.C. and A.G.; review and editing, E.C., A.G., M.G.C., G.B. and G.L.; supervision, G.B. and G.L.; funding acquisition, G.L. All authors have read and agreed to the published version of the manuscript.

Funding: Ministero dell'Università e della Ricerca: PRIN 2022 "2022RCTY7M—BiTMaP—Coupling the power of bioinformatics and experimental tools for accelerating the production, structural elucidation, and target identification of marine natural products" (PI: Gianluigi Lauro).

Institutional Review Board Statement: Not applicable.

Informed Consent Statement: Not applicable.

Data Availability Statement: No new data were created or analyzed in this study. Data sharing is not applicable to this article.

Conflicts of Interest: The authors declare no conflicts of interest. The funders had no role in the design of the study, in the collection, analysis, or interpretation of data, in the writing of the manuscript, or in the decision to publish the results.

References

1. Altmann, K.-H. Drugs from the oceans: Marine natural products as leads for drug discovery. *Chimia* **2017**, *71*, 646. [CrossRef] [PubMed]
2. Perry, N.B.; Ettouati, L.; Litaudon, M.; Blunt, J.W.; Munro, M.H.; Parkin, S.; Hope, H. Alkaloids from the antarctic sponge Kirkpatrickia varialosa.: Part 1: Variolin b, a new antitumour and antiviral compound. *Tetrahedron* **1994**, *50*, 3987–3992. [CrossRef]
3. Lu, W.-Y.; Li, H.-J.; Li, Q.-Y.; Wu, Y.-C. Application of marine natural products in drug research. *Biorg. Med. Chem.* **2021**, *35*, 116058. [CrossRef] [PubMed]
4. Mayer, A.M.S.; Glaser, K.B.; Cuevas, C.; Jacobs, R.S.; Kem, W.; Little, R.D.; McIntosh, J.M.; Newman, D.J.; Potts, B.C.; Shuster, D.E. The odyssey of marine pharmaceuticals: A current pipeline perspective. *Trends Pharmacol. Sci.* **2010**, *31*, 255–265. [CrossRef]
5. Bergmann, W.; Feeney, R.J. Contributions to the study of marine products. XXXII. The nucleosides of sponges. I. *J. Org. Chem.* **1951**, *16*, 981–987. [CrossRef]
6. Löwenberg, B.; Pabst, T.; Vellenga, E.; van Putten, W.; Schouten, H.C.; Graux, C.; Ferrant, A.; Sonneveld, P.; Biemond, B.J.; Gratwohl, A. Cytarabine dose for acute myeloid leukemia. *N. Engl. J. Med.* **2011**, *364*, 1027–1036. [CrossRef]
7. Murphy, T.; Yee, K.W. Cytarabine and daunorubicin for the treatment of acute myeloid leukemia. *Expert Opin. Pharmacother.* **2017**, *18*, 1765–1780. [CrossRef]
8. Chhikara, B.S.; Parang, K. Development of cytarabine prodrugs and delivery systems for leukemia treatment. *Expert Opin. Drug Deliv.* **2010**, *7*, 1399–1414. [CrossRef]
9. Moser, A.M.; Adamson, P.C.; Gillespie, A.J.; Poplack, D.G.; Balis, F.M. Intraventricular concentration times time (C × T) methotrexate and cytarabine for patients with recurrent meningeal leukemia and lymphoma. *Cancer* **1999**, *85*, 511–516. [CrossRef]
10. Ganjoo, K.N.; Patel, S. Trabectedin: An anticancer drug from the sea. *Expert Opin. Pharmacother.* **2009**, *10*, 2735–2743. [CrossRef]
11. Huryn, D.; Wipf, P. Natural product chemistry and cancer drug discovery. *Cancer Drug Des. Discov.* **2014**, *2*, 91–120.

12. Pettit, G.R.; Kamano, Y.; Herald, C.L.; Tuinman, A.A.; Boettner, F.E.; Kizu, H.; Schmidt, J.M.; Baczynskyj, L.; Tomer, K.B.; Bontems, R.J. The isolation and structure of a remarkable marine animal antineoplastic constituent: Dolastatin 10. *J. Am. Chem. Soc.* **1987**, *109*, 6883–6885. [CrossRef]
13. Turner, T.; Jackson, W.H.; Pettit, G.R.; Wells, A.; Kraft, A.S. Treatment of human prostate cancer cells with dolastatin 10, a peptide isolated from a marine shell-less mollusc. *Prostate* **1998**, *34*, 175–181. [CrossRef]
14. Prabhu, R.H.; Patravale, V.B. Marine-derived pharmaceuticals for oncotherapy: Clinical trial and FDA-approved compounds. In *Encyclopedia of Marine Biotechnology*; John Wiley & Sons, Ltd.: Hoboken, NJ, USA, 2020; Volume 4, pp. 2607–2618.
15. Kobayash, J.I.; Cheng, J.-F.; Nakamura, H.; Ohizumi, Y.; Hirata, Y.; Sasaki, T.; Ohta, T.; Nozoe, S. Ascididemin, a novel pentacyclic aromatic alkaloid with potent antileukemic activity from the okinawan tunicate didemnum sp. *Tetrahedron Lett.* **1988**, *29*, 1177–1180. [CrossRef]
16. Dassonneville, L.; Wattez, N.; Baldeyrou, B.; Mahieu, C.; Lansiaux, A.; Banaigs, B.; Bonnard, I.; Bailly, C. Inhibition of topoisomerase II by the marine alkaloid ascididemin and induction of apoptosis in leukemia cells. *Biochem. Pharmacol.* **2000**, *60*, 527–537. [CrossRef]
17. Bonnard, I.; Bontemps, N.; Lahmy, S.; Banaigs, B.; Combaut, G.; Francisco, C.; Colson, P.; Houssier, C.; Waring, M.; Bailly, C. Binding to DNA and cytotoxic evaluation of ascididemin, the major alkaloid from the Mediterranean ascidian Cystodytes dellechiajei. *Anti-Cancer Drug Des.* **1995**, *10*, 333–346.
18. Dirsch, V.M.; Kirschke, S.O.; Estermeier, M.; Steffan, B.; Vollmar, A.M. Apoptosis signaling triggered by the marine alkaloid ascididemin is routed via caspase-2 and JNK to mitochondria. *Oncogene* **2004**, *23*, 1586–1593. [CrossRef] [PubMed]
19. Duc, D.X.; Quoc, N.V. Isolation, Bioactivities, and Synthesis of Lamellarin Alkaloids: A Review. *Curr. Org. Chem.* **2022**, *26*, 961–990. [CrossRef]
20. Dias, N.; Vezin, H.; Lansiaux, A.; Bailly, C. Topoisomerase inhibitors of marine origin and their potential use as anticancer agents. In *DNA Binders and Related Subjects*; Springer: Berlin/Heidelberg, Germany, 2005; pp. 89–108.
21. Chittchang, M.; Batsomboon, P.; Ruchirawat, S.; Ploypradith, P. Cytotoxicities and structure–activity relationships of natural and unnatural lamellarins toward cancer cell lines. *ChemMedChem* **2009**, *4*, 457–465. [CrossRef]
22. Ballot, C.; Kluza, J.; Lancel, S.; Martoriati, A.; Hassoun, S.M.; Mortier, L.; Vienne, J.-C.; Briand, G.; Formstecher, P.; Bailly, C. Inhibition of mitochondrial respiration mediates apoptosis induced by the anti-tumoral alkaloid lamellarin D. *Apoptosis* **2010**, *15*, 769–781. [CrossRef]
23. Dembitsky, V.M.; Gloriozova, T.A.; Poroikov, V.V. Novel antitumor agents: Marine sponge alkaloids, their synthetic analogs and derivatives. *Mini Rev. Med. Chem.* **2005**, *5*, 319–336. [CrossRef]
24. Anderson, R.J.; Hill, J.B.; Morris, J.C. Concise total syntheses of variolin B and deoxyvariolin B. *J. Org. Chem.* **2005**, *70*, 6204–6212. [CrossRef] [PubMed]
25. Walker, S.R.; Carter, E.J.; Huff, B.C.; Morris, J.C. Variolins and related alkaloids. *Chem. Rev.* **2009**, *109*, 3080–3098. [CrossRef] [PubMed]
26. Simone, M.; Erba, E.; Damia, G.; Vikhanskaya, F.; Di Francesco, A.M.; Riccardi, R.; Bailly, C.; Cuevas, C.; Sousa-Faro, J.M.F.; D'Incalci, M. Variolin B and its derivate deoxy-variolin B: New marine natural compounds with cyclin-dependent kinase inhibitor activity. *Eur. J. Cancer* **2005**, *41*, 2366–2377. [CrossRef] [PubMed]
27. Bettayeb, K.; Tirado, O.M.; Marionneau-Lambot, S.; Ferandin, Y.; Lozach, O.; Morris, J.C.; Mateo-Lozano, S.; Drueckes, P.; Schächtele, C.; Kubbutat, M.H.; et al. Meriolins, a new class of cell death–inducing kinase inhibitors with enhanced selectivity for cyclin-dependent kinases. *Cancer Res.* **2007**, *67*, 8325–8334. [CrossRef]
28. Imperatore, C.; Aiello, A.; D'Aniello, F.; Senese, M.; Menna, M. Alkaloids from marine invertebrates as important leads for anticancer drugs discovery and development. *Molecules* **2014**, *19*, 20391–20423. [CrossRef]
29. Baeza, A.; Mendiola, J.; Burgos, C.; Alvarez-Builla, J.; Vaquero, J. Palladium-mediated C–N, C–C, and C–O functionalization of azolopyrimidines: A new total synthesis of Variolin B. *Tetrahedron Lett.* **2008**, *49*, 4073–4077. [CrossRef]
30. Baeza, A.; Mendiola, J.; Burgos, C.; Alvarez-Builla, J.; Vaquero, J.J. Application of Selective Palladium-Mediated Functionalization of the Pyrido [3′,2′:4,5] pyrrolo [1,2-c] pyrimidine Heterocyclic System for the Total Synthesis of Variolin B and Deoxyvariolin B. *EurJoc* **2010**, *1*, 607–5618. [CrossRef]
31. Ishibashi, F.; Miyazaki, Y.; Iwao, M. Total syntheses of lamellarin D and H. The first synthesis of lamellarin-class marine alkaloids. *Tetrahedron* **1997**, *53*, 5951–5962. [CrossRef]
32. Komatsubara, M.; Umeki, T.; Fukuda, T.; Iwao, M. Modular synthesis of lamellarins via regioselective assembly of 3,4,5-differentially arylated pyrrole-2-carboxylates. *J. Org. Chem.* **2014**, *79*, 529–537. [CrossRef]
33. Li, Q.; Jiang, J.; Fan, A.; Cui, Y.; Jia, Y. Total synthesis of lamellarins D, H, and R and ningalin B. *Org. Lett.* **2011**, *13*, 312–315. [CrossRef] [PubMed]
34. Handy, S.T.; Zhang, Y. Approaches to the synthesis of the lamellarins and related natural products. A review. *Org. Prep. Proced. Int.* **2005**, *37*, 411–445. [CrossRef]

35. Imbri, D.; Tauber, J.; Opatz, T. Synthetic approaches to the lamellarins—A comprehensive review. *Mar. Drugs* **2014**, *12*, 6142–6177. [CrossRef] [PubMed]
36. Sivaganesan, P.; VL, S.; Sahoo, A.; Elanchezhian, C.; Nataraj, G.; Chaudhuri, S. A Comprehensive Review of Synthetic Approaches Toward Lamellarin D and its Analogous. *ChemistrySelect* **2024**, *9*, e202403112. [CrossRef]
37. Theppawong, A.; Ploypradith, P.; Chuawong, P.; Ruchirawat, S.; Chittchang, M. Facile and divergent synthesis of lamellarins and lactam-containing derivatives with improved drug likeness and biological activities. *Chem. Asian J.* **2015**, *10*, 2631–2650. [CrossRef]
38. Manjappa, K.B.; Syu, J.-R.; Yang, D.-Y. Visible-light-promoted and Yb (OTf) 3-catalyzed constructions of coumarin-pyrrole-(iso) quinoline-fused pentacycles: Synthesis of lamellarin core, lamellarin D trimethyl ether, and lamellarin H. *Org. Lett.* **2016**, *18*, 332–335. [CrossRef]
39. Manjappa, K.B.; Lin, J.-M.; Yang, D.-Y. Construction of pentacyclic lamellarin skeleton via Grob reaction: Application to total synthesis of lamellarins H and D. *J. Org. Chem.* **2017**, *82*, 7648–7656. [CrossRef]
40. Lade, D.M.; Pawar, A.B.; Mainkar, P.S.; Chandrasekhar, S. Total synthesis of lamellarin D trimethyl ether, lamellarin D, and lamellarin H. *J. Org. Chem.* **2017**, *82*, 4998–5004. [CrossRef]
41. Mei, R.; Zhang, S.-K.; Ackermann, L. Concise Synthesis of Lamellarin Alkaloids by C–H/N–H Activation: Evaluation of Metal Catalysts in Oxidative Alkyne Annulation. *Synlett* **2017**, *28*, 1715–1718. [CrossRef]
42. Shirley, H.J.; Koyioni, M.; Muncan, F.; Donohoe, T.J. Synthesis of lamellarin alkaloids using orthoester-masked α-keto acids. *Chem. Sci.* **2019**, *10*, 4334–4338. [CrossRef]
43. Liang, L.F.; Guo, Y.W. Terpenes from the soft corals of the genus Sarcophyton: Chemistry and biological activities. *Chem. Biodivers.* **2013**, *10*, 2161–2196. [CrossRef]
44. Hamel, E.; Sackett, D.L.; Vourloumis, D.; Nicolaou, K. The coral-derived natural products eleutherobin and sarcodictyins A and B: Effects on the assembly of purified tubulin with and without microtubule-associated proteins and binding at the polymer taxoid site. *Biochemistry* **1999**, *38*, 5490–5498. [CrossRef] [PubMed]
45. Pietra, F. Fighting cancer with microtubule-stabilizing agents: A computational investigation of the complex between β-tubulin and the microtubule-stabilizing, antitumor marine diterpenoid sarcodictyin A. *Struct. Chem.* **2020**, *31*, 927–935. [CrossRef]
46. Risinger, A.L.; Giles, F.J.; Mooberry, S.L. Microtubule dynamics as a target in oncology. *Cancer Treat. Rev.* **2009**, *35*, 255–261. [CrossRef] [PubMed]
47. Nicolaou, K.; Pfefferkorn, J.; Xu, J.; Winssinger, N.; Ohshima, T.; Kim, S.; Hosokawa, S.; Vourloumis, D.; Van Delft, F.; Li, T. Total synthesis and chemical biology of the sarcodictyins. *Chem. Pharm. Bull.* **1999**, *47*, 1199–1213. [CrossRef]
48. Lindel, T.; Jensen, P.R.; Fenical, W.; Long, B.H.; Casazza, A.M.; Carboni, J.; Fairchild, C.R. Eleutherobin, a new cytotoxin that mimics paclitaxel (Taxol) by stabilizing microtubules. *J. Am. Chem. Soc.* **1997**, *119*, 8744–8745. [CrossRef]
49. Sosonyuk, S.E.; Peshich, A.; Tutushkina, A.V.; Khlevin, D.A.; Lozinskaya, N.A.; Gracheva, Y.A.; Glazunova, V.A.; Osolodkin, D.I.; Semenova, M.N.; Semenov, V.V. Synthesis and cytotoxicity of novel simplified eleutherobin analogues as potential antitumour agents. *Org. Biomol. Chem.* **2019**, *17*, 2792–2797. [CrossRef]
50. Su, J.-H.; Tseng, S.-W.; Lu, M.-C.; Liu, L.-L.; Chou, Y.; Sung, P.-J. Cytotoxic C21 and C22 terpenoid-derived metabolites from the sponge Ircinia sp. *J. Nat. Prod.* **2011**, *74*, 2005–2009. [CrossRef]
51. Nicolaou, K.; Winssinger, N.; Vourloumis, D.; Ohshima, T.; Kim, S.; Pfefferkorn, J.; Xu, J.-Y.; Li, T. Solid and solution phase synthesis and biological evaluation of combinatorial sarcodictyin libraries. *J. Am. Chem. Soc.* **1998**, *120*, 10814–10826. [CrossRef]
52. Driedger, D.; Fers-Lidou, A.; Schroeder, M.; Elisia, I.; Krystal, G.; Britton, R. An Expedient Synthesis of the Antimitotic Natural Products Sarcodictyin and Eleutherobin, and Carbohydrate Analogues. *J. Am. Chem. Soc.* **2025**, *147*, 28117–28126. [CrossRef]
53. Zhao, H.; McMillan, A.J.; Constantin, T.; Mykura, R.C.; Julia, F.; Leonori, D. Merging halogen-atom transfer (XAT) and cobalt catalysis to override E2-selectivity in the elimination of alkyl halides: A mild route toward contra-thermodynamic olefins. *J. Am. Chem. Soc.* **2021**, *143*, 14806–14813. [CrossRef]
54. Nicolaou, K.; Van Delft, F.; Ohshima, T.; Vourloumis, D.; Xu, J.; Hosokawa, S.; Pfefferkorn, J.; Kim, S.; Li, T. Total synthesis of eleutherobin. *Angew. Chem. Int. Ed. Engl.* **1997**, *36*, 2520–2524. [CrossRef]
55. Nicolaou, K.; Xu, J.-Y.; Kim, S.; Ohshima, T.; Hosokawa, S.; Pfefferkorn, J. Synthesis of the tricyclic core of eleutherobin and sarcodictyins and total synthesis of sarcodictyin A. *J. Am. Chem. Soc.* **1997**, *119*, 11353–11354. [CrossRef]
56. Chen, X.-T.; Bhattacharya, S.K.; Zhou, B.; Gutteridge, C.E.; Pettus, T.R.; Danishefsky, S.J. The total synthesis of eleutherobin. *J. Am. Chem. Soc.* **1999**, *121*, 6563–6579. [CrossRef]
57. Mowat, J.S. Studies Towards the Total Synthesis of Eleutherobin and Other Marine Natural Products. Ph.D. Thesis, Simon Fraser University, Vancouver, BC, Canada, 2012.
58. Carter, R.; Hodgetts, K.; McKenna, J.; Magnus, P.; Wren, S. Studies on the stereoselective synthesis of the marine antitumor agent eleutherobin. *Tetrahedron* **2000**, *56*, 4367–4382. [CrossRef]
59. Hickford, S.J.; Blunt, J.W.; Munro, M.H. Antitumour polyether macrolides: Four new halichondrins from the New Zealand deep-water marine sponge *Lissodendoryx* sp. *Biorg. Med. Chem.* **2009**, *17*, 2199–2203. [CrossRef]

60. Dissanayake, D.S.; Nagahawatta, D.P.; Lee, J.-S.; Jeon, Y.-J. Immunomodulatory effects of halichondrin isolated from marine sponges and its synthetic analogs in oncological applications. *Mar. Drugs* **2024**, *22*, 426. [CrossRef]
61. Newman, D.J. Drug discovery from natural sources. *Curr. Pharmacol. Rep.* **2023**, *9*, 67–89. [CrossRef]
62. Corley, D.G.; Herb, R.; Moore, R.E.; Scheuer, P.J.; Paul, V.J. Laulimalides. New potent cytotoxic macrolides from a marine sponge and a nudibranch predator. *J. Org. Chem.* **1988**, *53*, 3644–3646. [CrossRef]
63. Mooberry, S.L.; Tien, G.; Hernandez, A.H.; Plubrukarn, A.; Davidson, B.S. Laulimalide and isolaulimalide, new paclitaxel-like microtubule-stabilizing agents. *Cancer Res.* **1999**, *59*, 653–660.
64. Mooberry, S.L.; Randall-Hlubek, D.A.; Leal, R.M.; Hegde, S.G.; Hubbard, R.D.; Zhang, L.; Wender, P.A. Microtubule-stabilizing agents based on designed laulimalide analogues. *Proc. Natl. Acad. Sci. USA* **2004**, *101*, 8803–8808. [CrossRef]
65. Prota, A.E.; Bargsten, K.; Northcote, P.T.; Marsh, M.; Altmann, K.H.; Miller, J.H.; Díaz, J.F.; Steinmetz, M.O. Structural basis of microtubule stabilization by laulimalide and peloruside A. *Angew. Chem. Int. Ed.* **2014**, *53*, 1621–1625. [CrossRef]
66. Horton, P.A.; Koehn, F.E.; Longley, R.E.; McConnell, O.J. Lasonolide A, a new cytotoxic macrolide from the marine sponge *Forcepia* sp. *J. Am. Chem. Soc.* **1994**, *116*, 6015–6016. [CrossRef]
67. Isbrucker, R.A.; Guzman, E.A.; Pitts, T.P.; Wright, A.E. Early effects of lasonolide A on pancreatic cancer cells. *J. Pharmacol. Exp. Ther.* **2009**, *331*, 733–739. [CrossRef] [PubMed]
68. Zhang, Y.-W.; Ghosh, A.K.; Pommier, Y. Lasonolide A, a potent and reversible inducer of chromosome condensation. *Cell Cycle* **2012**, *11*, 4424–4435. [CrossRef] [PubMed]
69. West, L.M.; Northcote, P.T.; Battershill, C.N. Peloruside A: A potent cytotoxic macrolide isolated from the New Zealand marine sponge *Mycale* sp. *J. Org. Chem.* **2000**, *65*, 445–449. [CrossRef]
70. Liao, X.; Wu, Y.; De Brabander, J.K. Total synthesis and absolute configuration of the novel microtubule-stabilizing agent peloruside A. *Angew. Chem.* **2003**, *42*, 1648–1652. [CrossRef]
71. McGowan, M.A.; Stevenson, C.P.; Schiffler, M.A.; Jacobsen, E.N. An enantioselective total synthesis of (+)-peloruside A. *Angew. Chem.* **2010**, *49*, 6147–6151. [CrossRef]
72. Jin, M.; Taylor, R.E. Total synthesis of (+)-peloruside A. *Org. Lett.* **2005**, *7*, 1303–1305. [CrossRef]
73. Ghosh, A.K.; Xu, X.; Kim, J.-H.; Xu, C.-X. Enantioselective total synthesis of peloruside A: A potent microtubule stabilizer. *Org. Lett.* **2008**, *10*, 1001–1004. [CrossRef]
74. Wilmes, A.; Bargh, K.; Kelly, C.; Northcote, P.T.; Miller, J.H. Peloruside A synergizes with other microtubule stabilizing agents in cultured cancer cell lines. *Mol. Pharm.* **2007**, *4*, 269–280. [CrossRef]
75. Aicher, T.D.; Buszek, K.R.; Fang, F.G.; Forsyth, C.J.; Jung, S.H.; Kishi, Y.; Matelich, M.C.; Scola, P.M.; Spero, D.M.; Yoon, S.K. Total synthesis of halichondrin B and norhalichondrin B. *J. Am. Chem. Soc.* **1992**, *114*, 3162–3164. [CrossRef]
76. Jackson, K.L.; Henderson, J.A.; Motoyoshi, H.; Phillips, A.J. A total synthesis of norhalichondrin B. *Angew. Chem. Int. Ed.* **2009**, *48*, 2346–2350. [CrossRef] [PubMed]
77. Yamamoto, A.; Ueda, A.; Brémond, P.; Tiseni, P.S.; Kishi, Y. Total synthesis of halichondrin C. *J. Am. Chem. Soc.* **2012**, *134*, 893–896. [CrossRef] [PubMed]
78. Yahata, K.; Ye, N.; Ai, Y.; Iso, K.; Kishi, Y. Unified, Efficient, and Scalable Synthesis of Halichondrins: Zirconium/Nickel-Mediated One-Pot Ketone Synthesis as the Final Coupling Reaction. *Angew. Chem.* **2017**, *129*, 10936–10940. [CrossRef]
79. Ueda, A.; Yamamoto, A.; Kato, D.; Kishi, Y. Total synthesis of halichondrin A, the missing member in the halichondrin class of natural products. *J. Am. Chem. Soc.* **2014**, *136*, 5171–5176. [CrossRef]
80. Wang, Y.; Habgood, G.J.; Christ, W.J.; Kishi, Y.; Littlefield, B.A.; Yu, M.J. Structure–activity relationships of halichondrin B analogues: Modifications at C. 30–C. 38. *Bioorg. Med. Chem. Lett.* **2000**, *10*, 1029–1032. [CrossRef]
81. Nicolaou, K.; Pan, S.; Shelke, Y.; Das, D.; Ye, Q.; Lu, Y.; Sau, S.; Bao, R.; Rigol, S. A reverse approach to the total synthesis of halichondrin B. *J. Am. Chem. Soc.* **2021**, *143*, 9267–9276. [CrossRef]
82. Yoshimura, T.; Yakushiji, F.; Kondo, S.; Wu, X.; Shindo, M.; Shishido, K. Total synthesis of (+)-lasonolide A. *Org. Lett.* **2006**, *8*, 475–478. [CrossRef]
83. Trost, B.M.; Stivala, C.E.; Hull, K.L.; Huang, A.; Fandrick, D.R. A concise synthesis of (−)-lasonolide A. *J. Am. Chem. Soc.* **2014**, *136*, 88–91. [CrossRef]
84. Kang, S.H.; Kang, S.Y.; Choi, H.-W.; Kim, C.M.; Jun, H.-S.; Youn, J.-H. Stereoselective total synthesis of the natural (+)-lasonolide A. *Synthesis* **2004**, *2004*, 1102–1114. [CrossRef]
85. Ghosh, A.K.; Gong, G. Total Synthesis of Potent Antitumor Agent (−)-Lasonolide A: A Cycloaddition-Based Strategy. *Chem. Asian J.* **2008**, *3*, 1811–1823. [CrossRef] [PubMed]
86. Song, H.Y.; Joo, J.M.; Kang, J.W.; Kim, D.-S.; Jung, C.-K.; Kwak, H.S.; Park, J.H.; Lee, E.; Hong, C.Y.; Jeong, S.; et al. Lasonolide A: Structural revision and total synthesis. *J. Org. Chem.* **2003**, *68*, 8080–8087. [CrossRef] [PubMed]
87. Ghosh, A.K.; Gong, G. Enantioselective total synthesis of macrolide antitumor agent (−)-lasonolide A. *Org. Lett.* **2007**, *9*, 1437–1440. [CrossRef] [PubMed]

88. Kang, S.H.; Kang, S.Y.; Kim, C.M.; Choi, H.-W.; Jun, H.-S.; Lee, B.M.; Park, C.M.; Jeong, J.W. Total synthesis of natural (+)-lasonolide A. *Angew. Chem.* **2003**, *115*, 4927–4930. [CrossRef]
89. Trost, B.M.; Stivala, C.E.; Fandrick, D.R.; Hull, K.L.; Huang, A.; Poock, C.; Kalkofen, R. Total synthesis of (−)-lasonolide A. *J. Am. Chem. Soc.* **2016**, *138*, 11690–11701. [CrossRef]
90. Trost, B.M.; Cregg, J.J. Ruthenium-catalyzed alkene–alkyne coupling of disubstituted olefins: Application to the stereoselective synthesis of trisubstituted enecarbamates. *J. Am. Chem. Soc.* **2015**, *137*, 620–623. [CrossRef]
91. Pettit, G.R.; Kamano, Y.; Fujii, Y.; Herald, C.L.; Inoue, M.; Brown, P.; Gust, D.; Kitahara, K.; Schmidt, J.M.; Doubek, D.L. Marine animal biosynthetic constituents for cancer chemotherapy. *J. Nat. Prod.* **1981**, *44*, 482–485. [CrossRef]
92. Pettit, G.R.; Kamano, Y.; Dufresne, C.; Cerny, R.L.; Herald, C.L.; Schmidt, J.M. Isolation and structure of the cytostatic linear depsipeptide dolastatin 15. *J. Org. Chem.* **1989**, *54*, 6005–6006. [CrossRef]
93. Pettit, G.R.; Smith, T.H.; Arce, P.M.; Flahive, E.J.; Anderson, C.R.; Chapuis, J.-C.; Xu, J.-P.; Groy, T.L.; Belcher, P.E.; Macdonald, C.B. Antineoplastic agents. 599. Total synthesis of dolastatin 16. *J. Nat. Prod.* **2015**, *78*, 476–485. [CrossRef]
94. Pika, J.; Faulkner, D.J. A reinvestigation of the didemnaketals from the Palauan ascidian *Didemnum* sp. *Nat. Prod. Lett.* **1995**, *7*, 291–296. [CrossRef]
95. Potts, B.C.; Faulkner, D.J.; Chan, J.A.; Simolike, G.C.; Offen, P.; Hemling, M.E.; Francis, T.A. Didemnaketals A and B, HIV-1 protease inhibitors from the ascidian *Didemnum* sp. *J. Am. Chem. Soc.* **1991**, *113*, 6321–6322. [CrossRef]
96. Nicolaou, K.; Bella, M.; Chen, D.Y.K.; Huang, X.; Ling, T.; Snyder, S.A. Total synthesis of diazonamide A. *Angew. Chem.* **2002**, *114*, 3645–3649. [CrossRef]
97. Nicolaou, K.; Bheema Rao, P.; Hao, J.; Reddy, M.V.; Rassias, G.; Huang, X.; Chen, D.Y.K.; Snyder, S.A. The second total synthesis of diazonamide A. *Angew. Chem. Int. Ed.* **2003**, *42*, 1753–1758. [CrossRef]
98. Knowles, R.R.; Carpenter, J.; Blakey, S.B.; Kayano, A.; Mangion, I.K.; Sinz, C.J.; MacMillan, D.W. Total synthesis of diazonamide A. *Chem. Sci.* **2010**, *2011*, 308–320. [CrossRef] [PubMed]
99. Saxena, S. *Applied Microbiology*; Springer: Berlin/Heidelberg, Germany, 2015.
100. Erba, E.; Bergamaschi, D.; Ronzoni, S.; Faretta, M.; Taverna, S.; Bonfanti, M.; Catapano, C.; Faircloth, G.; Jimeno, J.; D'incalci, M. Mode of action of thiocoraline, a natural marine compound with anti-tumour activity. *Br. J. Cancer* **1999**, *80*, 971–980. [CrossRef] [PubMed]
101. Dahiya, R.; Dahiya, S.; Fuloria, N.K.; Jankie, S.; Agarwal, A.; Davis, V.; Sahadeo, V.; Radhay, V.; Ramsubhag, Y.; Mullings, W. Natural Thiazoline-based cyclodepsipeptides from marine cyanobacteria: Chemistry, bioefficiency and clinical aspects. *Curr. Med. Chem.* **2021**, *28*, 7887–7909. [CrossRef] [PubMed]
102. Boger, D.L.; Ichikawa, S. Total syntheses of thiocoraline and BE-22179: Establishment of relative and absolute stereochemistry. *J. Am. Chem. Soc.* **2000**, *122*, 2956–2957. [CrossRef]
103. Dahiya, R.; Dahiya, S.; Kumar, P.; Kumar, R.V.; Dahiya, S.; Kumar, S.; Saharan, R.; Basu, P.; Mitra, A.; Sharma, A. Structural and biological aspects of natural bridged macrobicyclic peptides from marine resources. *Arch. Pharm.* **2021**, *354*, 2100034. [CrossRef]
104. Edler, M.C.; Fernandez, A.M.; Lassota, P.; Ireland, C.M.; Barrows, L.R. Inhibition of tubulin polymerization by vitilevuamide, a bicyclic marine peptide, at a site distinct from colchicine, the vinca alkaloids, and dolastatin 10. *Biochem. Pharmacol.* **2002**, *63*, 707–715. [CrossRef]
105. Wipf, P.; Reeves, J.T.; Day, B.W. Chemistry and biology of curacin A. *Curr. Pharm. Des.* **2004**, *10*, 1417–1437. [CrossRef]
106. Rinehart, K.; Fregeau, N.; Warwick, R.; Garcia Gravalos, D.; Avila, J.; Faircloth, G. Spisulosine Compounds Having Antitumor Activity. PCT WO0052521 A, 31 August 1999. Volume 1, p. 19991021.
107. Ganesher, A.; Chaturvedi, P.; Sahai, R.; Meena, S.; Mitra, K.; Datta, D.; Panda, G. New Spisulosine Derivative promotes robust autophagic response to cancer cells. *Eur. J. Med. Chem.* **2020**, *188*, 112011. [CrossRef]
108. Gonda, J.; Fazekašová, S.; Martinková, M.; Mitríková, T.; Roman, D.; Pilátová, M.B. Synthesis and biological activity of sphingosines with integrated azobenzene switches. *Org. Biomol. Chem.* **2019**, *17*, 3361–3373. [CrossRef]
109. Warabi, K.; Matsunaga, S.; van Soest, R.W.M.; Fusetani, N. Dictyodendrins A−E, the First Telomerase-Inhibitory Marine Natural Products from the Sponge Dictyodendrilla v erongiformis. *J. Org. Chem.* **2003**, *68*, 2765–2770. [CrossRef] [PubMed]
110. Gowan, S.M.; Harrison, J.R.; Patterson, L.; Valenti, M.; Read, M.A.; Neidle, S.; Kelland, L.R. A G-quadruplex-interactive potent small-molecule inhibitor of telomerase exhibiting in vitro and in vivo antitumor activity. *Mol. Pharmacol.* **2002**, *61*, 1154–1162. [CrossRef] [PubMed]
111. Fürstner, A.; Domostoj, M.M.; Scheiper, B. Total synthesis of dictyodendrin B. *J. Am. Chem. Soc.* **2005**, *127*, 11620–11621. [CrossRef] [PubMed]
112. Fürstner, A.; Domostoj, M.M.; Scheiper, B. Total syntheses of the telomerase inhibitors dictyodendrin B, C, and E. *J. Am. Chem. Soc.* **2006**, *128*, 8087–8094. [CrossRef]
113. Buchgraber, P.; Domostoj, M.M.; Scheiper, B.; Wirtz, C.; Mynott, R.; Rust, J.; Fürstner, A. Synthesis-driven mapping of the dictyodendrin alkaloids. *Tetrahedron* **2009**, *65*, 6519–6534. [CrossRef]

114. Okano, K.; Fujiwara, H.; Noji, T.; Fukuyama, T.; Tokuyama, H. Total synthesis of dictyodendrin A and B. *Angew. Chem. Int. Ed.* **2010**, *49*, 5925–5929. [CrossRef]
115. Tokuyama, H. Construction of N-heterocycles fused with a highly substituted benzene ring by a benzyne-mediated cyclization/functionalization cascade reaction and its application to the total synthesis of marine natural products. *Chem. Pharm. Bull.* **2021**, *69*, 707–716. [CrossRef]
116. Hirao, S.; Yoshinaga, Y.; Iwao, M.; Ishibashi, F. A formal total synthesis of the telomerase inhibitor dictyodendrin B. *Tetrahedron Lett.* **2010**, *51*, 533–536. [CrossRef]
117. Ayats, C.; Soley, R.; Albericio, F.; Alvarez, M. Synthesis of the pyrrolo [2,3-c] carbazole core of the dictyodendrins. *Org. Biomol. Chem.* **2009**, *7*, 860–862. [CrossRef] [PubMed]
118. Hirao, S.; Sugiyama, Y.; Iwao, M.; Ishibashi, F. Synthetic approach to telomerase inhibitor dictyodendrin B: Synthesis of the pyrrolo [2,3-c] carbazole core. *Biosci. Biotechnol. Biochem.* **2009**, *73*, 1764–1772. [CrossRef]
119. Liang, J.; Hu, W.; Tao, P.; Jia, Y. Total synthesis of dictyodendrins B and E. *J. Org. Chem.* **2013**, *78*, 5810–5815. [CrossRef] [PubMed]
120. Ghosal, P.; Shaw, A.K. An efficient total synthesis of the anticancer agent (+)-spisulosine (ES-285) from Garner's aldehyde. *Tetrahedron Lett.* **2010**, *51*, 4140–4142. [CrossRef]
121. Amarante, G.W.; Cavallaro, M.; Coelho, F. Highly diastereoselective total synthesis of the anti-tumoral agent (±)-Spisulosine (ES285) from a Morita–Baylis–Hillman adduct. *Tetrahedron Lett.* **2010**, *51*, 2597–2599. [CrossRef]
122. Dinda, S.K.; Das, S.K.; Panda, G. Asymmetric total syntheses of spisulosine, its diastereo-and regio-isomers. *Tetrahedron* **2010**, *66*, 9304–9309. [CrossRef]
123. Fabišíková, M.; Martinková, M.; Hirková, S.; Gonda, J.; Pilátová, M.B.; Gönciová, G. Total synthesis and the anticancer activity of (+)-spisulosine. *Carbohydr. Res.* **2016**, *435*, 26–36. [CrossRef]
124. Abushanab, E.; Vemishetti, P.; Leiby, R.W.; Singh, H.K.; Mikkilineni, A.B.; Wu, D.C.; Saibaba, R.; Panzica, R.P. The chemistry of L-ascorbic and D-isoascorbic acids. 1. The preparation of chiral butanetriols and-tetrols. *J. Org. Chem.* **1988**, *53*, 2598–2602. [CrossRef]
125. Pitts, A.K.; O'Hara, F.; Snell, R.H.; Gaunt, M.J. A Concise and Scalable Strategy for the Total Synthesis of Dictyodendrin B Based on Sequential C- H Functionalization. *Angew. Chem. Int. Ed.* **2015**, *54*, 5451–5455. [CrossRef]
126. Matsuoka, J.; Inuki, S.; Matsuda, Y.; Miyamoto, Y.; Otani, M.; Oka, M.; Oishi, S.; Ohno, H. Total Synthesis of Dictyodendrins A–F by the Gold-Catalyzed Cascade Cyclization of Conjugated Diyne with Pyrrole. *Chem. Eur. J.* **2020**, *26*, 11150–11157. [CrossRef]

marine drugs

MDPI

Article

Design, Synthesis, and Evaluation of Novel Thiazole-Containing Algicides Inspired by Bacillamide A

Xiaoxue Li [1,†], Huili Li [2,†], Lei Shi [1,†], Zuguang Yin [1], Yuguo Du [3], Hongxia Zhang [2], Xin Wang [2], Xinxin Wang [2], Kexin Xu [2], Weili Wang [4], Ronglian Xing [2,*] and Yi Liu [1,*]

[1] School of Chemistry and Chemical Engineering, Yantai University, Yantai 264005, China; lixiaoxue0829@163.com (X.L.); sl17865561083@163.com (L.S.); y18354896509@outlook.com (Z.Y.)
[2] School of Life Sciences, Yantai University, Yantai 264005, China; 13256952529@163.com (H.L.); zhxia128@163.com (H.Z.); j977158314@126.com (X.W.); twist991117@163.com (X.W.); 13256493559@163.com (K.X.)
[3] State Key Laboratory of Environmental Chemistry and Eco-Toxicology, Research Center for Eco-Environmental Sciences, Chinese Academy of Sciences, Beijing 100085, China; duyuguo@rcees.ac.cn
[4] School of Chemistry and Material Science, Ludong University, 186 Hongqi Middle Road, Yantai 264025, China; weili.wang@ldu.edu.cn
[*] Correspondence: xingronglian@163.com (R.X.); liuyi@ytu.edu.cn (Y.L.)
[†] The authors are equally contribute to this article.

Abstract: The pursuit of highly effective, low-toxicity, and eco-friendly algicides for controlling and eradicating harmful algal blooms (HABs) is of paramount importance. The natural allelochemical bacillamide A has displayed impressive algicidal activity against harmful algae with favorable safety profiles. However, the poor synthetic efficiency and large dose requirements of bacillamide A limit its further application. In this paper, 17 thiazole-containing bacillamide derivatives (BDs) were designed and synthesized in three linear steps as potential algicides. Eight compounds (**6a**, **6c**, **6j**, **7b**, **7c**, **7d**, **7e**, and **7g**) displayed potent inhibitory effects against *Prorocentrum minimum*, *Skeletonema costatum*, and *Alexandrium pacificum*, and they had similar or better activity than the positive control ($CuSO_4$) and bacillamide A. Compound **6a** exhibited the most potent algicidal activity against *S. costatum* (half-maximal effective concentration [EC_{50}] = 0.11 μg/mL), being 23-fold more potent than bacillamide A, 28-fold more potent than $CuSO_4$, and 39-fold more potent than Diuron. Compound **6j** exhibited significant algicidal activity against the toxic dinoflagellates *P. minimum* (EC_{50} = 1.0 μg/mL) and *A. pacificum* (EC_{50} = 0.47 μg/mL), being 3–5-fold more potent than natural bacillamide A, Diuron, and $CuSO_4$. Micrographs and SEM images revealed that **6j** induced cell wall rupture and cellular content leakage. Biochemical and physiological studies indicated that **6j** might partially disrupt the antioxidant and photosynthetic systems in algal cells, resulting in morphological changes, cell wall rupture, and inclusion leakage. Our work suggests that **6j** has a distinct mode of action from $CuSO_4$ and provides a promising candidate for the development of new algicides, worthy of further investigation.

Keywords: algicidal activity; harmful algal blooms; Bacillamide A; thiazole-containing derivatives; allelopathic algicide; SAR

1. Introduction

Annual harmful algal blooms (HABs) have caused continuous health and environmental concerns over the last decade, as they are associated with numerous adverse effects such as seafood poisoning, economic losses, environmental damage, and pandemics [1]. Global climate change stressors (e.g., increasing temperatures, water acidification, ocean deoxygenation) and anthropogenic factors (e.g., discharge from wastewater treatment plants, aquaculture, marine transportation, ballast water transfer) have broadened the geographic distribution and frequency of HABs [2,3].

Furthermore, HABs produce a variety of potent naturally occurring biotoxins, including neurotoxic shellfish toxins, diarrhetic shellfish toxins, and paralytic shellfish toxins (PSTs) [4]. Unavoidably, these toxins can accumulate in the tissues of bivalve shellfish, fish, and other marine creatures. The consumption of poisoned seafood leads to severe and potentially fatal poisoning [5]. HAB toxins are responsible for 50,000–500,000 cases of intoxication annually, and they contribute to a global mortality rate of approximately 1.5% each year [6]. Marine toxigenic dinoflagellates such as *Gymnodinium catenatum*, *Alexandrium spp.*, and *Pyrodinium bahamense var.* compressum are the major producers of PSTs [7]. In 2021, *A. pacificum* was identified as the major producer of PSTs in China [8].

To date, a number of biological, physical, and chemical control techniques have been investigated to control HABs [9]. Although some physical and chemical methods can efficiently control and remove HABs, they are limited by drawbacks such as high time consumption and costs, non-target toxicity, and secondary pollution from heavy metals. Biological algicidal methods have attracted significant attention as environmentally friendly alternatives [10]. However, most of these methods remain at the laboratory scale, and their effectiveness in managing natural HABs is unclear. Therefore, there is an urgent need for novel, environmentally friendly algicides to control and eradicate HABs.

Allelopathic algicides have attracted considerable attention because of their high selectivity, high sustainability, and negligible toxicity in controlling HABs [11]. In 2003, the thiazole-containing natural algicide bacillamide A was first isolated from marine bacterium *Bacillus* sp. SY-1 by Okada group [12]. Bacillamide A exhibited excellent and selective algicidal activity against harmful dinoflagellates, including *Cochlodinium polykrikoides* (50% lethal concentration [LC_{50}] = 3.2 μg/mL), *Gyrodinium impudicum* (LC_{50} = 2.3 μg/mL), *Alexandrium catenella* (LC_{50} = 9.4 μg/mL), *Prorocentrum micans* (LC_{50} = 4.4 μg/mL), and the raphidophytes *Heterosigma akashiwo* (LC_{50} = 1.6 μg/mL) and *Chattonella* sp. (LC_{50} = 3.7 μg/mL). Comparatively, bacillamide A did not display algicidal activities against other microalgae (e.g., diatoms, cyanobacteria, green algae) [12,13]. Further studies revealed that bacillamide A exhibited moderate antibacterial activity against Gram-positive bacteria (*Salmonella choleraesuis* and *Vibrio cholerae*) and slight antifungal activity against *Alternaria* sp. [14]. The potent algicidal activity of bacillamide A has attracted attention from synthetic chemists and biologists. Recently, several promising algaecides have been reported, including pyrimidin-4-amine (**4k**) [15], 1,3,4-thiadiazole-containing (A3) algicides [16], cyclo(Ala-Gly) [17], natural allelopathic algicides [18], and several Bacillamide derivatives (BDs) [19,20] (Figure 1).

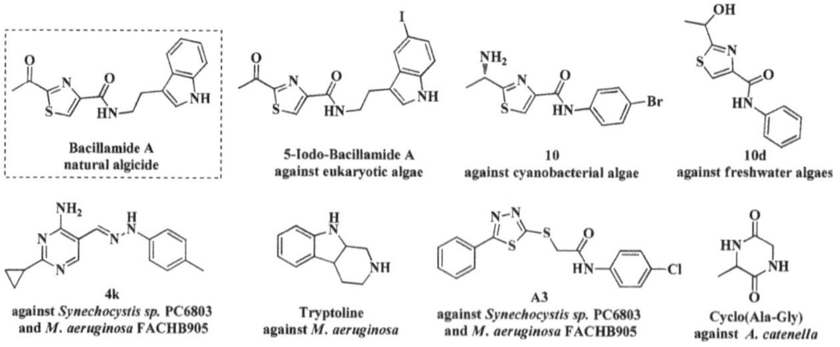

Figure 1. Bacillamide A and reported algicides.

Because of its high algicidal potency and distinct structure characteristics and our continuing focus on the total synthesis of thiazole-containing natural products, bacillamide A has attracted our attention [21]. However, large-scale preparation and structural modifications of bacillamide A have remained difficult. Therefore, structurally simplified and detailed structural modifications of bacillamide A would provide an opportunity for the development of highly effective, environmentally friendly algicides.

2. Results and Discussion

2.1. Chemical Synthesis

The natural algicide bacillamide A was prepared according to our previously reported synthesis route [21]. The synthesis route for BDs is presented in Scheme 1. The synthetic route of **6a–6k** began with the formation of the 2, 4-disubstituted thiazoles **3a–3k** following our reported cascade thiazole formation reaction, with the yields reaching 63–75% [22]. After saponification of **3a–3k**, the acids **4a–4k** were next reacted with tryptamine, generating BDs **6a–6k** in 45–67% yields. To explore the structure–activity relationship of the tryptamine unit, the thiazole **4a** was coupled with different amines to generate **7b–7g** in 44–51% yields for two steps. The structures of all synthesized BDs were characterized by ^{1}H and ^{13}C NMR spectra and high-resolution mass spectrometry (HRMS).

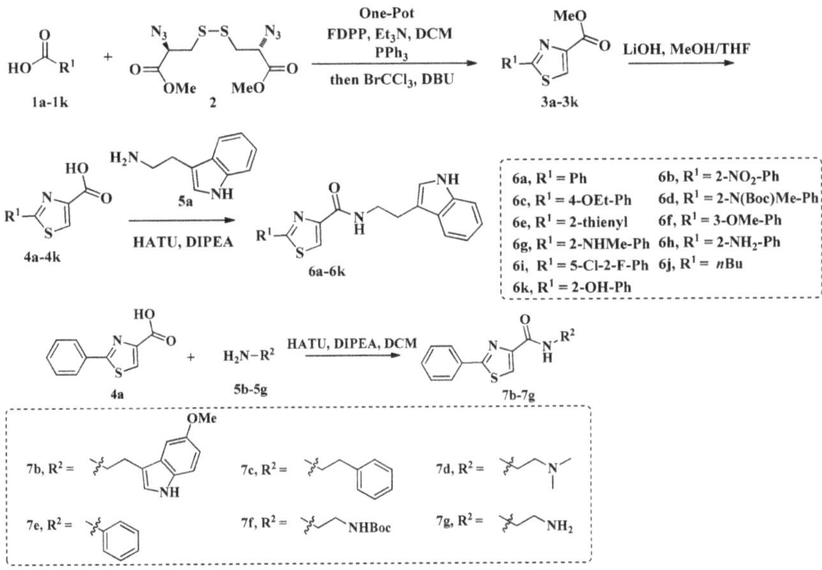

Scheme 1. General synthesis routes of bacillamide derivatives (**6a–6k** and **7b–7g**).

2.2. Algicidal Activity Assay and Structure–Activity Relationship Discussion

The inhibitory activities of bacillamide A and 17 BDs were preliminarily evaluated in three algae (*P. minimum, S. costatum, and A. pacificum*) to identify algicidal candidates. *S. costatum* is a single-celled diatom-type phytoplankton, whereas *P. minimum* and *A. pacificum* are toxic dinoflagellates. As presented in Figure 2, most of the synthesized BDs exhibited similar or better algicidal activity than bacillamide A and $CuSO_4$ after co-incubation for 24 h at a concentration of 50 mg/L. Notably, **6a**, **6c**, and **6j** exhibited >70% inhibition rates against *S. costatum* at 50 mg/L. Replacing the acetyl group of bacillamide A with 4-OEt-Ph (**6c**) or butyl (**6j**) significantly improved their inhibition rates (**6c**: 72.6%; **6j**: 81.7%) against *S. costatum*. However, substitution of phenyl groups or incorporation of the heteocyclic thiophene ring had little effect on their algicidal activity. Excluding the large steric hindrance of the Boc group (**7f**), replacing the tryptamine group in bacillamide A with 5-methoxytryptamine (**7b**), phenylethyl (**7c**), phenyl (**7e**), aminoethyl (**7g**), or dimethylaminoethyl (**7d**) did not result in significant decreases in algicidal activity, indicating that the thiazole unit was more important for maintaining algicidal potency.

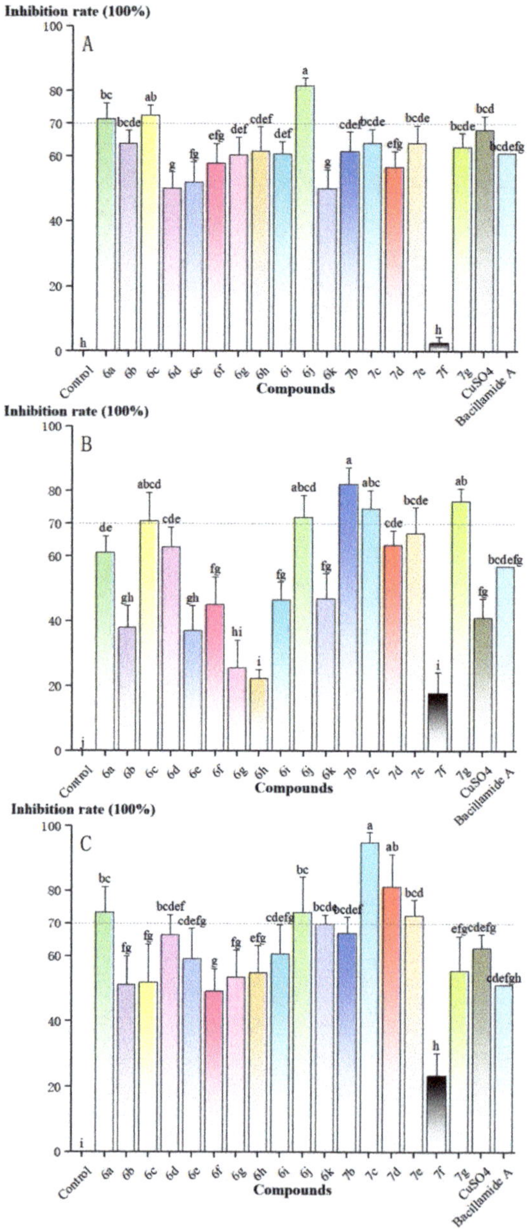

Figure 2. In vitro algicidal inhibition rates of synthesized BDs, bacillamide A, and $CuSO_4$ against the growth of *S. costatum* (**A**), *P. minimum* (**B**), and *A. pacificum* (**C**) at 50 mg/L for 24 h. Mean ± SD, n = 6. Different letters represent significant differences between groups, a > b > c > d > e > f > g > h > i > j ($p < 0.05$), and the same letters indicate no significant differences between groups.

As depicted in Figure 2B,C, the BDs with a thiazole skeleton also exhibited significant algicidal inhibition rates against the toxic dinoflagellates. Five thiazole-containing BDs all displayed inhibition rates exceeding 70% (**6c**: 70.8%; **6j**: 71.9%; **7b**: 82.3%; **7c**: 74.7%; and **7g**: 76.9%) against the growth of *P. minimum*. Compounds **6a, 6j, 7c, 7d,** and **7e** substantially inhibited *A. pacificum* growth with inhibition rates of 70–95%, exceeding those of bacillamide A (55.3%) and $CuSO_4$ (62.3%). After treatment for 24 h, **7c** displayed the most powerful inhibitory activity against *A. pacificum* at 50 mg/L. By contrast, **7f** lost most of its algicidal activity against *P. minimum* and *A. pacificum*. Notably, the inhibition rates of **6j** exceeded 70% for all three algal species. Regarding the suppression of dinoflagellates, the selectivity of **7b–7g** progressively increased, demonstrating that R^2 substitution resulted in better inhibition of dinoflagellate growth than did substitution at R^1.

To further evaluate algicidal efficacy of the synthesized BDs, those with inhibition rates exceeding 70% at 50 mg/L were selected for half-maximal effective concentration (EC_{50}) testing. As presented in Table 1, most of the synthesized BDs exhibited better algicidal activity than the commercial positive controls ($CuSO_4$ and Diuron). The BDs with the same tryptamine unit were analyzed, and the sequence of algicidal activity against *S. costatum* was **6a** (phenyl) > **6j** (butyl) > **6c** (4-OEt-phenyl). Compound **6a** exhibited the best algicidal activity against *S. costatum* (EC_{50} = 0.11 μg/mL), being 28-fold more potent than $CuSO_4$, 39-fold more potent than Diuron, and 23-fold more potent than bacillamide A. However, compared with **6a** and **6c**, **6j** exhibited better algicidal activity against *P. minimum* (EC_{50} = 1.0 μg/mL) and *A. pacificum* (EC_{50} = 0.47 μg/mL). Five synthesized phenylthiazole-containing BDs (**7b**, **7c**, **7d**, **7e**, and **7g**) exhibited good algicidal activity against *S. costatum* (EC_{50} = 0.24–2.28 μg/mL), *P. minimum* (EC_{50} = 1.32–3.38 μg/mL), and *A. pacificum* (EC_{50} = 0.53–3.42 μg/mL), demonstrating that the phenylthiazole unit was important for algicidal activity maintenance.

Table 1. The EC_{50} values of selected BDs against *S. costatum*, *P. minimum*, and *A. pacificum*.

N°	Compound	EC_{50} (μg/mL)		
		S. costatum	*A. pacificum*	*P. minimum*
6a	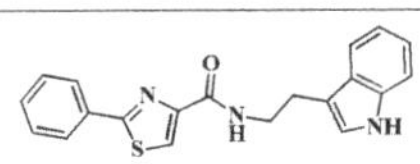	0.11 ± 0.02	3.32 ± 0.79	1.74 ± 0.40
6c	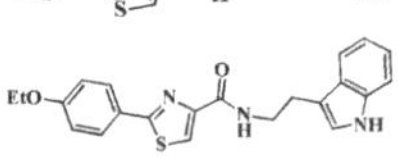	0.51 ± 0.04	2.43 ± 0.42	1.29 ± 0.08
6j	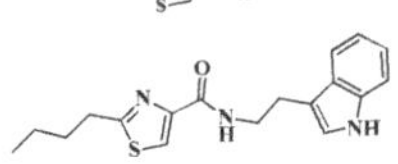	0.30 ± 0.02	0.47 ± 0.25	1.00 ± 0.11
7b	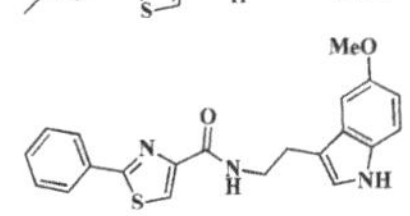	0.37 ± 0.07	0.72 ± 0.021	1.32 ± 0.38
7c	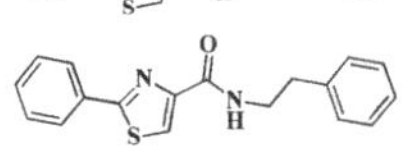	0.24 ± 0.058	0.53 ± 0.32	3.38 ± 0.84
7d	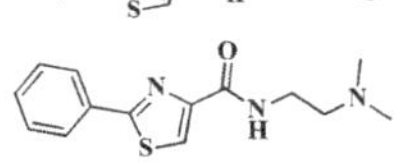	0.77 ± 0.21	2.02 ± 0.54	3.22 ± 0.39
7e	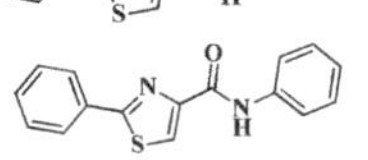	1.10 ± 0.31	0.69 ± 0.07	3.23 ± 0.39
7g	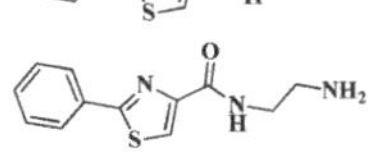	2.28 ± 0.37	3.42 ± 0.13	2.02 ± 0.27
bacillamide A	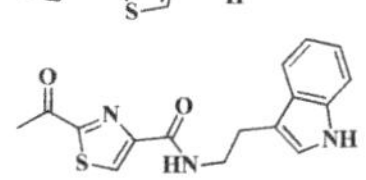	2.51 ± 0.09	2.17 ± 0.31	3.93 ± 0.28
Diuron	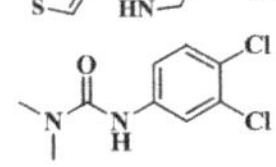	4.32 ± 0.14	5.69 ± 0.46	4.72 ± 0.41
$CuSO_4$	$CuSO_4$	3.12 ± 0.21	2.34 ± 0.06	3.61 ± 0.32

The full structure and the EC_{50} values of BDs are presented. Mean ± SD, n = 3.

2.3. Acute Toxicity Evaluation of BDs

To explore the safety profile of the synthesized BDs, the 2-phenylthiazole- and 2-butylthiazole-containing BDs (**6a** and **6j**) with the best algicidal activity were selected as representative compounds for further fish toxicity evaluation (Table S1). The Guide for Environmental Safety Assessment of Chemical Pesticides (GB/T31270.12) has documented the standards for toxicity ($LC_{50\,(96\,h)} > 10$ mg/L, low toxicity; $1.0 < LC_{50\,(96\,h)} \leq 10$ mg/L, moderate toxicity; $LC_{50\,(96\,h)} \leq 0.1$ mg/L, high toxicity). As seen in Table S1, after treatment with bacillamide A at 0.1 mg/L, 1 mg/L, and 10 mg/L for 0 h, 24 h, 48 h, 72 h, and 96 h, the zebrafish survival rates were 100%. Therefore, the acute toxicity of bacillamide A was classified as low. $CuSO_4$ at 10 mg/L all led to 100% zebrafish mortality within 48 h. Unfortunately, the acute toxicity of both **6a** and **6j** was classified as moderate. **6j** exhibited a better safety profile than **6a**. Although the survival rate of zebrafish after 24 h of treatment with **6j** at 10 mg/L was up to 80%, treatment with **6j** for more than 48 h also led to 100% mortality in zebrafish. These results suggest that bacillamide A has excellent biosafety in aquatic animals, and alkyl modification of the thiazole ring could represent a strategy for safe algicide development in the future.

2.4. Effects of BDs on the Cellular Morphology of P. minimum, S. costatum, and A. pacificum

Based on the excellent algicidal characteristics of **6j**, the effect on the cellular morphology of algae was next evaluated. As presented in Figure 3A,C,E, the three untreated algae (*S. costatum*, *P. minimum*, and *A. pacificum*) had well-defined shapes and smooth surfaces. After treatment with **6j** (10 mg/L), the micrographs illustrated that the cell walls of the treated algae (*S. costatum*, *P. minimum*, and *A. pacificum*) were broken or damaged or both and that there was leakage of the cytoplasm (Figure 3B,D,F).

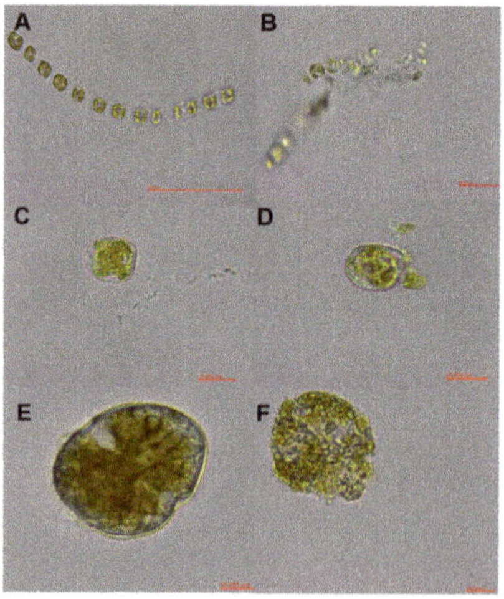

Figure 3. The effects of **6j** on the cell morphology of *S. costatum*, *P. minimum*, and *A. pacificum*. The algae cells were incubated with **6j** at the concentration of 10 mg/L for 4 h. The micrographs showing the effects of *S. costatum* (**A**), *P. minimum* (**C**), and *A. pacificum* (**E**) without treatment with **6j**. The micrographs showing the effects of **6j** on *S. costatum* (**B**), *P. minimum* (**D**), and *A. pacificum* (**F**).

Scanning electron microscope photographs showed that the untreated *S. costatum* and *P. minimum* also exhibited smooth surfaces, and the cells were arranged in orderly strings (Figure 4A,E). After incubation with **6j** (10 mg/L) for 4 h, **6j**-treated algal cells of *S. costatum* and *P. minimum* had rough and broken surfaces, and the disappearance of cytoplasm and nucleoid regions was observed (Figure 4C,G). The *P. minimum* cells had almost completely lysed, and they lost their integrity. Bacillamide A exhibited similar effects to that of **6j** on the morphology of algae cells, but the algae cell walls were broken down more severely by copper sulfate under SEM observation (Figure 4B,F,D,H). These results demonstrate that **6j** can cause significant cell wall damage and change the subcellular structure and morphology of *S. costatum* and *P. minimum* cells, highlighting its strong algicidal activity.

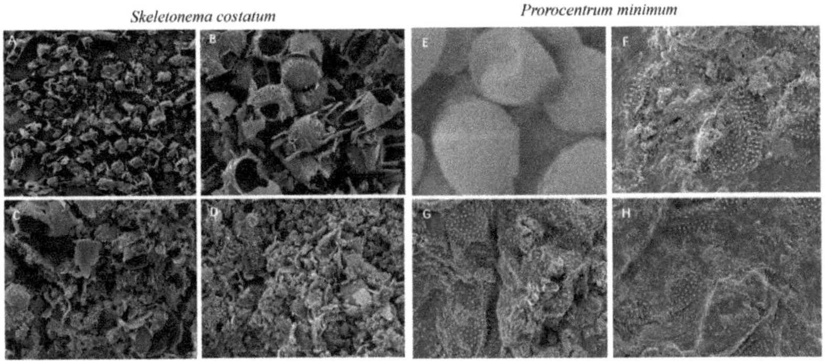

Figure 4. SEM images presenting the effects of treatment with DMSO (**A**), bacillamide A (**B**), **6j** (**C**), and $CuSO_4$ (**D**) on the cellular morphology of *S. costatum*. SEM images presenting the effects of treatment with DMSO (**E**), bacillamide A (**F**), **6j** (**G**), and $CuSO_4$ (**H**) on the cellular morphology of *P. minimum*. Scale bar = 10 μM.

2.5. *Preliminary Exploration of the Algicidal Action of* **6j**

In algal cells, photosystem II (PSII) was a crucial supramolecular complex located within thylakoid membranes. PSII is responsible for harvesting light energy, stimulating charge separation, and driving the electron transport process. These biological processes can effectively split the H_2O into protons and oxygen in algal cell under ambient temperature [23]. PSII dysfunction can lead to the failure to harvest light energy and lower the electron transfer rate across thylakoid membranes to photosystem I (PSI), resulting in the accumulation of reactive oxygen species (ROS).

As illustrated in Figure 5A,B, compared with the effects of the negative control, the quantum yield Fv/Fm of PSII in *P. minimum* and *S. costatum* decreased after treatment with 10 mg/L of **6j**, bacillamide A, and $CuSO_4$. After 72 h of exposure to bacillamide A or **6j**, the quantum yield Fv/Fm of PSIIin *S. costatum* decreased by 4- and 27-fold, respectively. Meanwhile, treatment with $CuSO_4$ led to a 48-fold reduction in the Fv/Fm. A similar tendency was observed in *P. minimum*, as treatment with bacillamide A and **6j** resulted in 2- and 3-fold decreases in the Fv/Fm of PSII after 72 h, respectively. However, $CuSO_4$ treatment caused a 20-fold decrease in the Fv/Fm. These results demonstrated that **6j** could reduce the efficiency of PSII, suggesting that the algicidal mechanism of BDs differs from that of $CuSO_4$.

Consistent with the reduction in the Fv/Fm, the ROS levels in *P. minimum* and *S. costatum* increased by 5.4- and 3-fold, respectively, after treatment with 10 mg/L of **6j** for 72 h (Figure 5C,D). A similar effect was observed after treatment with 10 mg/L of bacillamide A for 72 h. However, after treatment with 10 mg/L of $CuSO_4$ for 72 h, the ROS levels in *P. minimum* and *S. costatum* significantly increased by 9.6- and 7.7-fold, respectively. These results indicate that both **6j** and bacillamide A, similarly to $CuSO_4$, could increase ROS levels, leading to algal cell apoptosis.

Both microscopy and SEM revealed that treatment with **6j** lysed algal cells and destroyed their cell walls, prompting further exploration of its algicidal mechanism. Malondialdehyde (MDA) is the typical marker of lipid peroxidation [24]. As presented in Figure 5E,F, incubation with 10 mg/L of **6j** for 72 h increased MDA levels in *P. minimum* and *S. costatum* by 2.3- and 2.2-fold, respectively, versus the effects of the control (DMSO). Notably, bacillamide A treatment increased MDA levels by 2.0- and 2.6-fold, respectively, in these algal species. These findings suggest that the algicidal mode of action for both **6j** and bacillamide A involves reductions in the efficiency of PSII and increases in intracellular MDA and ROS levels, consequently causing algal cell rupture.

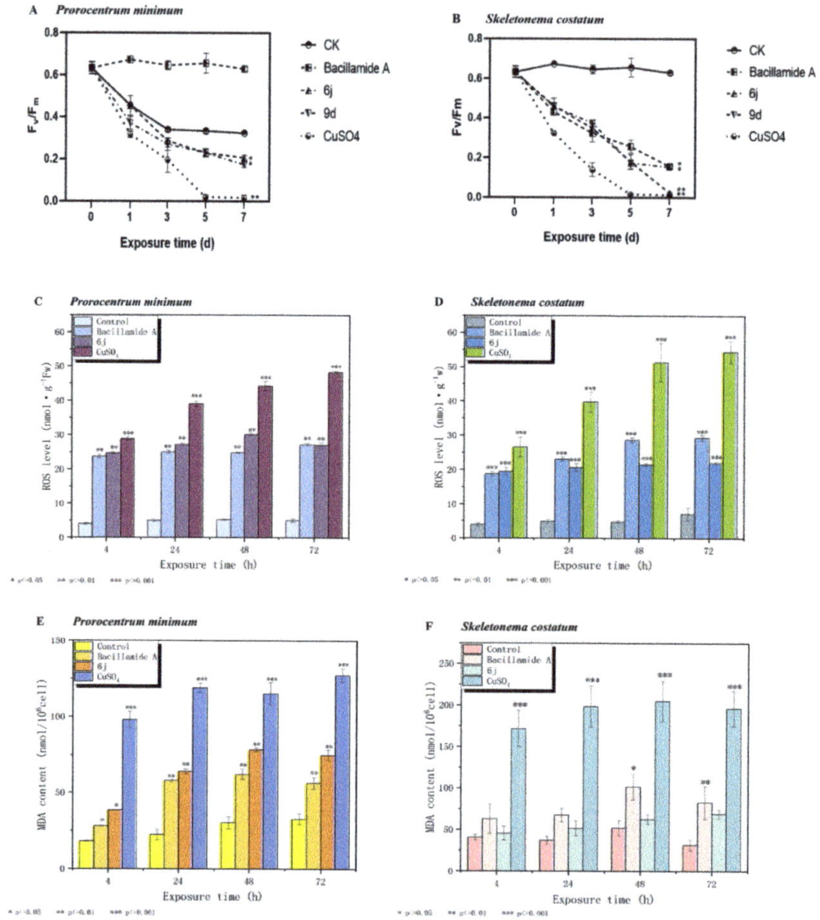

Figure 5. The effect of **6j** on the Fv/Fm of PSII in *P. minimum* (**A**) and *S. costatum* (**B**). (**C**) Effects of bacillamide A, DMSO, $CuSO_4$, and **6j** on ROS content levels in *P. minimum*. (**D**) Effects of bacillamide A, DMSO, $CuSO_4$, and **6j** on ROS content levels in *S. costatum*. (**E**) Effects of bacillamide A, DMSO, $CuSO_4$, and **6j** on MDA content levels in *P. minimum*. (**F**) Effects of bacillamide A, DMSO, $CuSO_4$, and **6j** on MDA content levels in *S. costatum*. DMSO was used as the negative control. $CuSO_4$ was used as the positive control. Mean ± SD, $n = 3$. * $p < 0.05$, ** $p < 0.01$, *** $p < 0.001$.

3. Materials and Methods

3.1. Instruments and Chemicals

Diuron (98% pure) and cupric sulfate anhydrous (98% pure) were supplied by China ACON Bitotech Co., Ltd. (Hangzhou, China). Tryptamine (98% pure) was supplied by China Heowns Biochem Technologies, LLC (Tianjin, China). Other chemicals (reagent grade) were purchased from commercial sources (InnoChem, Beijing, China). Flash chromatography (FC) silica gel (200–300 meshes, Qingdao Haiyang Chemical Go., Ltd., Qingdao, China) was used as the separating compound. The high-resolution mass spectra (HRMS), ^{1}H NMR, and ^{13}C NMR spectra (NMR in DMSO-d_6, $CDCl_3$ and CD_3OD with TMS as internal standard) were tested by using a Q-TOF analyzer (Thermo Fisher Scientific, BRE,

German), JEOL JNM-ECZ400S (400 MHz/100 MHz, Akishima, Japan) spectrometers, and Bruker spectrometers (500 and 125 MHz, Billerica, MA, USA), respectively. ^{1}H NMR and ^{13}C NMR spectra of BDs **6a–6k**, **7b–7g** were shown in Supplementary Materials. Compound **2** was obtained following our previous reported method [22]. Bacillamides A were prepared in 6 linear steps with 27% overall yield following our previous reported synthetic procedure [21].

3.2. *Algal Species*

P. minimum, *A. pacificum*, and *S. costatum* were purchased from Guangyu Biological Technology Co., Ltd. (Shanghai, China). The algae strain was cultured in F/2 medium ((12 h light: 12 h dark cycle), 20 ± 1 °C, 70 μmol m^{-2} s^{-1}). Purchased algae were transferred to sterile conical flasks for culture; after the algae proliferation was stabilized, the expanded culture was next carried out following standard conditions.

3.3. *Synthesis Procedure of BDs*

3.3.1. General Procedure for the Preparation of Thiazole Methyl Ester **3a–3k** [22,25]

A mixture of carboxylic acid **1** (6 mmol), pentafluorophenyl diphenylphosphinate (FDPP) (6 mmol), and triethylamine (TEA) (12 mmol) in 100 mL of CH_2Cl_2 were stirred at room temperature for 20 min. β-azido disulfide **2** (1.5 mmol) and PPh_3 (12 mmol) was subsequently added into the mixture and heated at 45 °C for 5 h. After cooling to 0 °C, bromotrichloromethane (12 mmol) and 1,8-diazabicycloundec-7-ene (DBU) (16 mmol) were added into the solution via syringe over 20 min. The mixture was stirred for 1 h until reaction was complete. Reaction was quenched by 100 mL of saturated NH_4Cl solution, and the mixture was extracted with DCM (200 mL × 3). The combined organic layer was washed with brine and dried over anhydrous Na_2SO_4, filtered, concentrated in vacuo (below 45 °C), and purified by flash chromatography to produce compound **3a–3k**.

3.3.2. General Procedure for Hydrolysis of **3a–3k**

To a solution of LiOH (200 mg, 8.4 mmol) in H_2O (20 mL)/MeOH (50 mL)/THF (50 mL) was added thiazole methyl ester **3a–3k** (10 mmol), and the reaction mixture was stirred at room temperature for 3–5 h. After the addition of 20 mL of H_2O, the solution was acidified (pH 3–5) with 10% aqueous solution of 1.0 N HCl. The solution was diluted with EtOAc (50 mL × 3). The extracts were washed with saturated brine, dried (Na_2SO_4) and concentrated under reduced pressure to produce carboxylic acid **4a–4k**.

3.3.3. General Procedure the Preparation of BDs **6a–6k** and **7b–7g**

A solution of acid **3a–3k** (1.0 mmol), DIPEA (2.0 mmol), and HATU (1.5 mmol) in 20 mL of CH_2Cl_2 was stirred at room temperature for 20 min. Amine **5a–5g** (1.0 mmol) was then added into the reaction mixture at 0 °C and stirred overnight. The solution was quenched by saturated aqueous NH_4Cl and extracted with 30 mL of CH_2Cl_2 for 3 replicates. After that, the combined organic phase was washed with brine and dried (Na_2SO_4), and the solvent was removed by rotary evaporation. Crude residue was purified by flash chromatography to produce BDs **6a–6k** and **7b–7g**.

3.4. *Algicidal Activity Assay*

The stock solutions of bacillamide A and different BDs were prepared in dimethyl sulfoxide (DMSO) with the requisition amount. The initial cell density of three algae (*P. minimum, S. costatum, and A. pacificum*) was up to 1.0 × 10^6 cells/L. A total of 20 mL of algae solution was exposed to bacillamide A and BDs at concentrations of 50 mg/L for growth-inhibition rate measurement (24 h). The controls received the same volume of DMSO. The inhibitory activities of bacillamide A, different BDs, and positive controls were screened by 96 well microtiter plates at different concentrations. Inhibition ratios (IRs) of cupric sulfate (50 mg/L, positive control), bacillamide A (50 mg/L), and BDs (50 mg/L) were calculated on algae using Equation (1).

$$IR = \frac{C_{c0} - C_{ex}}{C_{c0}} \times 100\% \quad (1)$$

The C_{C0} and C_{ex}, respectively, represent the algal densities of the control and experimental groups.

The half-maximal effective concentration (EC_{50}) against three algae species were evaluated: 20 mL of algae solution was, respectively, exposed to Diuron (positive control), cupric sulfate (positive control), and BDs (concentration: 0.1 mg/L, 0.2 mg/L, 1 mg/L, 5 mg/L, and 10 mg/L, time: 0 d, 1 d, 3 d, 5 d, 7 d, 9 d, 11 d, and 13 d). Copper sulfate and Diuron were used as the positive controls. EC_{50} values were calculated according to the equation of the quantity–effect relationship in Equation (2) using the Hill model of Graph Pad Prism software (8.0.2).

$$Y = \frac{\text{Bottom} + (\text{Top} - \text{Bottom})}{1 + 10^{(\text{Log } EC_{50} - X) \times \text{Hill Slope}}} \quad (2)$$

The X and Y values represent the concentration (mg/L) and response values of the control and experimental groups, respectively. The Top, Bottom, and Hill Slope represent the maximum response, minimum response, and the curve slope, respectively. The EC50 represents half of the maximum effective concentration.

3.5. Zebrafish Acute Toxicity Assay of Bacillamide A and BDs

The Guide for Environmental Safety Assessment of Chemical Pesticides has documented the criteria for toxicity (GB/T31270.12, $LC_{50\,(96\,h)} > 10$ mg/L, low toxicity; $1.0 < LC_{50\,(96\,h)} \leq 10$ mg/L, moderate toxicity; $LC_{50\,(96\,h)} \leq 0.1$ mg/L, high toxicity). Zebrafish acute toxicity of bacillamide A and synthesized BDs were evaluated at 0.1 mg/L, 1 mg/L, and 10 mg/L, respectively. Diuron and $CuSO_4$ were used as positive controls. The commercial zebrafish (body length > 3.0 cm) were domesticated in aerated tap water for 24 h, fed once daily for seven consecutive days, and stopped being fed before the experiment.

3.6. Observation of Cellular Morphology

There were morphological changes of algae cells treated by bacillamide A, BDs, and the positive control ($CuSO_4$). Scanning electron microscopy (SEM) and an optical microscope were used to detect the morphological changes of treated algae cells, after treatment of bacillamide A, BDs, and the positive control ($CuSO_4$) at 10 mg/L for 4 h. Cell samples were centrifuged at 12,000 rpm for 10 min, collected, fixed, gradient-dehydrated, and freeze-dried after gold coating following the reported procedure [26]. The SEM analyses were performed by scanning electron microscopy (SEM, JSM-7900F, Hitachi High-Tech Corporation, Tokyo, Japan).

3.7. Determination of the Indicators of the Antioxidant System and the Photosynthetic System

P. minimum, *S. costatum*, and *A. pacificum* cells were cultured in F/2 medium. All flasks were cultivated under 12 h of light: 12 h of dark and 70 $\mu mol\ m^{-2}\ s^{-1}$ at 20 ± 1 °C. Algae solution (20 mL) was exposed to **6j**, bacillamide A, $CuSO_4$, and DMSO at concentrations of 10 mg/L, followed by centrifuge at 4000 r/min for 10 min. Finally, the algal cells were collected and diluted in 6 mL of phosphate buffer (pH = 7.8). A small amount of quartz sand was added into the algal cells under ice bath. The obtained homogenate was next poured into a centrifuge tube and centrifuged at 5000 r/min for 25 min at 4 °C. The obtained supernatant was placed in the refrigerator at 4 °C for the next step experiment.

Fv/Fm values were determined by using AquaPen handheld algae fluorescence meter (Nanjing Mingao Instrument Co., Ltd., Nanjing, China). The algae cells were darkened for 30 min and Fv/Fm values were measured.

The reactive oxygen species (ROS) assay kit was purchased from SolarBio Co., Ltd., Beijing, China. The 2′,7′-dichlorodihydrofluorescein diacetate (DCFH-DA) could be oxidized by reactive oxygen or nitrogen species (ROS/RNS) to generate high fluorescent 2′,7′-dichlorofluoroscein (DCF). DCF could be detected by Cyto-FLEX flow cytometry. The ROS values were measured using a fluorescent probe assay in algae treatment with or without **6j**, bacillamide A, $CuSO_4$, and DMSO.

The malondialdehyde (MDA) assay kit was purchased from Lvyuandade Biochemical Co, Ltd., Beijing, China. The MDA parameter was monitored according to the procedure provided by the manufacturer. A total of 1 mL of algal extract was mixed with thiobarbituric acid solution (2 mL, 0.6%). The solution was sealed and kept in a boiling water bath for 15 min, followed by being cooled and centrifuged at 4500 r/min for 10 min. The absorbance values of collected supernatant were measured and calculated by the Formula (3) at 600 nm, 532 nm, and 450 nm:

$$\text{MDA content } (\text{nmol}\cdot\text{mgprot}^{-1}) = 6.45 \times (A_{532} - A_{600}) - 0.56 \times A_{450} \quad (3)$$

3.8. Data Analysis

All experiment results were performed in triplicates unless otherwise specified. Results have been expressed as mean ± standard deviation (SD). Statistical analyses were conducted with SPSS. The differences were considered significant at $p < 0.05$. Graphs were plotted using Origin 2022 and Graph Pad Prism.

4. Conclusions

In summary, inspired by the natural algicide bacillamide A, 17 thiazole-containing derivatives were designed and synthesized, and their efficacy against three HAB species (*P. minimum*, *S. costatum*, and *A. pacificum*) was evaluated. Compound **6j** displayed comparable or superior algicidal activity to Diuron and $CuSO_4$. Preliminary evaluations into the algacidal mechanism of **6j** illustrated that it can reduce the Fv/Fm of PSII and increase ROS and MDA levels in algal cells, but its algicidal effect was weaker than that of $CuSO_4$. Bacillamide A and **6j** inhibited algal growth through different mechanisms than $CuSO_4$. Unfortunately, although bacillamide A was less toxic to zebrafish (low toxicity) than $CuSO_4$ (moderate toxicity), the acute toxicity of **6j** was classified as moderate. These findings suggest that both bacillamide A and **6j** have the potential to serve as lead candidates for the development of highly effective, environmentally friendly algicidal agents for controlling HABs.

Supplementary Materials: Additional experimental procedures, characterization of BDs **6a–6k**, **7b–7f**, the ^{1}H, and ^{13}C NMR spectra of **6a–6k**, **7b–7g**, and bacillamide A in JEPG format (JEPG). The following supporting information can be downloaded at https://www.mdpi.com/article/10.3390/md22110494/s1, Table S1.

Author Contributions: Conceptualization, Y.L. and R.X.; methodology, X.L., H.L. and L.S.; software, W.W. and H.Z.; validation, X.L., H.L. and K.X.; formal analysis, X.W. (Xin Wang) and Y.L.; investigation, X.L., H.L. and L.S.; resources, Y.L., R.X. and Y.D.; data curation, Z.Y. and X.W. (Xinxin Wang); writing—original draft preparation, X.L., H.L. and L.S.; writing—review and editing, Y.L.; visualization, X.L. and H.L.; supervision, Y.L. and R.X.; project administration, Y.L.; funding acquisition, Y.L., R.X. and Y.D. All authors have read and agreed to the published version of the manuscript.

Funding: This work was supported in part by Natural Science Foundation of Shandong Province (grant no. ZR2020MB105), National Natural Science Foundation of China (grant no. 42376155, 42076110, 21402192), and National Key Research and Development Program of China (2023YFC3709004 and 2023YFC3709001).

Institutional Review Board Statement: Not applicable.

Data Availability Statement: Data are contained within the article and Supplementary Materials.

Conflicts of Interest: The authors declare that they have no known competing financial interests or personal relationships that could have appeared to influence the work reported in this paper.

References

1. Griffith, A.W.; Gobler, C.J. Harmful algal blooms: A climate change co-stressor in marine and freshwater ecosystems. *Harmful Algae* **2020**, *91*, 101590. [CrossRef] [PubMed]
2. Gobler, C.J. Climate change and harmful algal blooms: Insights and perspective. *Harmful Algae* **2020**, *91*, 101731. [CrossRef] [PubMed]
3. Yan, Z.; Kamanmalek, S.; Alamdari, N.; Nikoo, M.R. Comprehensive insights into harmful algal blooms: A review of chemical, physical, biological, and climatological influencers with predictive modeling approaches. *J. Environ. Eng.* **2024**, *150*, 0312–4002. [CrossRef]
4. Yan, T.; Li, X.-D.; Tan, Z.-J.; Yu, R.-C.; Zou, J.-Z. Toxic effects, mechanisms, and ecological impacts of harmful algal blooms in China. *Harmful Algae* **2022**, *111*, 102148. [CrossRef]
5. Sulieman, A.M.E.; Alanazi, N.; Abdelgadir, A.M.; Haddad, A.; ELHag, G.A. Algal Toxins. In *Microbial Toxins in Food Systems: Causes, Mechanisms, Complications, and Metabolism*; Springer: Berlin/Heidelberg, Germany, 2024; pp. 427–443.
6. McGowan, S. Harmful algal blooms. In *Biological and Environmental Hazards, Risks, and Disasters*; Elsevier: Amsterdam, The Netherlands, 2023; pp. 9–53.
7. Hernández-Sandoval, F.E.; Bustillos-Guzmán, J.J.; Band-Schmidt, C.J.; Núñez-Vázquez, E.J.; López-Cortés, D.J.; Fernández-Herrera, L.J.; Poot-Delgado, C.A.; Moreno-Legorreta, M. Effect of different N: P ratios on the growth, toxicity, and toxin profile of *gymnodinium catenatum* (Dinophyceae) strains from the gulf of california. *Toxins* **2022**, *14*, 501. [CrossRef]
8. Liu, Y.; Chen, Z.; Gao, Y.; Zou, J.; Lu, S.; Zhang, L. Identifying the source organisms producing paralytic shellfish toxins in a subtropical bay in the South China Sea. *Environ. Sci. Technol.* **2021**, *55*, 3124–3135. [CrossRef]
9. Wells, M.L.; Karlson, B.; Wulff, A.; Kudela, R.; Trick, C.; Asnaghi, V.; Berdalet, E.; Cochlan, W.; Davidson, K.; De Rijcke, M. Future HAB science: Directions and challenges in a changing climate. *Harmful Algae* **2020**, *91*, 101632. [CrossRef]
10. Anabtawi, H.M.; Lee, W.H.; Al-Anazi, A.; Mohamed, M.M.; Aly Hassan, A. Advancements in biological strategies for controlling harmful algal blooms (HABs). *Water* **2024**, *16*, 224. [CrossRef]
11. Zhu, X.; Dao, G.; Tao, Y.; Zhan, X.; Hu, H. A review on control of harmful algal blooms by plant-derived allelochemicals. *J. Hazard. Mater.* **2021**, *401*, 123403. [CrossRef]
12. Jeong, S.-Y.; Ishida, K.; Ito, Y.; Okada, S.; Murakami, M. Bacillamide, a novel algicide from the marine bacterium, *Bacillus* sp. SY-1, against the harmful dinoflagellate, *Cochlodinium polykrikoides*. *Tetrahedron Lett.* **2003**, *44*, 8005–8007. [CrossRef]
13. Ivanova, V.; Kolarova, M.; Aleksieva, K.; Gräfe, U.; Dahse, H.M.; Laatsch, H. Microbiaeratin, a new natural indole alkaloid from a *Microbispora aerata* strain, isolated from Livingston Island, Antarctica. *Prep. Biochem. Biotechnol.* **2007**, *37*, 161–168. [CrossRef] [PubMed]
14. Vaca, J.; Salazar, F.; Ortiz, A.; Sansinenea, E. Indole alkaloid derivatives as building blocks of natural products from *Bacillus thuringiensis* and *Bacillus velezensis* and their antibacterial and antifungal activity study. *J. Antibiot.* **2020**, *73*, 798–802. [CrossRef] [PubMed]
15. Zhou, Y.; Qin, Y.; Zhou, H.; Zhang, T.; Feng, J.; Xie, D.; Feng, L.; Peng, H.; He, H.; Cai, M. Design, synthesis, high algicidal potency, and putative mode of action of new 2-cyclopropyl-4-aminopyrimidine hydrazones. *Pestic. Biochem. Phys.* **2022**, *184*, 105098. [CrossRef] [PubMed]
16. Huang, S.; Zuo, L.; Zhang, L.; Guo, X.; Cheng, C.; He, Y.; Cheng, G.; Yu, J.; Liu, Y.; Chen, R. Design, synthesis, and mode of action of thioacetamide derivatives as the algicide candidate based on active substructure splicing strategy. *J. Agr. Food Chem.* **2024**, *72*, 7021–7032. [CrossRef]
17. Ko, S.-R.; Jeong, Y.; Cho, S.-H.; Lee, E.; Jeong, B.-S.; Baek, S.H.; Oh, B.-H.; Ahn, C.-Y.; Oh, H.-M.; Cho, B.-K. Functional role of a novel algicidal compound produced by *Pseudoruegeria* sp. M32A2M on the harmful algae *Alexandrium catenella*. *Chemosphere* **2022**, *300*, 134535. [CrossRef]
18. Li, H.; Xing, R.; Ji, X.; Liu, Y.; Chu, X.; Gu, J.; Wang, S.; Wang, G.; Zhao, S.; Cao, X. Natural algicidal compounds: Strategies for controlling harmful algae and application. *Plant. Physiol. Bioch.* **2024**, *215*, 108981. [CrossRef]
19. Wang, Y.; Liu, Q.; Wei, Z.; Liu, N.; Li, Y.; Li, D.; Jin, Z.; Xu, X. Thiazole amides, a novel class of algaecides against freshwater harmful algae. *Sci. Rep.* **2018**, *8*, 8555. [CrossRef]
20. Wang, B.; Tao, Y.; Liu, Q.; Liu, N.; Jin, Z.; Xu, X. Algicidal activity of bacillamide alkaloids and their analogues against marine and freshwater harmful algae. *Mar. Drugs* **2017**, *15*, 247. [CrossRef]
21. Sun, X.; Liu, Y.; Liu, J.; Gu, G.; Du, Y. Synthesis and structural reconfirmation of bacillamide B. *Org. Biomol. Chem.* **2015**, *13*, 4271–4277. [CrossRef]
22. Liu, Y.; Li, Z.; Xie, Y.; He, P.; Qiao, J.; Fan, X.; Du, Y. Efficient one-pot synthesis of 2,4-disubstituted thiazoles and dimeric thiazoles directly from acyl chlorides and β-azido disulfides. *Synthesis* **2017**, *49*, 4876–4886. [CrossRef]
23. Wei, X.; Su, X.; Cao, P.; Liu, X.; Chang, W.; Li, M.; Zhang, X.; Liu, Z. Structure of spinach photosystem II–LHCII supercomplex at 3.2 Å resolution. *Nature* **2016**, *534*, 69–74. [CrossRef] [PubMed]
24. Del Rio, D.; Stewart, A.J.; Pellegrini, N. A review of recent studies on malondialdehyde as toxic molecule and biological marker of oxidative stress. *Nurt. Metab. Cardiovas.* **2005**, *15*, 316–328. [CrossRef]

25. Kumara, S.; Aggarwal, R. A concise and efficient route to the total synthesis of bacillamide A and its analogues. *Arkivoc* **2018**, 354–361. [CrossRef]
26. Wang, W.; Liu, Y.; Xue, Z.; Li, J.; Wang, Z.; Liu, X. Activity of the novel fungicide SYP-34773 against plant pathogens and its mode of action on *Phytophthora infestans*. *J. Agr. Food Chem.* **2021**, *69*, 11794–11803. [CrossRef] [PubMed]

marine drugs

MDPI

Article

Structure-Activity Relationship Study of Majusculamide D: Overcoming Metabolic Instability and Severe Toxicity with a Fluoro Analogue

Xiuhe Zhao [1], Xiaonan Xi [1,*], Mingxiao Zhang [1], Mengxue Lv [1], Xiang Zhang [2], Yaxin Lu [2], Liang Wang [2,*] and Yue Chen [2,3,*]

1 The State Key Laboratory of Medicinal Chemical Biology, College of Pharmacy, Nankai University, Tianjin 300350, China; 15522215338@163.com (X.Z.); x18716062989@163.com (M.Z.); 15615637301@163.com (M.L.)

2 College of Chemistry, Nankai University, Tianjin 300071, China; 2120231187@mail.nankai.edu.cn (X.Z.); yaxinlu@nankai.edu.cn (Y.L.)

3 Haihe Laboratory of Sustainable Chemical Transformations, Tianjin 300192, China

* Correspondence: xi_xiaonan@foxmail.com (X.X.); lwang@nankai.edu.cn (L.W.); yuechen@nankai.edu.cn (Y.C.)

Abstract: Majusculamide D, isolated from the marine cyanobacterium *Moorea producens*, is an anticancer lipopentapeptide consisting of fatty acid, tripeptide, and pyrrolyl proline moieties. In this work, by utilizing a convergent synthetic approach, late-stage modification, and bioisostere strategy, 26 majusculamide D analogues were synthesized, and two (**1i** and **1j**) demonstrated IC_{50} values < 1 nM against PANC-1 cancer cells. The results summarized a preliminary structure-activity relationship mainly at the C23, C4, C34, and C10 sites. A series of in vitro assays, including wound healing, transwell, clone formation, EdU, and western blot, confirmed that majusculamide D inhibited the migration, invasion, and proliferation of pancreatic cancer cells. The optimized fluorinated analogue **1n** demonstrated a notable enhancement in stability during the mouse plasma assay (>50% left after 24 h), exhibited tumor-suppressive effects (51.5% at a dosage of 5 mg/kg), and successfully mitigated the severe toxicity (no mouse dead) observed in the group treated with majusculamide D (3 mice dead) in a xenografted mouse model.

Keywords: structure-activity relationship; natural products; anticancer; pancreatic cancer; metastasis

1. Introduction

Pancreatic cancer, with a 5-year survival rate of merely 12.8% [1], remains a lethal disease [2,3] without promisingly increased life expectancy. Moreover, it is likely to become the second leading cause of cancer-related mortality in America by 2030 [2]. Pancreatic cancer patients who undergo surgical resection have a chance for a cure, and subsequent adjuvant chemotherapy has improved their prognosis [4]. Nonetheless, approximately 80–85% of pancreatic cancer patients are unresectable or show cancer metastasis [4]. Chemotherapy remains the primary treatment modality to palliate cancer-related symptoms and extend life [4]. Clinically, novel drugs for treating pancreatic cancer are in urgent demand.

Developing natural product-derived bioactive entities, including small molecules and conjugates (e.g., antibody-drug conjugates), is vital for cancer therapy [5–7]. Furthermore, natural product-derived probes serve as effective tools for mechanistic research, enabling the investigation of complex cancer pathology [8]. Marine cyanobacteria provide kinds of small molecules with promising anticancer properties [9,10]. Microcolins and majusculamide D, isolated from the marine cyanobacterium *Moorea producens* (formerly named *Lyngbya majuscula*), share analogous structures and demonstrated bioactivities, especially for anticancer activities [11–16]. In 2019, Gerwick et al. discovered that majusculamide D exhibited remarkable inhibitory activity and up to 4×10^3 selectivity against pancreatic cancer cells in vitro [17]. Meanwhile, they achieved a breakthrough by completing the first synthetic route to majusculamide D, which further facilitated the determination of its absolute configuration [17]. Wang et al. uncovered that microcolin H induced autophagic cell death and exhibited anti-proliferating activity by targeting PITPα/β [18]. Recently, the synthesis of majusculamide D, along with its eight analogues modified at the fatty acid moiety, the C10-OH group, and the C2–C3 unsaturated double bond, was completed [19]. The in vitro bioactivity data against PANC-1 cells revealed a preliminary structure-activity relationship (SAR) that C10-OH and C2–C3 unsaturated double bonds were crucial in maintaining the inhibitory activity while the fatty acid moiety was tolerable [19]. Moreover, majusculamide D was found to show inhibitory activities against several cancer cell lines [19]. Given the remarkable selectivity and potency of majusculamide D, further pharmacological and medicinal studies may offer new insights into its associated mechanistic signaling pathways and lead to the development of majusculamide D-derived candidates with enhanced activity. Herein, the syntheses of 26 majusculamide D analogues, primarily modified at the tripeptide moiety and pyrrolyl proline moiety, along with their in vitro and in vivo biological evaluations, are reported.

Retrosynthetically, the same convergent strategy previously employed by Gerwick was adopted [17]. The target lipo pentapeptides (**1**) were deconstructed into the fatty acid, tripeptide, and pyrrolyl proline moieties, which were combined through well-established amide condensation (Scheme 1). To enhance the metabolic stability, it was anticipated that the C23-OAc (R^1) of the tripeptide moiety would be replaced using the bioisostere strategy (e.g., NAc) [20]. The fluorine atom was considered to be introduced as it makes an impact on the potency, conformation, metabolism, and membrane permeability [21]. The *para*-substituted OMe (R^3) group in the tyrosine of the tripeptide was envisioned to be changed to F, H, OH, or Ph to evaluate its impact on the bioactivities. Regarding the pyrrolyl proline moiety, the configuration of C4 was intended to be switched, or the methyl group at C4 was to be directly trimmed, to investigate whether the naturally occurring C4-*R*-Me is necessary. Given the poor water solubility of majusculamide D, we also aimed to improve its water solubility. The comprehensive SAR could guide us in further structural simplification and optimization [22].

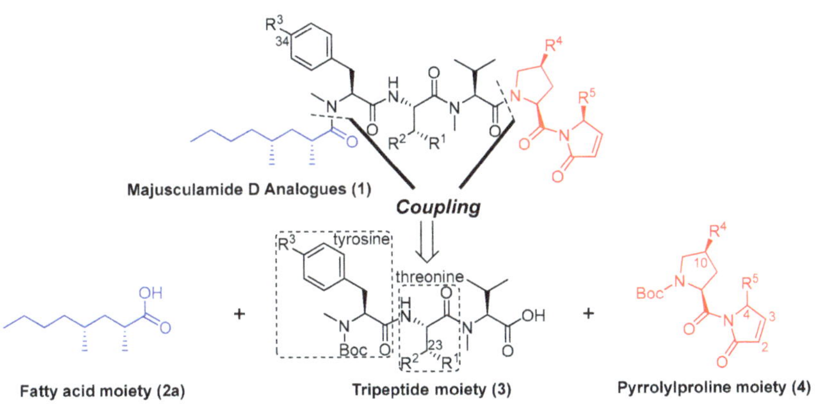

Scheme 1. Retrosynthetic analysis of majusculamide D analogues.

2. Results and Discussion

2.1. Syntheses and Inhibitory Activities of Majusculamide D Analogues

Syntheses toward the target compounds are depicted in Schemes 2 and 3. Moreover, the reaction conditions in these schemes closely parallel those previously reported by us. Compound **6c** was prepared employing the silver-mediated trifluoromethylation of alcohol developed by Qing et al. [23]. Meanwhile, the *N*-substituted R^1 at C23 in **6e** and **6f** was introduced via the Mitsunobu reaction using *L-allo*-threonine as the starting material. Following deprotection of the Boc group in compounds **6a–6f** with 4 N HCl (Scheme 2A), the resulting amines were coupled with compounds **7a–7e** employing a well-established coupling condition (HATU and DIPEA) to deliver **8a–8j**. Subsequent debenzylation of compounds **8a–8j** under the catalytic hydrogenation (Pd/C and H_2) condition provided 10 tripeptide analogues **3a–3j**. Next, the method developed by Gerwick [17] was employed to rapidly construct the pyrrolyl proline analogues **4a–4d** through a four-step sequence, which included activation of the carboxylic acid, imide formation, α-selenylation, and oxidation-triggered elimination (Scheme 2B).

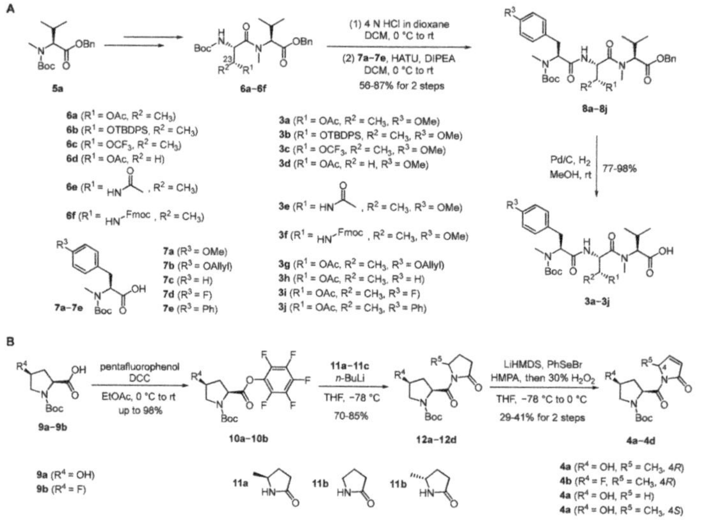

Scheme 2. (**A**) Synthesis of the tripeptide moiety. (**B**) Synthesis of the pyrrolylproline moiety.

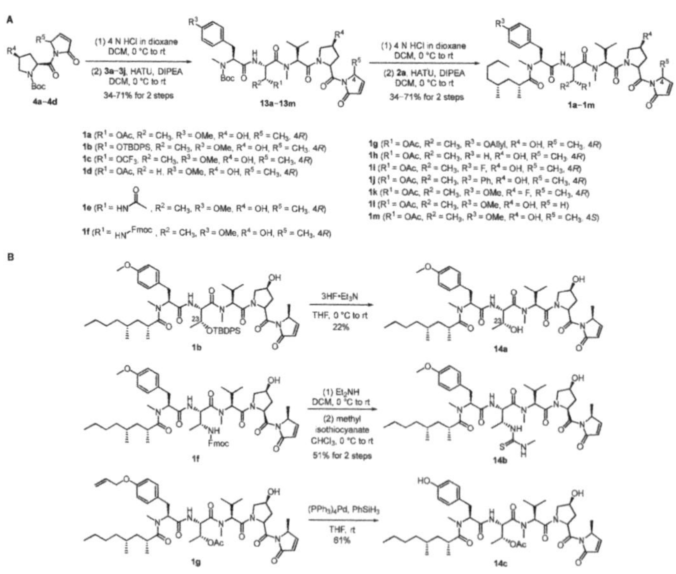

Scheme 3. (**A**) Syntheses of majusculamide D analogues **1a–1m**. (**B**) Syntheses of majusculamide D analogues **14a–14c**.

With building blocks in hand, we moved on to their coupling. The connection of the tripeptide and pyrrolyl proline moieties successfully delivered 13 advanced precursors, which were subsequently subjected to the final coupling with the fatty acid moiety **2a** to give compounds **1a–1m** (Scheme 3A). Direct deprotection of the TBDPS group of compound **1b** furnished **14a** (Scheme 3B) with an exposed hydroxy group at C23. Moreover, treating compound **1f** under the mild condition (Et_2NH) removed the Fmoc group, and the resulting amine was reacted with methyl isothiocyanate to produce a thiourea compound **14b**. The removal of the allyl group from compound **1g** resulted in the formation of phenolic compound **14c.**

For preliminary evaluation of anti-pancreatic cancer effects, 12 majusculamide D analogues (see Table 1) were tested against PANC-1 cancer cells. Meanwhile, it was noteworthy that the inhibitory activities of **14a** with C23-OH dropped dramatically (IC_{50} = 1162 nM), while the OCF_3 (**1c**), NAc (**1e**), and thiourea (**14b**) analogues, as well as the C23-demethyl analogue (**1d**), exhibited promising IC_{50} values ranging from 1.06−2.94 nM. These results indicated that the replacement of OAc with other groups at C23 was tolerable, while the exposed C23-OH deteriorated the inhibitory activity. When the methyl group of the *O*-Me tyrosine segment was removed (**14c**), the IC_{50} value of **14c** was 5.31 nM. Replacing the *O*-Me tyrosine with phenylalanine (**1h**), the IC_{50} value significantly decreased to 72.02 nM. Given that the O-Me group in anisole is a potentially metabolically unstable site, the OMe group with fluorine (**1i**) or phenyl (**1j**) were replaced, whose IC_{50} values maintained a nanomolar level (0.41 nM for **1i** and 0.70 nM for **1j**). As for the pyrrolyl proline moiety, compound **1k**, with the C10-OH on proline replaced by a fluorine atom, exhibited an IC_{50} value of 2.55 nM. Interestingly, the activity of C4 demethyl compound **1l** dropped significantly (134.2 nM), while the C4-*S* configured compound **1m** exhibited a comparable IC_{50} value (4.68 nM), demonstrating that the methyl group at C4 could not be removed directly.

Table 1. Inhibitory activities of majusculamide D analogues against PANC-1 cells.

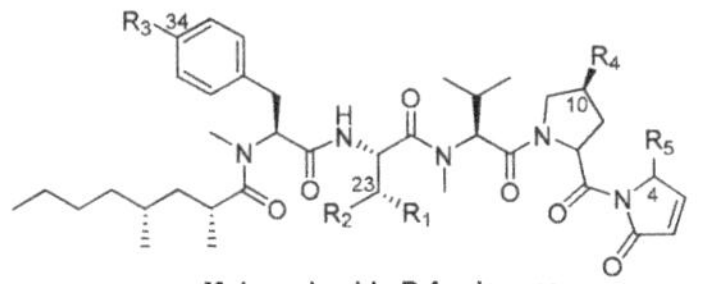

Majusculamide D Analogues

Compound	R[1]	R[2]	R[3]	R[4]	R[5]	IC_{50} (nM) [1]
1a (Majusculamide D)	OAc	CH_3	OMe	OH	CH_3 (*R*)	1.88 ± 0.82
14a	OH	CH_3	OMe	OH	CH_3 (*R*)	1162 ± 194.9
1c	OCF_3	CH_3	OMe	OH	CH_3 (*R*)	2.07 ± 0.67
1d	OAc	H	OMe	OH	CH_3 (*R*)	2.15 ± 0.37
1e	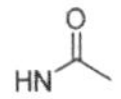	CH_3	OMe	OH	CH_3 (*R*)	2.94 ± 0.93
14b	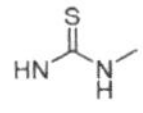	CH_3	OMe	OH	CH_3 (*R*)	1.06 ± 0.35
14c	OAc	CH_3	OH	OH	CH_3 (*R*)	5.31 ± 1.46
1h	OAc	CH_3	H	OH	CH_3 (*R*)	72.02 ± 21.88
1i	OAc	CH_3	F	OH	CH_3 (*R*)	0.41 ± 0.08
1j	OAc	CH_3	Ph	OH	CH_3 (*R*)	0.70 ± 0.07
1k	OAc	CH_3	OMe	F	CH_3 (*R*)	2.55 ± 0.55
1l	OAc	CH_3	OMe	OH	H	134.20 ± 78.18
1m	OAc	CH_3	OMe	OH	CH_3 (*S*)	4.68 ± 0.59

[1] IC_{50} values shown represent mean ± SD for n = 3. The cells were treated with the compound and incubated for an additional 72 h.

2.2. Syntheses and Inhibitory Activities of Majusculamide D Analogues Conjugated with One Extra Amino Acid

With ample amounts of the key intermediate **1f** available, attention was also directed towards late-stage modifications to enhance the water solubility of majusculamide D by attaching amino acids [24]. The intermediate prepared from the deprotection of compound **1f** was reacted with various protected amino acids in the presence of HATU and DIPEA to give **15a–15m**, which were ultimately converted into compounds **16a–16m** through treatment with TFA. (Scheme 4).

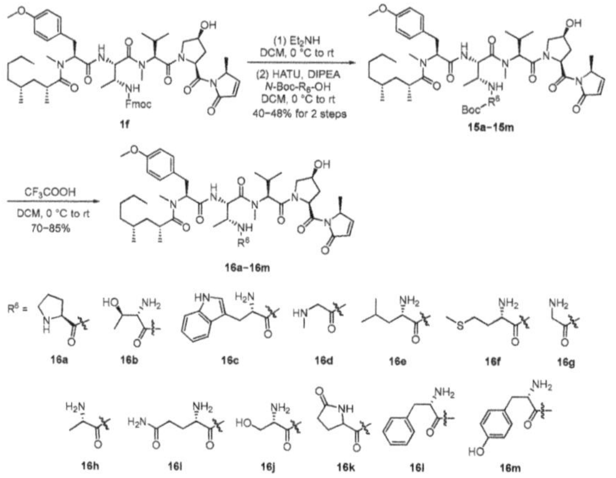

Scheme 4. Syntheses of majusculamide D analogues conjugated with one extra amino acid.

Compared to majusculamide D (**1a**), compounds **16a–16m** exhibited improved water solubility (Table 2). Among them, compound **16d** (solubility: 0.81 mg/mL) exhibited the highest water solubility. However, the IC_{50} value of compounds **16a–16m** decreased to deca−multihecto nanomolar levels. It is speculated that the addition of an extra amino acid may alter the spatial conformation, potentially affecting the ability to bind to the target or reducing membrane permeability, thereby leading to a decrease in activity.

Table 2. Inhibitory activities against PANC-1 cells and water solubility of compounds **16a–16m**.

Compound	IC_{50} (nM) [1]	Solubility (mg/mL) [2]
1a (Majusculamide D)	1.99 ± 0.68	Insoluble
16a	40.76 ± 14.06	0.21
16b	116.18 ± 53.97	0.41
16c	34.36 ± 4.50	0.20
16d	16.16 ± 6.72	0.81
16e	34.21 ± 6.36	0.23
16f	13.07 ± 6.30	0.17
16g	43.14 ± 29.8	0.16
16h	79.93 ± 45.89	0.36
16i	739.80 ± 712.91	0.53
16j	184.15 ± 33.25	0.36
16k	471.58 ± 69.72	0.33
16l	55.41 ± 14.73	0.13
16m	278.4 ± 14.95	0.16

[1] IC_{50} values shown represent mean ± SD for $n = 3$. The cells were treated with the compound and incubated for an additional 72 h. [2] Preliminary solubility tests: Weigh a specific amount of the compound **16a–16m** and place it in a fixed volume of water at 25 °C. After ultrasonic treatment for 30 min, the solution was observed. If no visible solute particles remain, the compound was considered completely dissolved, and the solubility was calculated based on the mass of the sample and the volume of water used.

2.3. Synthesis, Inhibitory Activity, Metabolic Stability Assay, and In Vivo Antitumor Activity of Majusculamide D Analogue 1n

According to the results of SAR and previous research, a target molecule (**1n**) was further designed in which the C23-OAc and C34-OMe groups were replaced with OCF3 and F groups, respectively, and one methyl group at C40 in the fatty acid chain was retained. Compound **1n** was successfully synthesized based on the previous procedure (Scheme 5). The biological results demonstrated that the IC_{50} value of compound **1n** against PANC-1 cells was 3.83 nM.

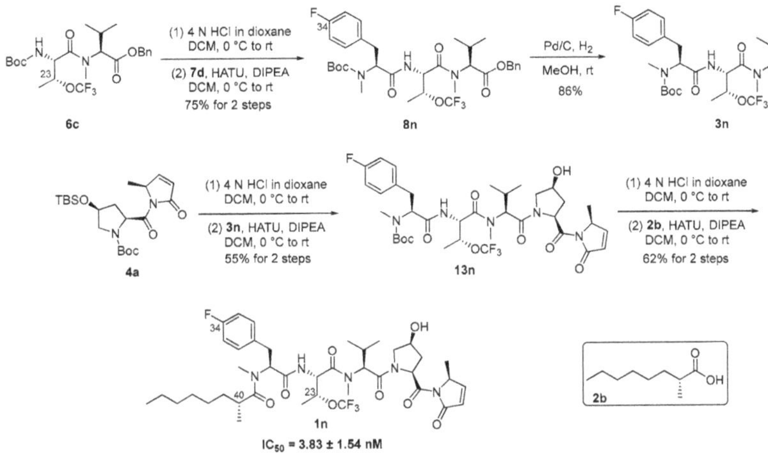

Scheme 5. Synthesis and inhibitory activity of optimized majusculamide D analogue **1n** against PANC-1 cells.

In the meantime, a series of in vitro assays, including wound healing, transwell, clone formation, EdU, and western blot, confirmed that majusculamide D inhibited the migration, invasion, and proliferation of pancreatic cancer cells and may function by suppressing the Wnt signaling pathway and the EMT process [25–31] (for experimental details, see the Supplementary Materials, Biological experiment part, and Figure S225). To determine whether the replacement of C23-OAc enhances metabolic stability, metabolic stability assays were conducted using **1a, 1c**, and **1n** in mouse plasma (Figure 1A). The results indicated that natural product **1a** vanished rapidly, with 54.7% left after 2 h. The metabolic instability may hinder its further in vivo medicinal applications. In sharp contrast, compounds **1c** and **1n** demonstrated significantly superior stability compared to **1a**, particularly **1n**, which retained more than half of its presence in the mouse plasma assay even after 24 h.

Furthermore, a xenografted murine subcutaneous tumor model was employed to evaluate the effects of majusculamide D and the optimized analogues **1c** and **1n** (Figure 1B). PANC1-bearing BALB/c nude mice were separated randomly, with a total of six mice in each group. Gemcitabine was chosen as the positive drug; the mice were then administered intravenous doses of **1c** (5 mg/kg), **1n** (5 mg/kg), **1a** (5 mg/kg), and gemcitabine (20 mg/kg) every other day for 24 days. Based on the monitoring of mouse body weight, **1n** had a lesser impact on weight gain compared to **1a**, indicating that **1n** may possess a higher safety profile (Figure 1C). Measurements of tumor volume and tumor weight revealed that **1n** demonstrated a tumor inhibition rate comparable to that of gemcitabine. In contrast, although the **1a**-treated group exhibited a high tumor inhibition rate, it was accompanied by a 50% mortality rate among the mice (Figure 1D–G).

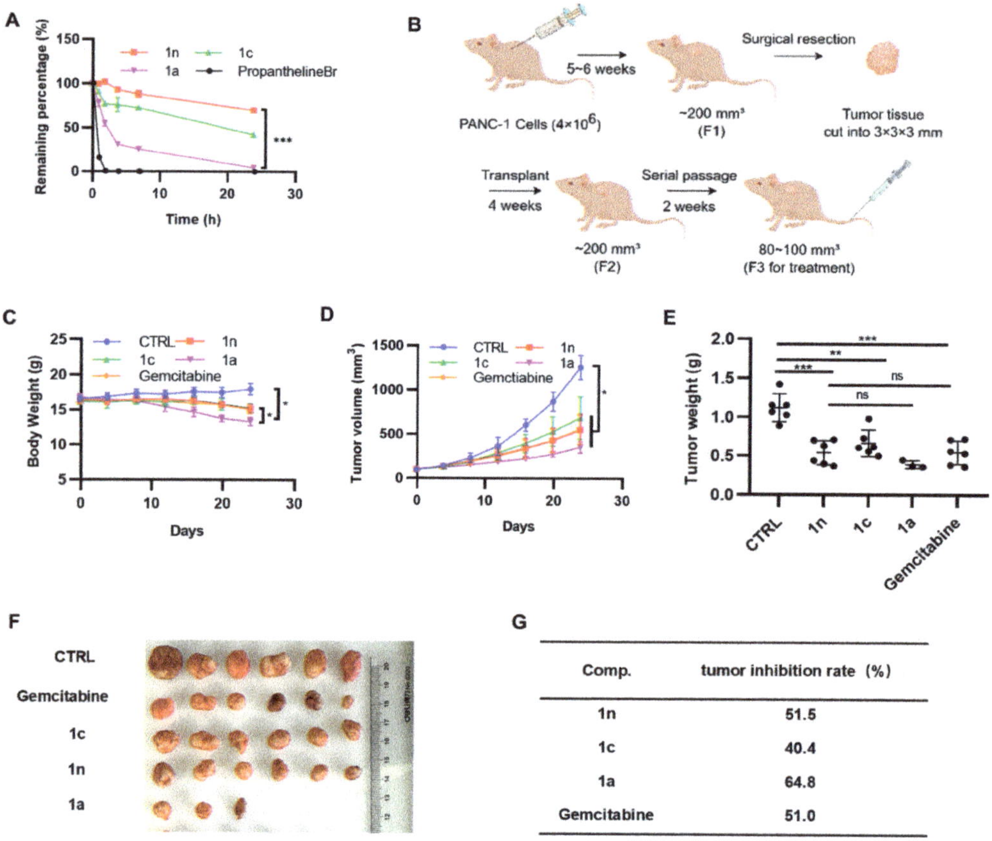

Comp.	tumor inhibition rate (%)
1n	51.5
1c	40.4
1a	64.8
Gemcitabine	51.0

Figure 1. Metabolic stability assays in mouse plasma and in vivo antitumor activity of **1a**, **1c**, and **1n**. (**A**) Curves of the remaining of **1a**, **1c**, and **1n** in mouse plasma. (**B**) Schematic illustration of the procedures for xenograft models established in mice. (**C**) Curves of the average mouse weight in different groups. (**D**) Growth curves of average tumor volume in different groups. (**E**) Tumor weight in different groups on the day mice were sacrificed. (**F**) Images of tumors dissected from each mouse in different groups on the day mice were sacrificed. (**G**) Tumor inhibition rate in different groups. Data are presented as mean ± SD, $n = 6$, ns = not significant, * $p < 0.05$, ** $p < 0.01$, *** $p < 0.001$.

In the biochemical and histological assays, **1n** (5 mg/kg) and **1a** (5 mg/kg) were administered to mice every other day, with the control group receiving an equivalent dose of saline. Following 14 days, mouse serum was collected for biochemical analysis, and organs were fixed for histological examination. Accordingly, serum biochemical analysis illustrated that ALT and AST levels were substantially elevated in the **1a**-treated group compared to the control group, indicating its potential hepatotoxicity. In contrast, no significant differences were observed between the **1N**-treated group and the control group (Figure 2A). Histological examination of liver and kidney tissues using H&E staining revealed that the liver tissues in the **1a**-treated group showed signs of hepatocyte necrosis and disruption of the hepatic cord structure. In comparison, the liver tissues of the **1n**-treated and control groups were normal. Additionally, H&E staining of kidney tissues revealed no significant pathological differences in any group (Figure 2B).

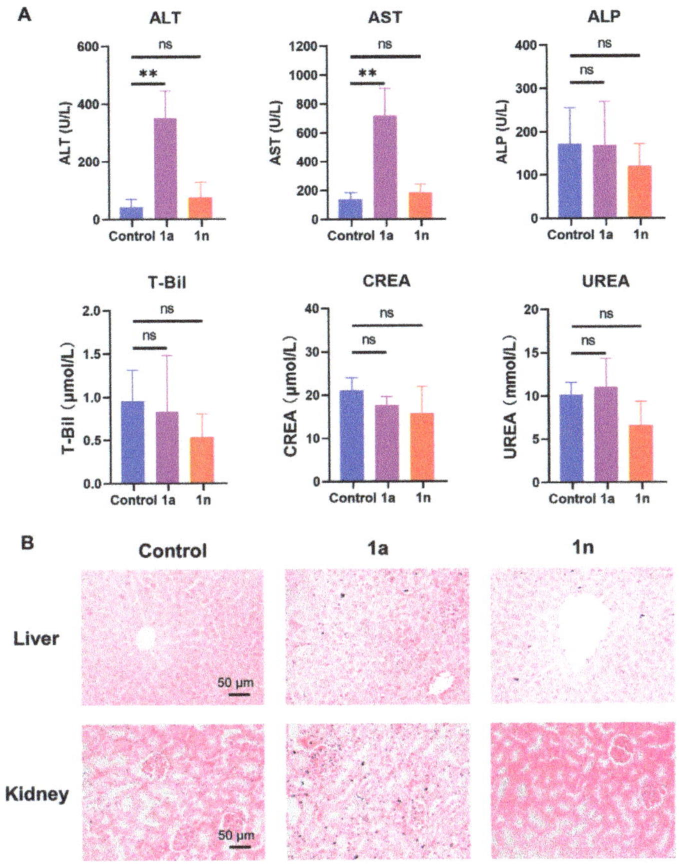

Figure 2. (**A**) Serum biochemical analysis of mice administered with **1a** and **1n**. Data are presented as mean ± SD, $n = 3$, ns = not significant, ** $p < 0.01$. (**B**) Representative images of hematoxylin and eosin (H&E) staining of liver and kidney tissues from mice administered with **1a** and **1n**.

3. Materials and Methods

3.1. Chemistry

Reagents were purchased from the Experimental Reagents and Technology Management Platform of Nankai University without further purification, unless otherwise stated. Dry solvents such as tetrahydrofuran (THF), dimethylformamide (DMF), and dichloromethane (DCM) were purified by solvent purification systems (Innovative Technology) or purchased directly as ultradry solvents. Reactions were monitored by thin layer chromatography (TLC) performed on silica gel plates using UV light as a visualizing agent and aqueous phosphomolybdic acid or basic aqueous potassium permanganate as a developing agent; 200–300 mesh silica gel was used for column chromatography.

^{1}H NMR (TMS as the internal standard), ^{19}F NMR spectra ($CFCl_3$ as the outside standard and low field is positive), and ^{13}C NMR spectra were recorded on a Bruker AV 400 instrument and calibrated by using internal references and solvent signals $CDCl_3$ (δ_H 7.26, δ_C 77.16), DMSO-*d6* (δ_H 2.50, δ_C 39.52), or Acetone-*d6* (δ_H 2.05, δ_C 206.26, 29.84). ^{1}H NMR data are reported as follows: chemical shift, multiplicity (s, singlet; d, doublet; t, triplet; q, quartet; br, broad; m, multiplet), coupling constants, and integration. High-resolution mass spectra (HRMS) were obtained with a Thermo ScientificTM Q Exactive Focus mass spectrometer (Orbitrap spec). Optical rotations were recorded on an Insmark

IP 120 digital polarimeter. The synthesis of compounds **1a–13a** and **2b** has been reported in previous studies [19].

Chemistry experimental procedures, except for compound **8n**, are available in the Supplementary Materials, which include synthetic procedures and characterization data (pages 5–59), NMR spectra (Figures S1–S221), and HPLC analysis (Figures S222–S224).

3.1.1. General Procedure for the Synthesis of **8b–8j** and **8n** (Take **8n** for Example)

To the solution of **6c** (3.23g, 6.58 mmol) in THF (20 mL) was added 4 N HCl in dioxane (32.9 mL, 131.70 mmol) at 0 °C. The mixture was allowed to reach room temperature, stirred for 1 h, and concentrated under reduced pressure to provide a white solid. To this salt was added a solution of **7d** (1.96 g, 6.58 mmol) and HATU (3.76 g, 9.88 mmol) in DCM (50 mL), then DIPEA (3.3 mL, 19.75 mmol) was added dropwise at 0 °C. The reaction was allowed to reach room temperature and stirred overnight. The mixture was concentrated, diluted with EtOAc (100 mL), and washed with aqueous 5% $NaHSO_4$ (3 × 100 mL) and brine (100 mL), dried (Na_2SO_4), filtered, concentrated in vacuo, and purified by column chromatography (25/1 to 2/1 petroleum ether/EtOAc) to provide compound **8n** (3.31 g, 75%) as a white solid. $[\alpha]_D^{22}$ = −87.7 (*c* = 0.5, $CHCl_3$). ^{1}H NMR (400 MHz, $CDCl_3$) δ 7.30 (d, *J* = 2.7 Hz, 5H), 7.13 (m, 2H), 7.00–6.65 (m, 3H), 5.20–5.02 (m, 2H), 5.01 (d, *J* = 7.9 Hz, 1H), 4.83 (dd, *J* = 29.8, 9.3 Hz, 2H), 4.50 (*p*, *J* = 6.4 Hz, 1H), 3.27 (dd, *J* = 14.4, 6.4 Hz, 1H), 3.02 (s, 1H), 2.97–2.82 (m, 3H), 2.71 (d, *J* = 25.0 Hz, 3H), 2.27–2.13 (m, 1H), 1.35 (d, *J* = 18.2 Hz, 9H), 1.18 (d, *J* = 6.3 Hz, 3H), 1.02–0.93 (m, 3H), 0.79–0.67 (m, 3H). ^{13}C NMR (100 MHz, $CDCl_3$) δ 170.2, 169.3, 163.0, 160.5, 156.2, 135.4, 133.2, 130.7, 130.6, 130.5, 128.7, 128.7, 128.6, 128.6, 128.5, 128.2, 122.9, 120.3, 115.3, 115.1, 80.8, 75.2, 67.1, 66.9, 61.9, 59.8, 52.3, 52.2, 33.3, 32.0, 31.6, 31.0, 29.8, 29.7, 29.4, 28.3, 28.2, 28.1, 28.1, 27.3, 22.8, 19.8, 19.7, 18.7, 18.6, 17.3, 14.2. ^{19}F NMR (376 MHz, $CDCl_3$) δ−57.9, −58.3, −58.4, −116.3, −116.6 (rotamer). HRMS (ESI) *m*/*z*: calculated for $C_{33}H_{43}N_3O_7F_4Na^+$ $[M + Na]^+$: 692.2929, found: 692.2923.

3.1.2. General Procedure for the Synthesis of **3b–3j** and **3n** (Take **3n** for Example)

To the solution of 8n (4.70 g, 7.02 mmol) in EtOH (50 mL) was added Pd/C 10% Wt (470 mg) at 0 °C. The reaction vessel was evacuated/backfilled with argon three times first, and then the reaction vessel was evacuated/backfilled with H_2 three times and stirred under this atmosphere overnight. The mixture was filtered through a pad of celite, washed with MeOH, and concentrated in vacuo and purified by column chromatography (100/1 to 25/1 DCM/MeOH) to provide compound 3n (3.50 g, 86%) as a white solid. $[\alpha]_D^{22}$ = −87.3 (*c* = 0.5, $CHCl_3$). ^{1}H NMR (400 MHz, $CDCl_3$) δ 7.60 (s, 1H), 7.18–7.07 (m, 3H), 6.98–6.83 (m, 2H), 5.18–5.05 (m, 1H), 4.90–4.72 (m, 2H), 4.57 (t, *J* = 6.5 Hz, 1H), 3.25 (dd, *J* = 14.4, 7.0 Hz, 1H), 3.06 (d, *J* = 46.7 Hz, 3H), 2.89 (d, *J* = 5.5 Hz, 1H), 2.74 (d, *J* = 21.3 Hz, 3H), 2.31–2.12 (m, 1H), 1.33 (d, *J* = 23.8 Hz, 12H), 1.09–0.98 (m, 3H), 0.76 (dd, *J* = 33.2, 6.1 Hz, 3H). ^{13}C NMR (100 MHz, $CDCl_3$) δ 173.6, 172.1, 170.7, 170.4, 169.6, 169.3, 163.0, 160.6, 156.6, 156.3, 133.0, 130.8, 130.7, 130.5, 125.4, 122.9, 120.4, 115.6, 115.4, 115.2, 81.3, 81.1, 75.2, 65.0, 62.4, 61.1, 59.7, 59.6, 52.4, 33.5, 33.1, 32.3, 31.0, 30.4, 29.8, 29.6, 28.2, 28.2, 27.5, 27.3, 19.9, 19.7, 18.8, 18.2, 17.5. ^{19}F NMR (376 MHz, $CDCl_3$) δ −57.9, −58.2, −116.3, −116.6. (rotamer). HRMS (ESI) *m*/*z*: calculated for $C_{26}H_{37}N_3O_7F_4Na^+$ $[M + Na]^+$: 602.2460, found: 602.2448.

3.1.3. General Procedure for the Synthesis of **13b–13n** (Take **13n** for Example)

To the solution of 4a (8.3 g, 19.53 mmol) in DCM (50 mL) was added 4 N HCl in dioxane (97.7 mL, 390.70 mmol) at 0 °C. The mixture was allowed to reach room temperature, stirred for 30 min, and concentrated under reduced pressure to provide a white solid. To this salt was added a solution of 3n (10.19 g, 17.58 mmol) and HATU (11.14 g, 19.30 mmol) in DCM (50 mL), then DIPEA (9.7 mL, 58.60 mmol) was added dropwise at 0 °C. The reaction was allowed to reach room temperature and stirred overnight. The mixture was concentrated, diluted with EtOAc (100 mL), and washed with aqueous 5% $NaHSO_4$ (3 × 100 mL) and brine (100 mL), dried (Na_2SO_4), filtered, concentrated in vacuo, and purified by column chromatography (3/1 to 1/2 DCM/EtOAc) to provide compound 13n (7.42 g, 55%) as a white foamed solid. $[\alpha]_D^{22}$ = −105.3 (c = 0.5, $CHCl_3$). ^{1}H NMR (400 MHz, $CDCl_3$) δ 7.28 (d, J = 2.0 Hz, 1H), 7.17–7.12 (m, 2H), 7.02–6.80 (m, 3H), 6.08 (dd, J = 6.0, 1.6 Hz, 1H), 5.59 (dd, J = 10.1, 2.0 Hz, 1H), 5.10–4.99 (m, 2H), 4.85–4.71 (m, 2H), 4.57 (q, J = 6.0 Hz, 1H), 4.37 (s, 1H), 3.92 (d, J = 11.6 Hz, 1H), 3.82 (dd, J = 11.6, 4.4 Hz, 1H), 3.29 (dd, J = 14.4, 6.4 Hz, 1H), 3.12–2.90 (m, 4H), 2.75 (d, J = 39.8 Hz, 4H), 2.39 (ddd, J = 14.6, 10.1, 4.7 Hz, 1H), 2.24 (s, 1H), 2.02 (d, J = 13.4 Hz, 1H), 1.45 (d, J = 6.7 Hz, 3H), 1.37 (d, J = 20.7 Hz, 9H), 1.32 (d, J = 2.7 Hz, 3H), 0.99 (d, J = 6.3 Hz, 3H), 0.85–0.69 (m, 3H). ^{13}C NMR (100 MHz, $CDCl_3$) δ 174.6, 170.4, 170.0, 169.0, 163.0, 160.6, 156.2, 154.4, 133.3, 130.7, 130.7, 125.4, 122.9, 120.3, 115.4, 115.2, 80.9, 74.9, 71.9, 60.3, 59.5, 58.6, 58.3, 57.2, 52.5, 52.2, 38.8, 36.7, 33.4, 31.6, 30.6, 29.8, 28.3, 27.4, 18.9, 18.4, 17.9, 17.0. ^{19}F NMR (376 MHz, $CDCl_3$) δ−58.3, −58.5, −116.3, −116.6 (rotamer). HRMS (ESI) m/z: calculated for $C_{36}H_{49}N_5O_9F_4Na^+$ $[M + Na]^+$: 794.3359, found: 794.3352.

3.1.4. General Procedure for the Synthesis of **1b–1n** (Take **1n** for Example)

To the solution of 13n (7.42 g, 9.61 mmol) in DCM (50 mL) was added 4 N HCl in dioxane (96.1 mL, 384.60 mmol) at 0 °C. The mixture was allowed to reach room temperature, stirred for 2 h, and concentrated under reduced pressure to provide a white solid. To this salt was added a solution of 2b (4.56 g, 28.84 mmol) and HATU (10.97 g, 28.84 mmol) in DCM (50 mL), then DIPEA (9.5 mL, 57.68 mmol) was added dropwise at 0 °C. The reaction was allowed to reach room temperature and stirred overnight. The mixture was concentrated, diluted with EtOAc (30 mL), and washed with aqueous 5% $NaHSO_4$ (3 × 100 mL) and brine (100 mL), dried (Na_2SO_4), filtered, concentrated in vacuo, and purified by column chromatography (2/1 to 1/3 DCM/EtOAc) to provide compound 1n (4.83 g, 62%) as a white foamed solid. $[\alpha]_D^{22}$ = −122.7 (c = 0.5, $CHCl_3$). ^{1}H NMR (400 MHz, $CDCl_3$) δ 7.28 (d, J = 2.0 Hz, 1H), 7.20–7.10 (m, 2H), 6.97–6.87 (m, 3H), 6.07 (dd, J = 6.1, 1.6 Hz, 1H), 5.58 (dd, J = 10.1, 2.1 Hz, 1H), 5.46 (dd, J = 9.8, 6.6 Hz, 1H), 5.09–4.98 (m, 2H), 4.79 (qt, J = 6.7, 1.8 Hz, 1H), 4.53 (p, J = 6.2 Hz, 1H), 4.36 (d, J = 4.7 Hz, 1H), 3.91 (d, J = 11.9 Hz, 1H), 3.84 (dd, J = 11.6, 4.4 Hz, 1H), 3.22 (dd, J = 14.8, 6.5 Hz, 1H), 3.00 (s, 3H), 2.95 (d, J = 5.1 Hz, 1H), 2.88 (s, 3H), 2.53 (h, J = 6.8 Hz, 1H), 2.39 (ddd, J = 14.6, 10.1, 4.8 Hz, 1H), 2.22 (dq, J = 10.9, 6.6 Hz, 1H), 2.01 (dd, J = 14.5, 1.9 Hz, 1H), 1.45 (d, J = 6.8 Hz, 3H), 1.42–1.36 (m, 1H), 1.30 (d, J = 6.2 Hz, 3H), 1.25–1.09 (m, 8H), 1.04 (d, J = 6.7 Hz, 3H), 0.99 (d, J = 6.5 Hz, 3H), 0.97–0.90 (m, 2H), 0.86 (t, J = 7.2 Hz, 3H), 0.75 (d, J = 6.7 Hz, 3H). ^{13}C NMR (100 MHz, $CDCl_3$) δ 178.2, 174.4, 170.1, 169.9, 169.0, 168.9, 168.8, 168.8, 162.9, 160.5, 154.3, 132.5, 132.5, 130.5, 130.4, 125.3, 122.7, 120.2, 115.4, 115.2, 74.8, 74.8, 71.7, 59.3, 58.5, 58.2, 57.0, 56.9, 52.2, 36.6, 36.1, 34.0, 32.8, 31.6, 30.9, 30.5, 29.2, 27.3, 27.1, 22.6, 18.8, 18.4, 17.9, 16.9, 14.0. ^{19}F NMR (376 MHz, $CDCl_3$) δ −58.3, −116.2. HRMS (ESI) m/z: calculated for $C_{40}H_{57}N_5O_8F_4Na^+$ $[M + Na]^+$: 834.4035, found: 834.4029.

3.2. *Experimental Cells and Animals*

PANC-1 was purchased from the National Experimental Cell Resource Sharing Platform. PANC-1 was cultured in DMEM medium containing 10% serum. The 4-week-old BALB/C nude mice were purchased from Beijing Vital River Laboratory Animal Technology Co., Ltd. and raised at the Animal Resources Center of Nankai University. The animal experiments have been approved by the Ethics Committee of Nankai University (2022-SYDWLL-000025, 2024-SYDWLL-000762).

3.3. *MTT Cell Activity Assay*

A total of 3000 PANC-1 cells were resuspended in 200 μL of culture medium and seeded into 96-well plates. After 24 h, the cells were treated with the compound and incubated for an additional 72 h. Following the incubation, 20 μL of 5 mg/mL MTT solution (Solarbio, China) was added to each well in the dark, and the cells were incubated for another 4 h. After incubation, the culture medium was discarded, and the wells were washed with PBS to remove any residual medium. Then, 200 μL of DMSO was added to each well to fully dissolve the formazan crystals, and the solution was mixed thoroughly.

The absorbance was measured at 492 nm/570 nm, and the data were analyzed using GraphPad Prism.

3.4. Stability in Mouse Plasma Assay

Thaw plasma at room temperature and vortex for 3–5 s. Centrifuge at 3000 rpm at 10 °C for 10 min, and carefully transfer the supernatant to a new Eppendorf tube. Preincubate the plasma at 37 °C for 10 min. Prepare a series of test substances by adding 3 μL of the compound (100 μM) to 297 μL of plasma to achieve a final concentration of 1 μM, ensuring that the DMSO concentration in plasma is 1%. Propantheline bromide is used as a positive control. Incubate the mixture at 37 °C, and at specified time points (0, 1, 2, 4, and 24 h), take 50 μL of the plasma sample. To terminate the reaction, add 250 μL of acetonitrile (containing an internal standard), vortex thoroughly, and centrifuge at 16,000 rcf (4 °C) for 10 min. Collect 130 μL of the supernatant and dilute with 70 μL of pure water for LC-MS/MS analysis. The concentration of the test substances in plasma samples was determined using LC-MS/MS. The stability of the test substance in plasma was evaluated by measuring the remaining percentage of the compound in the plasma over time. For example, the remaining percentage of bromopropyl in the plasma of CD-1 mice after a 2-h incubation was 0.90%, demonstrating that the testing system is suitable for evaluating the stability of test substances in plasma.

3.5. In Vivo Antitumor Activity

A total of 4×10^6 PANC-1 cells suspended in 100 μL PBS were subcutaneously injected into the right shoulder region of BALB/c nude mice. When the tumor volume reached approximately 200 mm^3, the mice were euthanized, and the tumor tissues were harvested and designated as F1 generation. Tumor tissues were then cut into small cubes measuring approximately $3 \times 3 \times 3$ mm, which were implanted into new BALB/c mice to propagate the tumors. This procedure was repeated to obtain the F2 generation of tumors. Finally, mice bearing F3 generation transplant tumors were used for drug treatment experiments. When the tumor volume reached approximately 80–100 mm^3, the mice were randomly divided into five groups ($n = 6$): control group, 5 mg/kg compound **1a** group, 5 mg/kg compound **1c** group, 5 mg/kg compound **1n** group, and 20 mg/kg gemcitabine group. The compounds **1a**, **1c**, and **1n** were dissolved in DMSO and then diluted with 0.9% physiological saline to achieve a final concentration of 0.5 mg/mL as the dosing concentration. Gemcitabine was dissolved directly in 0.9% saline to achieve a final concentration of 2 mg/mL as the dosing concentration. The compounds were administered intravenously every two days, alternating between the left and right tail veins to minimize vein damage. Injections were performed using ultra-fine syringes (30G needles) to reduce stress and ensure consistent delivery. The body weight and tumor volume of the mice were measured every four days. On day 24, the mice were euthanized, and the tumor weights were recorded. Tumor volume (V) was calculated using the formula: $V = (ab^2)/2$, with "a" representing the long diameter of the tumor and "b" representing the short diameter of the tumor. Tumor volume measurements showed that the **1n**-treated group exhibited a tumor inhibition rate comparable to that of gemcitabine, with tumor volumes of 553.3 $\pm$ 166.8 mm^3 and 561.1 $\pm$ 177.3 mm^3, respectively. The **1a**-treated group demonstrated a significantly smaller tumor volume of 353.0 $\pm$ 66.7 mm^3, indicating a high tumor inhibition rate, although this group experienced a 50% mortality rate among mice. In contrast, the control group displayed a much larger tumor volume of 1262 $\pm$ 137.7 mm^3 (Figure 1D). Similarly, tumor weight measurements supported these findings. The **1n** and gemcitabine-treated groups showed comparable tumor weights of 0.542 $\pm$ 0.156 g and 0.548 $\pm$ 0.153 g, respectively. The **1a**-treated group had a significantly lower tumor weight of 0.393 $\pm$ 0.049 g, while the control group exhibited the highest tumor weight of 1.118 $\pm$ 0.177 g (Figure 1E,F). Tumor weight was used to calculate the tumor inhibition rate (Figure 1G).

3.6. H&E Staining

Mice were euthanized, and liver and kidney tissues were collected and fixed in 10% neutral-buffered formalin for 48 h. The fixed tissues were processed for paraffin embedding, including dehydration in a graded ethanol series, clearing with xylene, and infiltration with molten paraffin wax. Paraffin blocks were sectioned into 4 μm slices using a rotary microtome, and the sections were mounted onto glass slides. The slides were dried at 60 °C for 4 h to ensure proper tissue adhesion. Following deparaffinization and rehydration, staining was performed according to the manufacturer's instructions for the H&E staining kit (Solarbio, China). The sections were immersed in a hematoxylin solution for 3 min to stain the nuclei and then rinsed under running tap water for 1 minute to remove excess stain. Differentiation was achieved by briefly immersing the slides in a 1% hydrochloric acid-ethanol solution, followed by neutralization in 0.6% ammonia water until the nuclei appeared blue. Eosin staining was applied for 30 s to stain cytoplasmic and extracellular components, imparting a pink coloration. The slides were rinsed under running tap water for 30 s to remove excess eosin. Finally, the sections were dehydrated through a graded ethanol series, cleared with xylene, and coverslipped with a neutral resin mounting medium to preserve the stained tissues for microscopic examination.

4. Conclusions

The syntheses of 26 majusculamide D analogues were successfully completed and subsequently evaluated for their anti-pancreatic cancer activity. Among them, two compounds (**1i** and **1j**) demonstrated IC_{50} values < 1 nM. The biological results indicate that the C23-OAc could be replaced with OCF_3. The removal of the C4-Me group and the acetyl group of C23-OAc both resulted in a significant decrease in activity. However, replacing the C10-OH and C34-OMe with an F atom was well tolerated. Although attaching one extra amino acid at C23 enhanced the water solubility of natural products, their activities diminished dramatically. A series of in vitro assays, including wound healing, transwell, clone formation, EdU, and western blot, were conducted for the purpose of evaluating the inhibitory effects of majusculamide D on migration, invasion, and proliferation against pancreatic cancer cell lines. The results indicated that majusculamide D inhibited the migration and proliferation of pancreatic cancer cells and may be involved in the epithelial-mesenchymal transition (EMT) process.

The designed analog **1n** exhibited an apparent improvement in the mouse plasma stability assay compared to majusculamide D. The in vivo data of **1n** demonstrated therapeutic benefit compared to the control group. Above all, **1n** overcame the severe toxicity of mouse death arising in the natural product-treated group at a dosage of 5 mg/kg. The serum biochemical analysis indicated potential hepatotoxicity of the natural product, as evidenced by elevated ALT and AST levels. Histological examination of liver and kidney tissues with H&E staining further confirmed hepatocyte necrosis and disruption of hepatic cord structure in the natural product-treated group. In contrast, the **1n**-treated group showed no significant differences in serum biochemical parameters compared to the control group, and liver tissue appeared normal. The results collectively suggested that natural products may have higher toxicity, and our modification effectively reduced the severe toxicity, such as mouse death, of natural products while maintaining a good tumor inhibition rate. However, the current results only demonstrate that **1n** is less toxic than natural products, with the underlying mechanisms remaining unclear. Further studies, particularly on its exact mode of action and pharmacokinetics, are necessary. Efforts to expand the therapeutic window through strategies such as prodrugs, antibody-drug conjugates, peptide-drug conjugates, and other innovative approaches are ongoing, and additional findings will be reported in due course.

Supplementary Materials: The following supporting information can be downloaded at: https://www.mdpi.com/article/10.3390/md22120537/s1, Part 1: Synthetic procedures and characterization data (pages 5–59); Figures S1–S221: ^{1}H and ^{13}C NMR spectra; Figures S222–S224: HPLC analysis; Figure S225: Compound **1a** inhibited the migration, invasion, and proliferation of pancreatic cancer cells.

Author Contributions: X.Z. (Xiuhe Zhao), X.X., Y.L., L.W. and Y.C. devised the project; X.Z. (Xiuhe Zhao), M.Z. and M.L. synthesized the compounds; X.X. carried out the biological studies; X.Z. (Xiuhe Zhao) and X.Z. (Xiang Zhang) analyzed the data; X.Z. (Xiuhe Zhao) and L.W. wrote the manuscript. All authors have read and agreed to the published version of the manuscript.

Funding: This study was supported by the National Natural Science Foundation of China (Grant No. 82073695 to L.W., 82303509 to X.X.), the Fundamental Research Funds for the Central Universities (63243109 to L.W., 63241203 to L.W.), the Hundred Young Academic Leaders Program of Nankai University to L.W. (Nankai University), the Frontiers Science Center for New Organic Matter (63181206), and the China Postdoctoral Science Foundation (2022M711711 to X.X.).

Institutional Review Board Statement: The 4-week-old BALB/C nude mice were purchased from Beijing Vital River Laboratory Animal Technology Co., Ltd. and raised at the Animal Resources Center of Nankai University. The animal experiments have been approved by the Ethics Committee of Nankai University (2022-SYDWLL-000025, 2024-SYDWLL-000762).

Data Availability Statement: The data are contained within the article or Supplementary Materials; further inquiries can be directed to the corresponding author.

Acknowledgments: We would like to thank Home for Researchers for providing us with schematic elements (license number: ASTOSc171c).

Conflicts of Interest: The authors declare no conflicts of interest.

References

1. Cancer Stat Facts: Pancreatic Cancer. Available online: https://seer.cancer.gov/statfacts/html/pancreas.html (accessed on 8 August 2024).
2. Wood, L.D.; Canto, M.I.; Jaffee, E.M.; Simeone, D.M. Pancreatic cancer: Pathogenesis, screening, diagnosis, and treatment. *Gastroenterology* **2022**, *163*, 386–402. [CrossRef]
3. Siegel, R.L.; Miller, K.D.; Fuchs, H.E.; Jemal, A. Cancer statistics, 2021. *CA Cancer J. Clin.* **2021**, *71*, 7–33. [CrossRef] [PubMed]
4. Mizrahi, J.D.; Surana, R.; Valle, J.W.; Shroff, R.T. Pancreatic cancer. *Lancet* **2020**, *395*, 2008–2020. [CrossRef] [PubMed]
5. Newman, D.J.; Cragg, G.M. Natural products as sources of new drugs over the nearly four decades from 01/1981 to 09/2019. *J. Nat. Prod.* **2020**, *83*, 770–803. [CrossRef]
6. Newman, D.J. Natural products and drug discovery. *Natl. Sci. Rev.* **2022**, *9*, nwac206. [CrossRef] [PubMed]
7. Atanasov, A.G.; Zotchev, S.B.; Dirsch, V.M.; Supuran, C.T. Natural products in drug discovery: Advances and opportunities. *Nat. Rev. Drug Discov.* **2021**, *20*, 200–216. [CrossRef] [PubMed]
8. Luo, H.; Tian, L.; Zhang, Y.; Wu, Y.; Li, B.; Liu, J. Recent advances in molecular and nanoparticle probes for fluorescent bioanalysis. *Nano Res.* **2024**, *17*, 6443–6474. [CrossRef]
9. Carroll, A.R.; Copp, B.R.; Grkovic, T.; Keyzers, R.A.; Prinsep, M.R. Marine natural products. *Nat. Prod. Rep.* **2024**, *41*, 162–207. [CrossRef] [PubMed]
10. Ren, X.; Xie, X.; Chen, B.; Liu, L.; Jiang, C.; Qian, Q. Marine natural products: A potential source of anti-hepatocellular carcinoma drugs. *J. Med. Chem.* **2021**, *64*, 7879–7899. [CrossRef] [PubMed]
11. Koehn, F.E.; Longley, R.E.; Reed, J.K. Microcolins A and B, new immunosuppressive peptides from the blue-green alga Lyngbya majuscula. *J. Nat. Prod.* **1992**, *55*, 613–619. [CrossRef] [PubMed]
12. Moore, R.E.; Entzeroth, M. Majusculamide D and deoxymajusculamide D, two cytotoxins from Lyngbya majuscula. *Phytochemistry* **1988**, *27*, 3101–3103. [CrossRef]
13. Takamatsu, S.; Nagle, D.G.; Gerwick, W.H. Secondary metabolites from marine cyanobacteria and algae inhibit LFA-1/ICAM-1 mediated cell adhesion. *Planta Med.* **2004**, *70*, 127–131. [PubMed]
14. Meickle, T.; Matthew, S.; Ross, C.; Luesch, H.; Paul, V. Bioassay-guided isolation and identification of Desacetylmicrocolin B from Lyngbya cf. polychroa. *Planta Med.* **2009**, *75*, 1427–1430. [CrossRef] [PubMed]
15. Guzmán, E.A.; Harmody, D.; Pitts, T.P.; Vera-Diaz, B.; Winder, P.L.; Yu, Y.; Wright, A.E. Inhibition of IL-8 secretion on BxPC-3 and MIA PaCa-2 cells and induction of cytotoxicity in pancreatic cancer cells with marine natural products. *Anti-Cancer Drugs* **2017**, *28*, 153–160. [CrossRef]
16. Yu, H.-B.; Glukhov, E.; Li, Y.; Iwasaki, A.; Gerwick, L.; Dorrestein, P.C.; Jiao, B.-H.; Gerwick, W.H. Cytotoxic Microcolin lipopeptides from the marine cyanobacterium *Moorea producens*. *J. Nat. Prod.* **2019**, *82*, 2608–2619. [CrossRef] [PubMed]
17. Caro-Diaz, E.J.E.; Valeriote, F.A.; Gerwick, W.H. Highly convergent total synthesis and assignment of absolute configuration of Majusculamide D, a potent and selective cytotoxic metabolite from *Moorea* sp. *Org. Lett.* **2019**, *21*, 793–796. [CrossRef] [PubMed]
18. Yang, H.; Zhang, X.; Wang, C.; Zhang, H.; Yi, J.; Wang, K.; Hou, Y.; Ji, P.; Jin, X.; Li, C.; et al. Microcolin H, a novel autophagy inducer, exerts potent antitumour activity by targeting PITPα/β. *Signal Transduct. Target. Ther.* **2023**, *8*, 428. [CrossRef]

19. Zhao, X.; Lv, M.; Xi, X.; Lu, Y.; Wang, L.; Chen, Y. Synthesis of anti-pancreatic cancer natural product Majusculamide D and analogues reveals a preliminary structure-activity relationships. *Chin. J. Chem.* **2024**, *42*, 605–610. [CrossRef]
20. Patani, G.A.; LaVoie, E.J. Bioisosterism: A Rational Approach in Drug Design. *Chem. Rev.* **1996**, *96*, 3147–3176. [CrossRef]
21. Meanwell, N.A. Fluorine and fluorinated motifs in the design and application of bioisosteres for drug design. *J. Med. Chem.* **2018**, *61*, 5822–5880. [CrossRef]
22. Wang, S.; Dong, G.; Sheng, C. Structural simplification of natural products. *Chem. Rev.* **2019**, *119*, 4180–4220. [CrossRef]
23. Liu, J.; Xu, X.; Qing, F. Silver-mediated oxidative trifluoromethylation of alcohols to alkyl trifluoromethyl ethers. *Org. Lett.* **2015**, *17*, 5048–5051. [CrossRef] [PubMed]
24. Chen, S.; Bi, K.; Wu, S.; Li, Y.; Huang, Y.; Sheng, C.; Dong, G. Water-soluble derivatives of evodiamine: Discovery of evodiamine-10-phosphate as an orally active antitumor lead compound. *Eur. J. Med. Chem.* **2021**, *220*, 113544. [CrossRef]
25. Wang, Z.; Li, Z.; Ji, H. Direct targeting of β-catenin in the Wnt signaling pathway: Current progress and perspectives. *Med. Res. Rev.* **2021**, *41*, 2109–2129. [CrossRef]
26. Valenta, T.; Hausmann, G.; Basler, K. The many faces and functions of β-catenin. *EMBO J.* **2012**, *31*, 2714–2736. [CrossRef] [PubMed]
27. Liu, M.; Yang, J.; Zhang, Y.; Zhou, Z.; Cui, X.; Zhang, L.; Fung, K.-M.; Zheng, W.; Allard, F.D.; Yee, E.U.; et al. ZIP4 promotes pancreatic cancer progression by repressing ZO-1 and Claudin-1 through a ZEB1-dependent transcriptional mechanism. *Clin. Cancer Res.* **2018**, *24*, 3186–3196. [CrossRef]
28. Singh, A.B.; Sharma, A.; Smith, J.J.; Krishnan, M.; Chen, X.; Escheich, S.; Washington, M.K.; Yeatman, T.J.; Beauchamp, R.D.; Dhawan, P. Claudin-1 up-regulates the repressor ZEB-1 to inhibit E-Cadherin expression in colon cancer cells. *Gastroenterology* **2011**, *141*, 2140–2153. [CrossRef] [PubMed]
29. Tan, E.J.; Kahata, K.; Idås, O.; Thuault, S.; Heldin, C.H.; Moustakas, A. The high mobility group A2 protein epigenetically silences the *Cdh1* gene during epithelial-to-mesenchymal transition. *Nucleic Acids Res.* **2015**, *43*, 162–178. [CrossRef]
30. Zhou, Z.; Qutaish, M.; Han, Z.; Schur, R.M.; Liu, Y.; Wilson, D.L.; Lu, Z.-R. LMRI detection of breast cancer micrometastases with a fibronectin-targeting contrast agent. *Nat. Commun.* **2015**, *6*, 7984. [CrossRef] [PubMed]
31. Sara, M.R.; Vera, M.G.; Catarina, G.T.; Cláudia, M.L.; João, L.; Diana, M.; Paula, C.D.; Helene, N.K.; Isabelle, B.P.; Rui, H.; et al. Vimentin epigenetic deregulation in bladder cancer associates with acquisition of invasive and metastatic phenotype through epithelial-to-mesenchymal transition. *Int. J. Biol. Sci.* **2023**, *19*, 1–12.

marine drugs

MDPI

Article

Total Synthesis of the Marine Cyclic Depsipeptide Lagunamide D

Huiru Nan [1], Xiong-En Long [1], Jianfei He [1], Hailiang Xing [1], Min-Jing Cheng [4], Jin-Bao Peng [1], Tao Ye [2,3,*], Jia-Lei Yan [1,*] and Junyang Liu [1,2,*]

1 School of Pharmacy and Food Engineering, Wuyi University, Jiangmen 529020, China; huiru_nan@foxmail.com (H.N.); wananlxe@163.com (X.-E.L.); 18230816752@163.com (J.H.); 18255186096@163.com (H.X.); pengjb_05@126.com (J.-B.P.)
2 State Key Laboratory of Chemical Oncogenomics, Key Laboratory of Chemical Genomics, Peking University Shenzhen Graduate School, Shenzhen, 518055, China
3 Qian Yan (Shenzhen) Pharmatech. Ltd., Shenzhen 518172, China
4 Center for Bioactive Natural Molecules and Innovative Drugs, and Guangdong Province Key Laboratory of Pharmacodynamic Constituents of TCM and New Drugs Research, College of Pharmacy, Jinan University, Guangzhou 510632, China; chengmj1235@jnu.edu.cn
* Correspondence: yet@pkusz.edu.cn (T.Y.); yanjialei@wyu.edu.cn (J.-L.Y.); liujy@wyu.edu.cn (J.L.)

Abstract: Lagunamide D is a structurally distinct 26-membered cytotoxic cyclic depsipeptide, originally isolated from a marine cyanobacterium. It exhibits potent antiproliferative activity in the low nanomolar range against A549 human lung adenocarcinoma cells and HCT116 colon cancer cells. A significant challenge associated with lagunamide D is its propensity for intramolecular acyl migration, which leads to the formation of a contracted 24-membered analog, lagunamide D′. This structural rearrangement complicates its isolation, characterization, and synthesis. In this study, the total synthesis of lagunamide D was achieved in a 14-step longest linear sequence, starting from the known intermediate **17**, with an overall yield of 4.6%. The synthetic strategy involved several key transformations, including Ghosh's $TiCl_4$-promoted anti-aldol reaction, Corey–Bakshi–Shibata reduction (CBS reduction), cross-metathesis, Pinnick oxidation, and Yamaguchi esterification. Furthermore, this synthetic effort unambiguously confirmed the stereochemistry of the natural product.

Keywords: lagunamide D; marine natural products; depsipeptide; total synthesis

1. Introduction

Natural products and their derivatives have long been recognized as invaluable sources of pharmaceuticals, playing a pivotal role in drug discovery and development. Many modern medicines are derived from natural compounds, demonstrating their significant contribution to human health [1]. While terrestrial plants, animals, and microorganisms have traditionally served as primary sources for natural product-based drugs, marine-derived compounds have garnered increasing attention due to their exceptional chemical diversity, unique structural features, and promising pharmacological potential [2–4]. The harsh and competitive marine environment has driven the evolution of highly specialized secondary metabolites with novel mechanisms of action, making them particularly attractive candidates for pharmaceutical development.

Several marine-derived drugs have already received regulatory approval for the treatment of various diseases, including cancer, chronic pain, and neurodegenerative disorders such as Alzheimer's disease. Notable examples include Cytarabine (Cytosar-U®), an antileukemic agent; Trabectedin (Yondelis®), used in soft tissue sarcoma and ovarian cancer;

Ziconotide (Prialt®), a potent analgesic; Eribulin mesylate (Halaven®), a microtubule inhibitor for metastatic breast cancer; Plitidepsin (Aplidin®), with antiviral and anticancer properties; Brentuximab vedotin (Adcetris®), an antibody–drug conjugate for lymphomas; and Omega-3-Acid ethyl esters (Lovaza®), used in cardiovascular disease management [5]. Beyond these approved drugs, more than 20 marine-derived compounds are currently progressing through various phases of clinical trials, further highlighting their potential in therapeutic applications [6–8].

Despite their immense pharmaceutical promise, the development of marine natural products faces significant challenges, particularly regarding their limited natural availability. Many bioactive compounds are produced in minute quantities by marine organisms, making large-scale extraction impractical and unsustainable. To address this issue, researchers have explored alternative strategies such as total chemical synthesis, semi-synthesis, and microbial fermentation to ensure a reliable supply. While biosynthetic technologies, including genetic engineering and heterologous expression, offer promising avenues for sustainable production, these approaches also present technical and logistical challenges [9]. Continued advancements in synthetic methodologies and biotechnological innovations are therefore crucial for unlocking the full potential of marine-derived pharmaceuticals.

Lagunamide D, a novel cytotoxic cyclic depsipeptide, was first isolated in 2019 by Luesch's research group from a marine cyanobacterium collected at Loggerhead Key in Dry Tortugas, Florida. The compound was obtained in an extremely low isolation yield of 0.003% [10], highlighting the challenge of natural product extraction. Lagunamide D represents a new member of the lagunamide family, expanding the structural diversity within this class of bioactive molecules [11,12] (Figure 1).

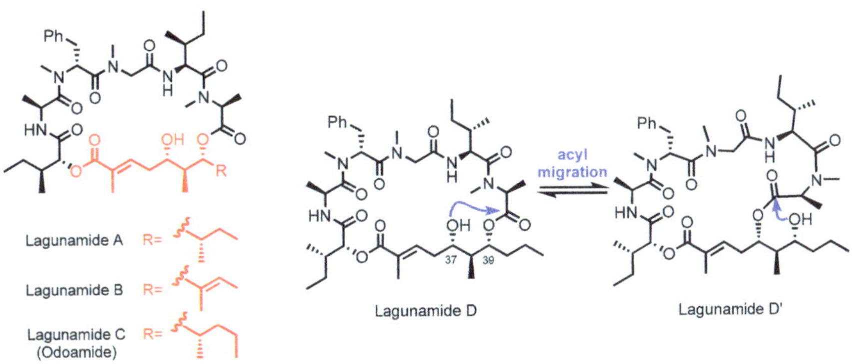

Figure 1. Structures of lagunamides A–D and D′.

The planar structure of lagunamide D was elucidated through a comprehensive analysis of 1D and 2D nuclear magnetic resonance (NMR) spectra, complemented by high-resolution mass spectrometry (HRMS) data. Notably, the absolute stereochemistry of the hydroxyl groups at positions C-37 and C-39 within the polyketide segment was determined using a modified Mosher method. Meanwhile, the configuration of the methyl group at position C-38 was deduced through a combination of Kishi's NMR database [13,14] and detailed comparisons of hydrogen peak shapes and splitting patterns in the ^{1}H NMR spectrum with those observed in lagunamide A. These rigorous structural studies provided valuable insight into the stereochemical framework of lagunamide D. A particularly intriguing observation was made during high-performance liquid chromatography (HPLC) separation, where intramolecular ester exchange led to the formation of a cyclization product, lagunamide D′. This transformation involved acyl migration within the macrocyclic core, converting the native 26-membered macrocycle into a contracted 24-membered analog [10] (Figure 1). Such structural rearrangements underscore the dynamic nature of cyclic depsipeptides and pose additional considerations for their synthetic and biological studies. In terms of biological activity, lagunamide D exhibits potent antiproliferative effects against human cancer cell lines. It demonstrates strong cytotoxicity towards A549 human lung adenocarcinoma cells (IC_{50} = 7.1 ± 1.7 nM) and HCT116 colon cancer cells (IC_{50} = 5.1 nM) [15], suggesting its potential as a promising lead compound for anticancer drug development. Given this remarkable bioactivity and its complex structural framework, we aim to undertake a total synthesis of lagunamide D. This effort will not only confirm its stereochemistry with absolute certainty but also provide a sustainable and scalable synthetic route to facilitate further medicinal chemistry investigations.

The key synthetic challenges associated with the lagunamide family primarily involve the construction of the anti-anti-syn configuration at the C37–C40 stereogenic centers and the incorporation of the unsaturated ester subunit within the fatty acid fragment (highlighted in red, Figure 1). In 2012, Ye and co-workers reported the first total synthesis and stereochemical revision of lagunamide A [16], highlighting the use of a double asymmetric Brown crotylboration to establish the required anti-anti-syn configuration of the C37–C40 stereogenic centers, as well as the Horner–Wadsworth–Emmons (HWE) reaction to install the α,β-unsaturated carboxylic acid unit within the polyketide chain. Lin's group achieved the second total synthesis of lagunamide A [17], employing an asymmetric Paterson anti-aldol condensation to establish the C38–C39 stereogenic centers, followed by stereoselective allylation to install the required C37 chiral center. Furthermore, the α,β-unsaturated carboxylic acid unit was constructed via a cross-metathesis (CM) reaction. In 2018, Kazmaier and co-workers reported the third total synthesis of lagunamide A [18], utilizing a sequence of six iterative Matteson homologation steps and subsequent oxidation to generate the C37–C40 stereogenic centers. This was followed by the installation of the α,β-unsaturated ester unit through an HWE reaction. In 2016, Oishi et al. reported the first total synthesis of odoamide (lagunamide C) [19,20], featuring the use of an Evans syn-aldol reaction to establish the C39–C40 stereocenters, followed by a substrate-controlled Mukaiyama aldol reaction and a subsequent Mitsunobu reaction to install the C37 chiral center and the α,β-unsaturated ester. Currently, no reports on the total synthesis of lagunamide D exist. For the total synthesis of lagunamide D, we envisioned that the C38–C39 chiral centers could be established through an alternative anti-aldol reaction, such as the $TiCl_4$-promoted protocol developed by Ghosh, while the C37 stereocenter could be installed via asymmetric reduction of the corresponding ketone. To the best of our knowledge, this approach has not been employed in previous lagunamide syntheses.

Our retrosynthetic analysis is illustrated in Scheme 1. The key transformation in our strategy is the macrocyclization between L-Ile and *N*-Me-L-Ala, which serves as the pivotal step in constructing the macrocyclic core of the target molecule. Following this, we implemented a strategic disconnection at the ester bond linking the α-hydroxy group of the 2-hydroxy-3-methylpentanoic acid moiety and the unsaturated acid. This approach effectively simplifies the molecule into two key intermediates: intermediate **2** and the polyketide subunit **3**, both possessing a comparable level of complexity. The formation of the ester bond in fragment **3** can be efficiently achieved through the reaction of an acyl chloride derivative with the corresponding alcohol. Meanwhile, the synthesis of the unsaturated acid is planned via a cross-metathesis reaction [21,22], enabling fragment **3** to be derived from a simpler precursor, the alcohol fragment **4**. The construction of fragment **4** is envisioned through a highly stereoselective route. Specifically, it can be assembled from intermediates **6** and **7** utilizing Ghosh's $TiCl_4$-promoted anti-aldol reaction [23], which plays a crucial role in establishing the stereogenic centers at C38 and C39 with high selectivity. Furthermore, the stereogenic center at C37 will be introduced through a stereoselective reduction of the corresponding ketone, ensuring precise control over the molecule's three-dimensional architecture. This retrosynthetic plan strategically leverages well-established reactions to achieve efficient and selective bond formations, paving the way for a streamlined synthesis of the target molecule.

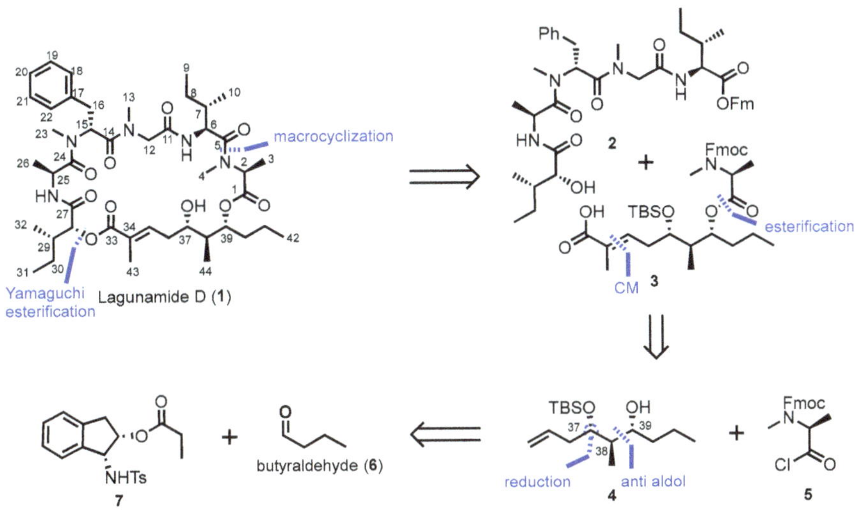

Scheme 1. Retrosynthetic analysis of lagunamide D (**1**).

2. Results and Discussion

The synthesis began with the preparation of the linear pentapeptide compound **2**, as depicted in Scheme 2. The process started with the coupling of *N*-Me-Gly-OMe·HCl (**8**) and Boc-*N*-Me-D-Phe-OH (**9**) using HATU(2-(7-Azabenzotriazol-1-yl)-*N*,*N*,*N*′,*N*′-tetramethyluronium hexafluorophosphate)/HOAt(3H-[1,2,3]-Triazolo [4,5-b] pyridin-3-ol)/DIPEA(*N*,*N*-Diisopropylethylamine)/DMF(*N*,*N*-Dimethylformamide) as the reaction conditions. This step efficiently produced the dipeptide **10** in an excellent yield of 93%. Next, the dipeptide **10** underwent hydrolysis with LiOH, converting the ester into a carboxylic acid. The resulting acid was then subjected to peptide coupling with amine **11** under similar conditions, affording the tripeptide **12** in an overall yield of 68% over two steps. Subsequent treatment of **12** with TFA (Trifluoroacetic acid) removed the Boc protecting group, generating a free amine. This intermediate was then coupled with Boc-LL-Ala-OH (**13**), forming the tetrapeptide **14** with a moderate yield of 61% over two steps. Finally, Boc deprotection of **14** using TFA yielded the corresponding amine **15**, which was coupled with α-hydroxy acid **16** under the same peptide coupling conditions. This step completed the synthesis of the pentapeptide **2** with an overall yield of 63% over the last two steps.

Upon successfully synthesizing pentapeptide **2**, we shifted our focus to obtaining the polyketide fragment **3**, as depicted in Scheme 3. Following established literature procedures [24], the anti-aldol product **17** was synthesized from butanal (**6**) under Ghosh's $TiCl_4$-promoted anti-aldol conditions [23]. This was followed by benzyl (Bn) protection using the Bn-TCAI (Benzyl 2,2,2-trichloroacetimidate) reagent and a catalytic amount of TfOH. Treatment of compound **17** with isopropyl magnesium chloride and *N*,*O*-dimethylhydroxylamine hydrochloride yielded the Weinreb amide in a moderate yield of 78%. Subsequent reaction with allyl magnesium bromide led to the formation of ketone **18**. Stereoselective reduction of ketone **18** was crucial to obtaining the desired 1,3-syn hydroxyl substrate. Initially, we adopted conditions previously used in the total synthesis of des-thiomethyllooekeyolide A [25], employing methanol as the solvent and $NaBH_4$ as the reducing agent at −30 °C. However, the stereoselectivity was inconsistent, ranging from 5:1 to 7:1 diastereomeric ratio (dr). Other conditions were tested, including the following: $MeOH/NaBH_4$ at −60 °C and −78 °C, $MeOH/NaBH_4/CeCl_3·7H_2O$ at −60 °C, KBH_4/THF at −78 °C, and LiAl(O*t*-Bu)$_3$H/THF at −78 °C. Despite these variations, the selectivity did not improve significantly. Ultimately, the best results were obtained using (*R*)-Me-CBS{(3aR)-1-Methyl-3,3-diphenyltetrahydro-1H,3H-pyrrolo[1,2-c][1,3,2]oxazaborole}/THF at −78 °C [26], achieving a remarkable selectivity of dr > 10:1 with an 89% yield. The resulting alcohol was treated with TBSOTf to afford product **20** in a high yield of 89%. Subsequent deprotection of the benzyl group at 50 °C using DDQ in a wet DCE solvent [27] yielded secondary alcohol **4** in a moderate yield of 69%. To confirm the relative stereochemistry at positions C37 and C39, the TBS protecting group in compound **4** was removed, followed by 1,3-diol acetonide protection to afford acetonide **21** in an excellent 93% yield. Analysis of the ^{13}C NMR chemical shift of acetonide **21** confirmed the anticipated 1,3-syn configuration based on the distinct shifts of the ketal methyl groups (19.6 and 30.2 ppm for equatorial and axial methyl groups, respectively) [28] and the ketal carbon (97.8 ppm). Next, compound **4** was subjected to esterification using freshly prepared Fmoc-L-(*N*-Me)Ala-Cl, yielding ester **22** with a 66% yield, without epimerization. An olefin cross-metathesis reaction between substrate **22** and methyl acrylate **23**, catalyzed by Grubbs II in DCM at 50 °C (sealed tube), proceeded smoothly, affording the desired aldehyde in an 81% yield. Finally, Pinnick oxidation of the resulting aldehyde using $NaClO_2$ successfully delivered the unsaturated carboxylic acid **3**.

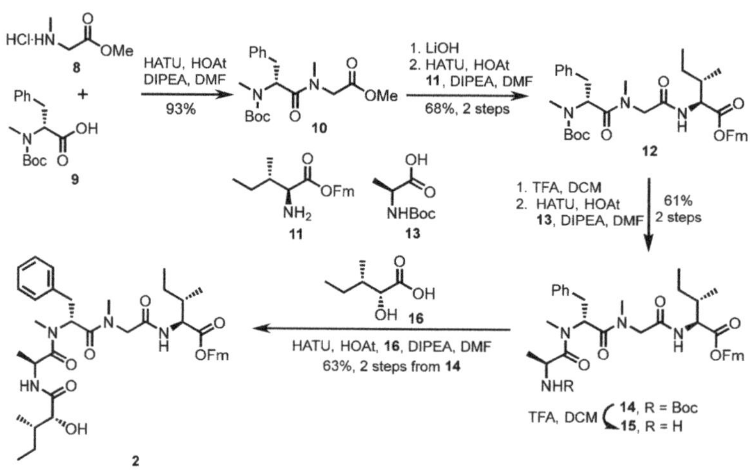

Scheme 2. Synthesis of pentapeptide **2**.

With pentapeptide **2** and carboxylic acid **3** in hand, we next focused on their esterification (Scheme 4). Despite multiple attempts using Yamaguchi esterification [29], Steglich esterification [30], Shiina esterification [31], and the Ghosez reagent [32], we were unable to obtain the desired product. We speculated that this failure was due to the relatively low reactivity of conjugate acid **3** compared to a saturated acid, as well as the inherent complexity of the flexible alcohol **2**. To overcome this challenge, we shifted our focus to coupling alcohol **25** with acid **3**. Under Yamaguchi conditions, this reaction successfully yielded the key intermediate **26** in an acceptable 68% yield. Subsequent deprotection of the allyl group from compound **26**, followed by condensation with amine **15** under HATU conditions, afforded cyclization precursor **27** in a satisfactory 73% overall yield.

Finally, after removing the Fm (9-Fluorenylmethyl) and Fmoc (Fluorenylmethoxycarbonyl) protecting groups using diethylamine, we investigated the macrocyclization reaction. Although HRMS confirmed the presence of the molecular ion peak corresponding to the target product, isolation of the cyclized compound proved challenging due to the low yield of this reaction.

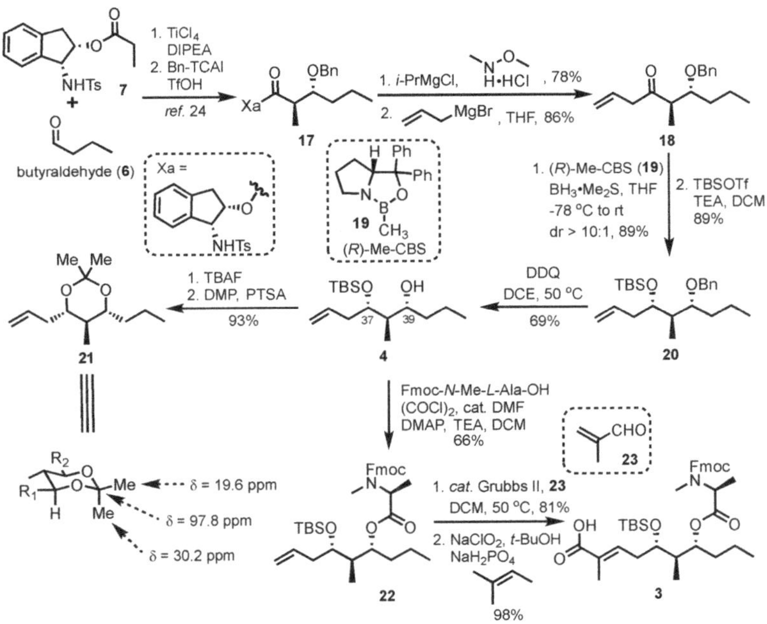

Scheme 3. Synthesis of carboxylic acid **3**.

To complete the total synthesis of lagunamide D, the macrocyclization site was reselected between the α-hydroxy acid and L-Ala moiety (Scheme 5). To achieve this, the Fm and Fmoc protecting groups of compounds **14** and **26** were removed, yielding acid **29** and amine **30**, respectively. These intermediates were then subjected to HATU/HOAt/DIPEA/DMF conditions, forming the cyclization precursor **31** with an overall yield of 44% over two steps. Notably, using DEPBT(3-(Diethoxyphosphoryloxy)-1,2,3- benzotriazin-4(3H)-one)/DIPEA/THF conditions [33,34] improved the yield to 53%. Subsequent deprotection of the allyl group using $Pd(PPh_3)_4$/NMA(*N*-methylaniline)/THF provided carboxylic acid **32**. Treatment with TFA removed the Boc and TBS protecting groups. Finally, macrocyclization under HATU/HOAt/2,4,6-collidine/DMF conditions yielded compound **1** with an overall yield of 67% over three steps, completing the synthesis of lagunamide D. Acyl migration between lagunamides D and D′ has been reported in common HPLC solvents like methanol and acetonitrile, complicating purification. Fortunately, no such structural transformations were observed during our synthesis. In our synthetic procedure, DMF was utilized in the macrolactamization, while purification was carried out using an ethyl acetate/petroleum ether system, with the exclusion of methanol at every stage. This stability of lagunamide D during these processes may be attributed to the different conformations of the substrate in various solvents, as proposed by Kimura and Oishi in their investigations on the acyl migration of kulokekahilide-2 [35] and odoamide [36], respectively. The ^{1}H and ^{13}C NMR spectra of synthetic lagunamide D matched those of the natural product (see Figure S1 and Table S1 in the Supporting Information). Additionally, the optical rotation was measured at $[\alpha]_D^{20.0} = -57.1$ (*c* 0.07, MeOH), which, while slightly higher than the reported value of $[\alpha]_D^{20.0} = -34.7$ (*c* 0.05, MeOH) [10], confirmed the absolute stereochemistry of lagunamide D, as shown in Figure 1.

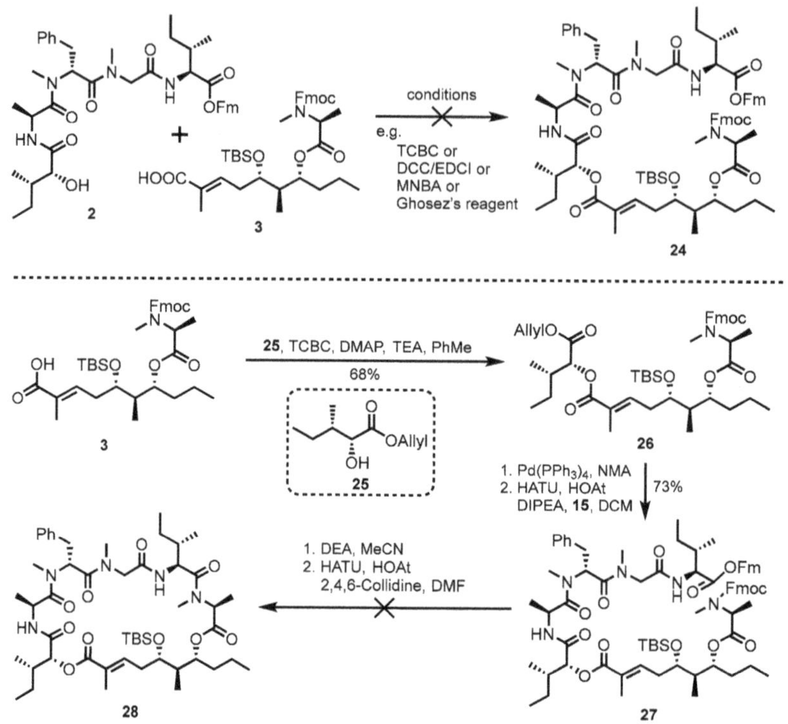

Scheme 4. Initial attempts towards the total synthesis of lagunamide D (**1**).

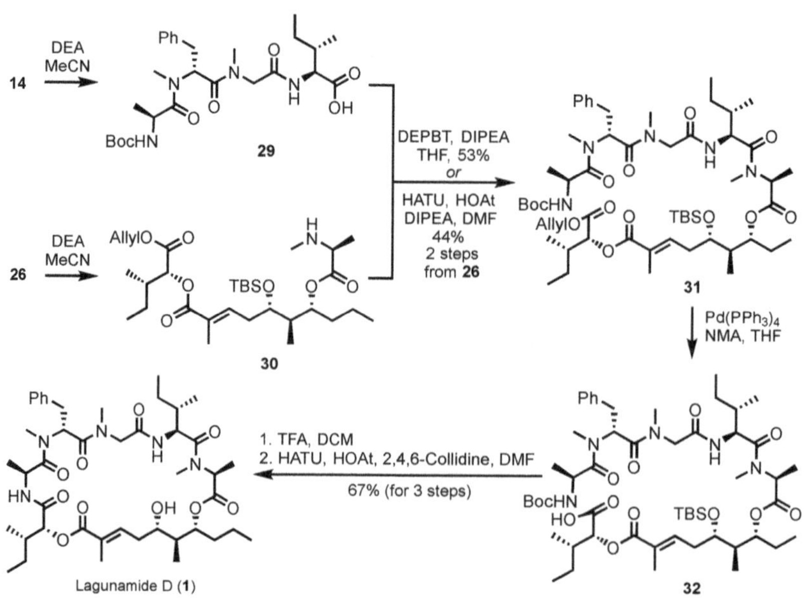

Scheme 5. Completion of the total synthesis of lagunamide D (**1**).

3. Materials and Methods

3.1. General Experiment

All reactions were conducted in flame-dried or oven-dried glassware under an atmosphere of dry nitrogen or argon. Oxygen- and/or moisture-sensitive solids and liquids were transferred appropriately. The concentration of solutions in vacuo was accomplished using a rotary evaporator fitted with a diaphragm vacuum pump. Residual solvents were removed under an oil vacuum pump (0.1–0.2 mm Hg). All reaction solvents were purified before use: Tetrahydrofuran (THF) was distilled from Na/benzophenone. Toluene was distilled over molten sodium metal. Dichloromethane (DCM), 1,2-dichloroethane (DCE), *N,N*-dimethylformamide (DMF), acetonitrile (MeCN), *N,N*-diisopropylethylamine (DIPEA), 2,4,6-collidine, and trimethylamine (Et_3N) were distilled from CaH_2. The reagents were purchased at the highest commercial quality and used without further purification unless otherwise stated. Flash column chromatography was performed using the indicated solvents on silica gel (100–200 mesh, Xinnuo, Yantai, China). Reactions were monitored using thin-layer chromatography (TLC), which was carried out using pre-coated sheets (Xinnuo silica gel coated with fluorescent indicator F254, 0.25 mm). Compounds were visualized with UV light, iodine, and ceric ammonium molybdate stainer phosphomolybdic acid in EtOH. The ^1H NMR spectra were recorded on 500 MHz or 600 MHz spectrometers (Bruker Avance, Karlsruhe, Germany). Chemical shifts are reported in parts per million (ppm), relative to either a tetramethylsilane (TMS) internal standard or the signals of the deuterated solvent. The following abbreviations are used to describe the spin multiplicity: s = singlet, d = doublet, t = triplet, q = quartet, m = multiplet, br = broad, dd = doublet of doublets, dt = doublet of triplets, dq = doublet of quartets, ddd = doublet of doublet of doublets; other combinations are derived from those listed above. Coupling constants (J) are reported in hertz (Hz) for the corresponding solutions, and chemical shifts are reported as parts per million (ppm) relative to residual $CHCl_3$ δH (7.26 ppm). ^{13}C-NMR nuclear magnetic resonance spectra were recorded at 126 MHz or 151 MHz for the corresponding solutions, and chemical shifts are reported as parts per million (ppm) relative to residual $CDCl_3$ δC (77.16 ppm). All high-resolution mass spectra (HRMS) were obtained by Thermo Scientific's UltiMate 3000 Series liquid system (Germering, Bavaria, Germany) and Thermo Scientific's Q-Exactive combined quadrupole Orbitrap mass spectrometer (Germering, Bavaria, Germany). Optical rotations were recorded on a Rudolph AutoPol-I polarimeter (Shanghai, China) at 589 nm with a 50 mm cell. Data are reported as follows: specific rotation (c (g/100 mL), solvent).

3.2. Synthesis of Dipeptide **10**

To a solution of Boc-*N*-Me-D-Phe-OH (1.00 g, 3.6 mmol) and *N*-Me-Gly-OMe·HCl (0.65 g, 4.7 mmol) in anhydrous DMF (5.0 mL), HOAt (0.10 g, 0.72 mmol), DIPEA (3.1 mL, 17.9 mmol), and HATU (2.72 g, 7.2 mmol) were added at room temperature, and the mixture was stirred overnight. The reaction mixture was quenched with saturated NH_4Cl (aq.), and the aqueous phase was extracted with ethyl acetate (20.0 mL × 3). The combined organic layers were then washed with water and brine, dried over anhydrous Na_2SO_4, filtered, and concentrated. The resulting residue was purified by flash chromatography on silica gel (PE(petroleum ether)/EA(Ethyl acetate) = 2:1), yielding dipeptide **10** (1.20 g, 93%) as a colorless oil. $[\alpha]_D^{25.0}$ = +110.7 (*c* 0.7, MeOH); ^1H NMR (500 MHz, $CDCl_3$) exists as rotational conformers: δ 7.31–7.11 (m, 5H), 5.33 (dd, *J* = 8.4, 6.7 Hz, 0.33H), 5.21 (dd, *J* = 9.1, 6.0 Hz, 0.17H), 5.02 (dd, *J* = 9.6, 5.1 Hz, 0.33H), 4.85 (dd, *J* = 9.2, 5.3 Hz, 0.17H), 4.39–4.14 (m, 1H), 4.04–3.90 (m, 0.67H), 3.78 (d, *J* = 17.2 Hz, 0.33H), 3.72 (s, 1H), 3.71 (s, 1H), 3.68 (s, 0.5H), 3.67 (s, 0.5H), 3.14 (dd, *J* = 13.9, 6.7 Hz, 0.5H), 3.07 (dd, *J* = 22.3, 5.7 Hz, 0.5H), 3.04–2.98 (m, 3H), 2.98–2.90 (m, 1H), 2.84 (s, 1H), 2.81 (s, 1H), 2.73 (s, 0.5H), 2.70 (s, 0.5H), 1.31 (s, 3H),

1.25 (s, 1.5H), 1.17 (s, 3H), 1.12 (s, 1.5H); ^{13}C NMR (126 MHz, $CDCl_3$) exists as rotational conformers: δ 170.9, 170.6, 170.5, 170.1, 169.5, 169.5, 169.4, 169.1, 155.2, 155.2, 154.3, 153.9, 138.1, 138.0, 137.6, 137.5, 129.5, 129.5, 129.5, 128.4, 128.4, 128.2, 126.4, 126.3, 80.4, 80.1, 80.1, 80.0, 58.1, 57.9, 55.8, 55.6, 52.3, 52.2, 52.1, 52.1, 50.7, 50.5, 50.0, 49.9, 36.0, 35.8, 35.1, 35.1, 29.6, 28.9, 28.9, 28.2, 28.1, 27.9, 27.7; HRMS (ESI-TOF) *m/z*: $C_{19}H_{28}N_2NaO_5^+$ [M + Na]$^+$: calcd: 387.1890; found: 387.1896.

3.3. *Synthesis of Tripeptide* **12**

Dipeptide **10** (2.97 g, 8.2 mmol) was dissolved in a mixture of THF-MeOH-H_2O (10.0 mL/10.0 mL/5.0 mL), and LiOH (1 M in H_2O, 16.5 mL, 16.5 mmol) was added at room temperature. The mixture was stirred for 2 h and then acidified to pH = 5 with 1 M HCl (aq.). The aqueous phase was extracted with ethyl acetate (30.0 mL × 3), and the combined organic phase was washed with brine, dried over anhydrous Na_2SO_4, filtered, and concentrated to yield the crude acid, which was not further purified. To a solution of the residue acid and amine **11** (3.62 g, 7.5 mmol) in anhydrous DMF (25.0 mL), HOAt (1.03 g, 7.5 mmol), DIPEA (9.2 mL, 52.7 mmol), and HATU (35.7 g, 15.1 mmol) were added at room temperature, and the mixture was stirred overnight. The reaction mixture was quenched with saturated NH_4Cl (aq.) and extracted with ethyl acetate (30.0 mL × 3). The combined organic layers were washed with saturated NH_4Cl (aq.) and brine, dried over anhydrous Na_2SO_4, filtered, and concentrated. The resulting residue was purified by flash chromatography on silica gel (PE/EA = 2:1), yielding tripeptide **12** (3.60 g, 68%) as a colorless oil. $[\alpha]_D^{20.0}$ = +35.8 (*c* 1.5, MeOH); ^{1}H NMR (500 MHz, $CDCl_3$) exists as rotational conformers: δ 7.85–7.74 (m, 2H), 7.66–7.55 (m, 2H), 7.46–7.38 (m, 2H), 7.38–7.31 (m, 2H), 7.30–7.14 (m, 5H), 6.82 (d, *J* = 8.1 Hz, 0.15H), 6.63 (d, *J* = 8.6 Hz, 0.3H), 6.56 (d, *J* = 8.6 Hz, 0.45H), 6.21 (d, *J* = 8.6 Hz, 0.1H), 5.37 (t, *J* = 7.6 Hz, 0.45H), 5.15 (t, *J* = 7.7 Hz, 0.15H), 5.06 (dd, *J* = 9.2, 5.4 Hz, 0.3H), 5.00 (dd, *J* = 10.4, 4.2 Hz, 0.1H), 4.64–4.51 (m, 3H), 4.28–4.17 (m, 1.5H), 4.09–3.95 (m, 0.8H), 3.95–3.80 (m, 0.3H), 3.75 (d, *J* = 15.3 Hz, 0.4H), 3.17 (dd, *J* = 14.0, 7.1 Hz, 0.45H), 3.12–3.06 (m, 0.45H), 3.07 (s, 1H), 3.06–3.02 (m, 1.55H), 3.02–2.93 (m, 1.55H), 2.89–2.81 (m, 3H), 1.88–1.75 (m, 1H), 1.42–1.32 (m, 1H), 1.35 (s, 3H), 1.31–1.26 (m, 1H), 1.25–1.13 (m, 1H), 1.20 (s, 3H), 1.11 (s, 1H), 1.03–0.91 (m, 1H), 0.88–0.75 (m, 6H); ^{13}C NMR (126 MHz, $CDCl_3$) exists as rotational conformers: δ 171.6, 171.5, 171.5, 171.2, 168.5, 168.3, 155.4, 154.3, 143.6, 143.4, 143.4, 141.4, 141.4, 137.9, 137.4, 129.5, 129.4, 128.5, 128.3, 128.3, 127.9, 127.2, 126.5, 126.5, 124.9, 124.8, 120.1, 80.3, 80.1, 66.7, 66.6, 57.8, 56.5, 56.5, 55.6, 53.5, 52.7, 52.5, 46.8, 37.6, 37.5, 36.4, 36.1, 35.3, 29.7, 29.1, 28.2, 28.1, 28.0, 27.7, 24.9, 24.9, 24.8, 15.3, 15.3, 11.6; HRMS (ESI-TOF) *m/z*: $C_{38}H_{48}N_3O_6^+$ [M + H]$^+$: calcd: 642.3538; found: 642.3542.

3.4. *Synthesis of Tetrapeptide* **14**

To a solution of tripeptide **12** (3.58 g, 5.6 mmol) in anhydrous CH_2Cl_2 (25.0 mL), TFA (5.0 mL) was added at room temperature. The mixture was stirred for 0.5 h and then concentrated under reduced pressure to yield the crude amine, which was not further purified. To a solution of the obtained amine and acid **13** in anhydrous DMF (25.0 mL), HOAt (0.68 g, 5.0 mmol), DIPEA (6.1 mL, 34.9 mmol), and HATU (3.79 g, 10.0 mmol) were added, and the mixture was stirred at room temperature overnight. The reaction mixture was quenched with saturated NH_4Cl (aq.), and the aqueous phase was extracted with ethyl acetate (50.0 mL × 3). The combined organic layers were then washed with saturated NH_4Cl (aq.), water, and brine, dried over anhydrous Na_2SO_4, filtered, and concentrated. The resulting residue was purified by flash chromatography on silica gel (PE/EA = 3:2), yielding tetrapeptide **14** (2.40 g, 61%) as a colorless oil. $[\alpha]_D^{25.0}$ = +7.7 (*c* 1.0, MeOH); ^{1}H NMR (500 MHz, $CDCl_3$) exists as rotational conformers: δ 7.85–7.75 (m, 2H), 7.65–7.58

(m, 2H), 7.45–7.38 (m, 2H), 7.33 (q, J = 7.8 Hz, 2H), 7.30–7.12 (m, 5H), 6.83 (d, J = 8.3 Hz, 0.3H), 6.64 (d, J = 8.7 Hz, 0.7H), 5.78 (dd, J = 9.2, 6.7 Hz, 0.7H), 5.62 (dd, J = 9.8, 6.2 Hz, 0.3H), 5.38 (d, J = 8.2 Hz, 0.7H), 5.30 (d, J = 7.8 Hz, 0.3H), 4.67–4.50 (m, 3H), 4.49–4.36 (m, 1H), 4.22 (t, J = 6.1 Hz, 1H), 4.17 (d, J = 17.0 Hz, 0.3H), 4.13 (d, J = 15.5 Hz, 0.7H), 3.87 (d, J = 15.5 Hz, 0.7H), 3.72 (d, J = 17.0 Hz, 0.3H), 3.23–3.14 (m, 1H), 3.14–3.06 (m, 1H), 3.04 (s, 3H), 3.00 (s, 3H), 1.90–1.77 (m, 1H), 1.44–1.34 (m, 9H), 1.22–1.13 (m, 1H), 1.04–0.95 (m, 1H), 0.88 (d, J = 6.8 Hz, 3H), 0.85–0.75 (m, 6H); ^{13}C NMR (126 MHz, $CDCl_3$) exists as rotational conformers: δ 173.9, 173.3, 171.7, 171.5, 171.1, 170.2, 168.2, 155.3, 143.5, 143.3, 141.4, 141.3, 136.4, 129.3, 129.2, 128.4, 127.9, 127.9, 127.2, 127.2, 126.8, 124.9, 124.8, 120.1, 79.6, 79.5, 66.7, 66.7, 56.7, 56.4, 53.9, 53.4, 52.5, 52.4, 46.8, 46.8, 46.6, 37.6, 37.6, 36.6, 35.5, 35.4, 35.2, 30.4, 29.7, 28.3, 28.3, 25.0, 24.8, 17.7, 17.5, 15.3, 15.3, 11.7, 11.6; HRMS (ESI-TOF) m/z: $C_{41}H_{52}N_4NaO_7^+$ $[M + Na]^+$: calcd: 735.3728; found: 735.3726.

3.5. Synthesis of Pentapeptide 2

To a solution of tripeptide **14** (2.45 g, 3.4 mmol) in anhydrous CH_2Cl_2 (15.0 mL), TFA (5.0 mL) was added at room temperature. The mixture was stirred for 30 min and then concentrated under reduced pressure to yield the crude amine, which was not further purified. To a solution of the obtained amine and compound **16** in anhydrous DMF (15.0 mL), HOAt (0.46 g, 3.4 mmol), DIPEA (4.1 mL, 23.7 mmol), and HATU (2.57 g, 6.8 mmol) were added, and the mixture was stirred at room temperature overnight. The reaction mixture was quenched with saturated NH_4Cl (aq.), and the aqueous phase was extracted with ethyl acetate (50.0 mL × 3). The combined organic layers were then washed with saturated NH_4Cl (aq.), water, and brine, dried over anhydrous Na_2SO_4, filtered, and concentrated. The resulting residue was purified by flash chromatography on silica gel (PE/EA = 1:5), yielding tetrapeptide **2** (1.58 g, 63%) as a colorless oil. $[\alpha]_D^{25.0}$ = +12.9 (c 0.9, MeOH); ^{1}H NMR (500 MHz, $CDCl_3$) exists as rotational conformers: δ 7.86–7.72 (m, 2H), 7.65–7.54 (m, 2H), 7.47–7.38 (m, 2H), 7.37–7.30 (m, 2H), 7.30–7.05 (m, 6H), 6.87 (d, J = 8.5 Hz, 0.3H), 6.63 (d, J = 8.7 Hz, 0.7H), 5.74 (t, J = 7.9 Hz, 0.7H), 5.61 (t, J = 8.0 Hz, 0.3H), 4.82 (q, J = 7.0 Hz, 0.7H), 4.72 (t, J = 7.0 Hz, 0.3H), 4.65–4.48 (m, 3H), 4.22 (t, J = 6.2 Hz, 1H), 4.20–4.09 (m, 1H), 4.09–4.02 (m, 1H), 3.88–3.76 (m, 1H), 3.23–3.13 (m, 1.3H), 3.12–3.02 (m, 4H), 3.01–2.92 (m, 3.7H), 1.91–1.74 (m, 2H), 1.53–1.42 (m, 1H), 1.35–1.24 (m, 1H), 1.24–1.13 (m, 1H), 1.09–0.96 (m, 1H), 0.96–0.88 (m, 6H), 0.88–0.71 (m, 9H); ^{13}C NMR (126 MHz, $CDCl_3$) δ exists as rotational conformers: 173.2, 173.1, 172.8, 171.8, 171.7, 170.9, 170.2, 168.1, 168.0, 143.5, 143.3, 141.4, 141.3, 136.3, 129.3, 129.1, 128.5, 127.9, 127.9, 127.2, 127.2, 126.9, 124.9, 124.8, 120.1, 73.9, 73.9, 66.8, 56.7, 56.4, 54.0, 53.4, 52.5, 52.3, 46.7, 45.5, 45.2, 38.6, 37.8, 37.6, 36.5, 35.4, 35.1, 30.6, 30.5, 29.7, 26.2, 25.0, 24.9, 17.6, 17.4, 15.3, 12.7, 12.6, 11.9, 11.7, 11.6; HRMS (ESI-TOF) m/z: $C_{42}H_{54}N_4NaO_7^+$ ccc$^+$: calcd: 749.3885; found: 749.3895.

3.6. Synthesis of Ketone 18

To a stirred solution of compound **17** (2.32 g, 4.4 mmol) and *N*,*O*-dimethylhydroxylamine hydrochloride (3.03 g, 31.1 mmol) in anhydrous THF (15.0 mL), *i*-PrMgCl (26.6 mL, 53.3 mmol) was added dropwise at −30 °C. After stirring for 1 h, the reaction mixture was warmed to −20 °C. After stirring for 1 h, the reaction mixture was warmed to 0 °C. After stirring for an additional hour, the reaction mixture was quenched with saturated NH_4Cl (aq.), and the aqueous phase was extracted with ethyl acetate (50.0 mL × 3). The combined organic layers were then washed with saturated NH_4Cl (aq.) and brine, dried over anhydrous Na_2SO_4, filtered, and concentrated. The resulting residue was purified by flash chromatography on silica gel (PE/EA = 4:1), yielding Weinreb amide **S1** (0.95 g, 78%) as a colorless oil. $[\alpha]_D^{25.0}$ = −8.0 (c 1.0, MeOH); ^{1}H NMR (500 MHz, $CDCl_3$) δ 7.43–7.25 (m, 5H), 4.54 (s, 2H), 3.75 (ddd, J = 8.7, 6.8, 3.1 Hz, 1H), 3.65 (s, 3H), 3.29–3.17 (m, 1H), 3.22 (s, 3H), 1.69–1.58 (m, 1H), 1.58–1.40 (m, 3H),

1.10 (d, J = 6.9 Hz, 3H), 0.95 (t, J = 7.1 Hz, 3H); ^{13}C NMR (126 MHz, $CDCl_3$) δ 176.4, 139.0, 128.2, 127.8, 127.3, 81.0, 72.8, 61.4, 39.1, 33.5, 32.0, 18.0, 14.4, 13.5; HRMS (ESI-TOF) m/z: $C_{16}H_{25}NNaO_3^+$ [M + Na]$^+$: calcd: 302.1727; found: 302.1737.

To a stirred solution of compound **S1** (1.50 g, 5.4 mmol) in anhydrous THF (20.0 mL), allylmagnesium bromide (13.6 mL, 13.6 mmol, 1.0 M in THF) was added at 0 °C, and the mixture was stirred for 0.5 h at room temperature. The reaction mixture was quenched with saturated NH_4Cl (aq.), and the aqueous phase was extracted with ethyl acetate (30.0 mL × 3). The combined organic layers were then washed with saturated NH_4Cl (aq.) and brine, dried over anhydrous Na_2SO_4, filtered, and concentrated. The resulting residue was purified by flash chromatography on silica gel (PE/EA = 30:1), yielding ketone **18** (1.23 g, 86%) as a colorless oil. $[\alpha]_D^{25.0} = -57.8$ (c 0.9, MeOH); ^{1}H NMR (500 MHz, $CDCl_3$) δ 7.40–7.27 (m, 5H), 5.95 (ddt, J = 17.1, 10.2, 6.9 Hz, 1H), 5.19 (dd, J = 10.2, 1.5 Hz, 1H), 5.10 (dd, J = 17.2, 1.6 Hz, 1H), 4.52 (d, J = 11.1 Hz, 1H), 4.43 (d, J = 11.0 Hz, 1H), 3.71 (ddd, J = 8.2, 6.0, 3.6 Hz, 1H), 3.28 (dd, J = 6.9, 1.7 Hz, 2H), 2.93 (dq, J = 8.3, 7.0 Hz, 1H), 1.58–1.39 (m, 4H), 1.05 (d, J = 7.0 Hz, 3H), 0.95 (t, J = 7.0 Hz, 3H); ^{13}C NMR (126 MHz, $CDCl_3$) δ 211.8, 138.4, 130.7, 128.3, 127.9, 127.6, 118.6, 81.0, 72.3, 49.0, 48.3, 33.1, 17.7, 14.3, 12.6; HRMS (ESI-TOF) m/z: $C_{17}H_{24}NaO_2^+$ [M + Na]$^+$: calcd: 283.1669; found: 283.1677.

3.7. Synthesis of Compound 20

To a solution of ketone **18** (0.40 g, 1.5 mmol) in anhydrous THF (20.0 mL), (R)-Me-CBS (2.3 mL, 2.3 mmol, 1.0 M in THF) was added under an argon atmosphere, and the mixture was stirred for 10 min at room temperature. After cooling the reaction mixture to −78 °C, $BH_3{\cdot}Me_2S$ (0.20 mL, 2.0 mmol, 10.0 M in THF) was added, and the mixture was stirred for 3 h. The reaction mixture was then warmed to −20 °C and stirred for 0.5 h. The reaction mixture was quenched with MeOH (0.10 mL) and saturated NH_4Cl (aq.) (5.0 mL) at 0 °C, and the aqueous phase was extracted with ethyl acetate (20.0 mL × 3). The combined organic layers were then washed with saturated NH_4Cl (aq.) and brine, dried over anhydrous Na_2SO_4, filtered, and concentrated. The resulting residue was purified by flash chromatography on silica gel (PE/EA = 30:1), yielding alcohol **S2** (0.40 g, 89%) as a colorless oil. $[\alpha]_D^{25.0}$ = +4.1 (c 1.0, MeOH); ^{1}H NMR (500 MHz, $CDCl_3$) δ 7.42–7.28 (m, 5H), 6.00–5.86 (m, 1H), 5.25–5.12 (m, 2H), 4.62–4.46 (m, 2H), 3.68–3.57 (m, 2H), 2.49–2.38 (m, 1H), 2.22–2.08 (m, 1H), 2.00–1.89 (m, 1H), 1.68–1.57 (m, 1H), 1.57–1.49 (m, 2H), 1.48–1.40 (m, 1H), 0.95 (t, J = 7.2 Hz, 3H), 0.88 (d, J = 7.0 Hz, 3H); ^{13}C NMR (126 MHz, $CDCl_3$) δ 138.5, 135.2, 128.4, 127.9, 127.6, 117.8, 82.2, 73.17, 7.35, 4.55, 39.2, 32.3 18.0, 14.4, 11.9; HRMS (ESI-TOF) m/z: $C_{17}H_{26}NaO_2^+$ [M + Na]$^+$: calcd: 285.1825; found: 285.1832.

To a solution of alcohol **S2** (2.22 g, 8.5 mmol) in anhydrous CH_2Cl_2 (20.0 mL), Et_3N (4.7 mL, 33.8 mmol) and TBSOTf (3.9 mL, 16.9 mmol) were added at room temperature under an argon atmosphere, and the mixture was stirred for 1 h. The reaction mixture was quenched with saturated NH_4Cl (aq.), and the aqueous phase was extracted with ethyl acetate (30.0 mL × 3). The combined organic layers were then washed with saturated NH_4Cl (aq.) and brine, dried over anhydrous Na_2SO_4, filtered, and concentrated under reduced pressure. The resulting residue was purified by flash chromatography on silica gel (PE/EA = 30:1), yielding compound **20** (2.80 g, 89%) as a colorless oil. $[\alpha]_D^{25.0}$ = +4.5 (c 0.9, MeOH); ^{1}H NMR (500 MHz, $CDCl_3$) δ 7.45–7.24 (m, 5H), 5.95–5.83 (m, 1H), 5.11–5.01 (m, 2H), 4.56–4.44 (m, 2H), 3.82 (td, J = 6.1, 4.5 Hz, 1H), 3.53 (ddd, J = 8.6, 5.7, 3.2 Hz, 1H), 2.39–2.26 (m, 1H), 2.26–2.18 (m, 1H), 2.11–1.99 (m, 1H), 1.63–1.54 (m, 1H), 1.54–1.42 (m, 2H), 1.42–1.28 (m, 1H), 0.94 (t, J = 6.9 Hz, 3H), 0.92 (s, 9H), 0.86 (d, J = 7.0 Hz, 3H), 0.08 (s, 3H), 0.05 (s, 3H); ^{13}C NMR (126 MHz, $CDCl_3$) δ 139.2, 135.4, 128.3, 127.8, 127.3, 116.7, 79.8, 72.8, 71.0, 40.2, 38.1, 32.3, 25.9, 18.9, 18.1, 14.5, 10.1, −4.0, −4.7; HRMS (ESI-TOF) m/z: $C_{23}H_{40}NaO_2Si^+$ [M + Na]$^+$: calcd: 399.2690; found: 399.2699.

3.8. Synthesis of Alcohol 4

To a solution of compound **20** (1.62 g, 4.3 mmol) in wet DCE (25.0 mL, analytically pure), 2,3-dichloro-5,6-dicyano-1,4-benzoquinone (3.89 g, 17.2 mmol) was added at 50 °C, and the mixture was stirred for 1 h. The reaction mixture was cooled to room temperature and quenched with saturated $Na_2S_2O_3$ (aq.) (20.0 mL), after which the aqueous phase was extracted with DCM (50.0 mL × 3). The combined organic layers were washed with 1 M NaOH (aq.)-saturated $Na_2S_2O_3$ (aq.) (V_{NaOH}: $V_{Na2S2O3}$ = 1:1) and brine, dried over anhydrous Na_2SO_4, filtered, and concentrated under reduced pressure. The resulting residue was purified by flash chromatography on silica gel (PE/EA = 20:1), yielding alcohol **4** (0.85 g, 69%) as a colorless oil. $[\alpha]_D^{25.0}$ = +3.3 (*c* 1.2, MeOH); ^{1}H NMR (500 MHz, $CDCl_3$) δ 5.94–5.82 (m, 1H), 5.18–4.99 (m, 2H), 3.80 (q, *J* = 5.4 Hz, 1H), 3.61–3.54 (m, 1H), 2.74 (s, 1H), 2.41–2.33 (m, 1H), 2.32–2.23 (m, 1H), 1.76–1.68 (m, 1H), 1.58–1.49 (m, 2H), 1.43–1.33 (m, 2H), 0.95 (t, *J* = 6.6 Hz, 3H), 0.93 (s, 9H), 0.84 (d, *J* = 7.0 Hz, 3H), 0.11 (s, 6H); ^{13}C NMR (126 MHz, $CDCl_3$) δ 135.0, 117.1, 75.9, 73.8, 43.1, 39.3, 36.5, 25.9, 18.6, 18.0, 14.2, 12.8, −4.2, −4.7; HRMS (ESI-TOF) *m/z*: $C_{16}H_{34}NaO_2Si^+$ [M + Na]$^+$: calcd: 309.2220; found: 309.2226.

3.9. Synthesis of Acetonide 21

To a solution of compound **4** (53.0 mg, 0.18 mmol) in anhydrous THF (3.0 mL), TBAF (0.4 mL, 0.4 mmol) was added at room temperature under an argon atmosphere, and the mixture was stirred for 30 min. The reaction mixture was concentrated under reduced pressure. The resulting residue was purified by flash chromatography on silica gel (PE/EA = 1:1), yielding diol **S4** as a colorless oil.

To a solution of the diol **S4** obtained above in anhydrous CH_2Cl_2 (1.0 mL), 2,2-dimethoxypropane (3.0 mL, 25.1 mmol) and PTSA (2.0 mg, 11.6 mmol) were added at room temperature under an argon atmosphere, and the mixture was stirred for 5 min. The reaction mixture was quenched with saturated Et_3N (0.5 mL, 3.6 mmol), and the solvent was concentrated under reduced pressure. The resulting residue was purified by flash chromatography on silica gel (PE/EA = 50:1), yielding acetonide **21** (36.7 mg, 93%) as a colorless oil. $[\alpha]_D^{20.0}$ = +14.7 (*c* 0.8, MeOH); ^{1}H NMR (500 MHz, $CDCl_3$) δ 5.93 (ddt, *J* = 17.2, 10.3, 6.8 Hz, 1H), 5.11–5.02 (m, 2H), 3.54 (ddd, *J* = 10.2, 7.0, 3.1 Hz, 1H), 3.46 (ddd, *J* = 10.3, 8.0, 2.4 Hz, 1H), 2.39 (dddd, *J* = 12.8, 6.5, 3.2, 1.6 Hz, 1H), 2.20 (dt, *J* = 14.6, 7.1 Hz, 1H), 1.60–1.48 (m, 2H), 1.43 (s, 3H), 1.39 (s, 3H), 1.37–1.29 (m, 3H), 0.91 (t, *J* = 7.0 Hz, 3H), 0.79 (d, *J* = 6.6 Hz, 3H); ^{13}C NMR (126 MHz, $CDCl_3$) δ 135.2, 116.2, 97.8, 74.1, 73.7, 37.7, 37.5, 35.2, 30.2, 19.6, 18.2, 14.0, 12.2.

3.10. Synthesis of Ester 22

To a solution of Fmoc-*N*-Me-L-Ala-OH (3.17 g, 9.8 mmol) in anhydrous CH_2Cl_2 (15.0 mL) at 0 °C, oxalyl chloride (2.8 mL, 32.5 mmol) and catalytic DMF (32 μL, 0.41 mmol) were added, and the mixture was warmed to room temperature. The reaction mixture was stirred for 1 h and then concentrated under reduced pressure to yield the crude acyl chloride, which was used directly in the subsequent step. To a solution of alcohol **4** (932 mg, 3.3 mmol) and DMAP (0.99 g, 8.1 mmol) in anhydrous CH_2Cl_2 (15.0 mL), Et_3N (4.5 mL, 32.5 mmol) was added at room temperature under an argon atmosphere. The reaction mixture was cooled to 0 °C, and a solution of the crude acyl chloride obtained above in anhydrous CH_2Cl_2 (15.0 mL) was added. The mixture was then warmed to room temperature and stirred for 1 h. The reaction was quenched with methanol (1.0 mL) and saturated NH_4Cl (aq.) (5.0 mL), and the aqueous phase was extracted with ethyl acetate (30.0 mL × 3). The combined organic layers were washed with 1 M HCl (aq.), saturated NH_4Cl (aq.), and brine and then dried over anhydrous Na_2SO_4, filtered, and concentrated. The resulting residue was purified by flash chromatography on silica gel (PE/EA

= 20:1), yielding ester **22** (1.26 g, 66%) as a colorless oil. $[\alpha]_D^{20.0}$ = −6.0 (*c* 0.7, MeOH); ^{1}H NMR (500 MHz, $CDCl_3$) exists as rotational conformers: δ 7.85–7.77 (m, 2H), 7.70–7.57 (m, 2H), 7.46–7.37 (m, 2H), 7.37–7.30 (m, 2H), 5.91–5.78 (m, 1H), 5.20–4.97 (m, 3H), 4.97–4.91 (m, 0.7H), 4.85–4.79 (m, 0.3H), 4.49–4.35 (m, 2H), 4.33–4.23 (m, 1H), 3.72–3.63 (m, 1H), 2.97–2.91 (m, 3H), 2.34–2.24 (m, 1H), 2.22–2.13 (m, 1H), 1.99–1.90 (m, 1H), 1.64–1.48 (m, 2H), 1.45 (d, *J* = 7.3 Hz, 3H), 1.40–1.20 (m, 2H), 1.00–0.82 (m, 15H), 0.12–0.01 (m, 6H); ^{13}C NMR (126 MHz, $CDCl_3$) exists as rotational conformers: δ 171.5, 171.3, 156.5, 155.9, 144.1, 144.9, 141.3, 135.4, 135.0, 127.7, 127.1, 125.1, 125.1, 120.0, 119.8, 116.9, 76.1, 76.0, 72.9, 67.9, 67.8, 54.2, 47.3, 41.6, 41.5, 37.9, 37.7, 32.8, 32.5, 30.4, 30.2, 25.9, 18.8, 18.7, 18.1, 15.4, 14.9, 14.1, 10.4, −4.1, −4.7; HRMS (ESI-TOF) *m*/*z*: $C_{35}H_{51}NNaO_5Si^+$ [M + Na]$^+$: calcd: 616.3429; found: 616.3436.

3.11. *Synthesis of Ester* **26**

In a sealed tube, α-methylacrolein (11.1 mL, 3.5 mmol) and Grubbs II catalyst (8.9 mg, 10.0 μmol) were added to a solution of ester **22** (1.22 g, 2.1 mmol) in anhydrous CH_2Cl_2 (10.0 mL) at room temperature. After purging with nitrogen gas for 30 min, the reaction mixture was warmed to 50 °C and stirred overnight. The mixture was then concentrated under reduced pressure. The resulting residue was purified by flash chromatography on silica gel (PE/EA = 10:1), yielding aldehyde **S3** (1.06 g, 81%) as a colorless oil. $[\alpha]_D^{25.0}$ = −21.3 (*c* 0.8, MeOH); ^{1}H NMR (500 MHz, $CDCl_3$) exists as rotational conformers: δ 9.38 (s, 0.73H), 9.35 (s, 0.27H), 7.87–7.74 (m, 2H), 7.68–7.55 (m, 2H), 7.52–7.41 (m, 2H), 7.41–7.30 (m, 2H), 6.67–6.48 (m, 1H), 5.14–5.00 (m, 1H), 4.94–4.81 (m, 1H), 4.52–4.33 (m, 2H), 4.33–4.20 (m, 1H), 3.95–3.79 (m, 1H), 2.96 (s, 2.2H), 2.92 (s, 0.8H), 2.59–2.42 (m, 2H), 2.02–1.93 (m, 1H), 1.74 (s, 3H), 1.65–1.51 (m, 2H), 1.49–1.42 (m, 3H), 1.41–1.22 (m, 2H), 0.99–0.84 (m, 15H), 0.13–−0.02 (m, 6H); ^{13}C NMR (126 MHz, $CDCl_3$) δ exists as rotational conformers: 195.3, 195.0, 171.9, 156.5, 152.0, 151.0, 144.0, 143.9, 141.3, 140.3, 127.7, 127.1, 127.1, 125.0, 120.0, 120.0, 76.0, 75.8, 71.6, 71.4, 68.0, 67.8, 54.2, 47.2, 42.6, 42.3, 33.4, 32.2, 30.2, 25.8, 18.6, 18.5, 18.0, 15.3, 14.9, 14.2, 14.1, 10.3, 10.2, 9.4. −4.4, −4.7; HRMS (ESI-TOF) *m*/*z*: $C_{37}H_{53}NNaO_6Si^+$ [M + Na]$^+$: calcd: 658.3534; found: 658.3541.

To a stirred solution of aldehyde **S3** (1.05 g, 1.7 mmol) and 2-methyl-2-butene (16 mL) in *t*-BuOH/pH = 7 phosphate buffer (2:1, 24.0 mL), $NaClO_2$ (4.33 g, 49.5 mmol) and NaH_2PO_4 (9.53 g, 61.1 mmol) were added at room temperature, and the mixture was stirred for 1 h. The reaction mixture was acidified to pH = 3 with 1 M HCl (aq.), and the aqueous phase was then extracted with ethyl acetate (30.0 mL × 3). The combined organic layers were washed with saturated NH_4Cl (aq.) and brine, dried over anhydrous Na_2SO_4, filtered, and concentrated. The resulting residue was purified by flash chromatography on silica gel (PE/EA = 1:1), yielding acid **3** (1.05 g, 98%) as a colorless oil.

To a solution of acid **3** (353 mg, 0.58 mmol), alcohol **25** (300 mg, 1.70 mmol), and DMAP (0.35 g, 2.90 mmol) in anhydrous PhMe (10.0 mL) at −20 °C, 2,4,6-trichlorobenzoyl chloride (0.30 mL, 1.70 mmol) was added, and the mixture was stirred for 0.5 h. The reaction mixture was then warmed to room temperature and stirred overnight. The mixture was acidified to pH = 3 with 1 M HCl (aq.), and the organic phase was extracted with ethyl acetate (30.0 mL × 3). The combined organic layers were washed with 1 M HCl (aq.), saturated $NaHCO_3$ (aq.), and brine, dried over anhydrous Na_2SO_4, filtered, and concentrated. The resulting residue was purified by flash chromatography on silica gel (PE/EA = 1:3), yielding ester **26** (318 mg, 68%) as a colorless oil. $[\alpha]_D^{25.0}$ = −25.0 (c 0.8, MeOH); ^{1}H NMR (600 MHz, $CDCl_3$) exists as rotational conformers: δ 7.84–7.76 (m, 2H), 7.72–7.56 (m, 2H), 7.48–7.39 (m, 2H), 7.39–7.31 (m, 2H), 7.00–6.88 (m, 1H), 5.91 (ddt, J = 16.5, 10.9, 5.6 Hz, 1H), 5.33 (d, J = 17.4 Hz, 1H), 5.24 (d, J = 10.3 Hz, 1H), 5.08 (d, J = 3.5 Hz, 1H), 5.07–5.03 (m, 1H), 4.95–4.86 (m, 0.66H), 4.83–4.79 (m, 0.34H), 4.75–4.60 (m, 2H), 4.49–4.36 (m, 2H), 4.32–4.23 (m, 1H),

3.86–3.79 (m, 1H), 2.93 (s, 2H), 2.91 (s, 1H), 2.42–2.30 (m, 2H), 2.10–2.00 (m, 1H), 2.00–1.91 (m, 1H), 1.88 (s, 2.5H), 1.85 (s, 0.5H), 1.63–1.51 (m, 3H), 1.51–1.39 (m, 4H), 1.37–1.23 (m, 2H), 0.99 (d, J = 6.9 Hz, 3H), 0.98–0.81 (m, 18H), 0.10–0.00 (m, 6H);^{13}C NMR (151 MHz, $CDCl_3$) exists as rotational conformers: δ 171.6, 171.2, 169.9, 167.4, 156.4, 155.8, 144.1, 143.9, 141.3, 141.3, 140.6, 140.2, 131.8, 127.7, 127.1, 125.1, 125.1, 120.0, 118.5, 76.2, 76.0, 74.8, 71.7, 71.6, 67.9, 67.8, 65.5, 54.3, 54.1, 47.2, 42.5, 42.4, 36.8, 33.4, 33.1, 32.4, 32.3, 30.2, 29.7, 26.1, 25.8, 18.5, 17.9, 15.3, 14.9, 14.5, 14.1, 12.7, 11.7, 10.4. −4.3, −4.7; HRMS (ESI-TOF) m/z: $C_{46}H_{67}NNaO_9Si^+$ $[M + Na]^+$: calcd: 828.4477; found: 828.4487.

3.12. Synthesis of Compound **27**

To a solution of compound **26** (0.14 g, 0.17 mmol) and $Pd(PPh_3)_4$ (19.6 mg, 17 µmol) in anhydrous THF (2.0 mL), PhNHMe (37.7 µL, 0.34 mmol) was added. The resulting mixture was stirred at room temperature for 1 h. The reaction was quenched with TFA (75.6 µL, 1.02 mmol), diluted with ethyl acetate (30.0 mL), and washed sequentially with 1 M HCl (aq.) (3.0 mL × 2). The organic phase was washed with brine, dried over anhydrous Na_2SO_4, filtered, and concentrated to afford the crude acid, which was used in the next step without further purification. The crude acid was dissolved in anhydrous DMF (5.0 mL); HOAt (22.74 mg, 0.17 mmol), DIPEA (0.29 mL, 1.7 mmol), amine **15** (0.11 g, 0.15 mmol), and HATU (0.12 g, 0.34 mmol) were added at room temperature; and the mixture was stirred overnight. The reaction mixture was quenched with saturated NH_4Cl (aq.), and the aqueous phase was extracted with ethyl acetate (20.0 mL × 3). The combined organic layers were then washed with water and brine, dried over anhydrous Na_2SO_4, filtered, and concentrated. The resulting residue was purified by flash chromatography on silica gel (PE/EA = 1:1), yielding compound **27** (0.17 g, 73%) as a colorless oil. $[\alpha]_D^{20.0}$ = −12.9 (*c* 0.6, MeOH); ^{1}H NMR (600 MHz, Chloroform-*d*) exists as rotational conformers: δ 7.83–7.74 (m, 4H), 7.66–7.53 (m, 4H), 7.49–7.38 (m, 4H), 7.37–7.30 (m, 4H), 7.27–7.15 (m, 5H), 6.95–6.89 (m, 1H), 6.65 (d, *J* = 7.4 Hz, 1H), 6.52 (d, *J* = 8.6 Hz, 1H), 5.84 (dd, *J* = 9.5, 6.5 Hz, 0.7H), 5.76 (t, *J* = 8.2 Hz, 0.3H), 5.23–5.18 (m, 1H), 5.07–4.98 (m, 1H), 4.93–4.87 (m, 1H), 4.75–4.68 (m, 1H), 4.59–4.51 (m, 3H), 4.45–4.37 (m, 2H), 4.30–4.20 (m, 2H), 4.06–3.94 (m, 2H), 3.90–3.82 (m, 1H), 3.22–3.12 (m, 2H), 3.12–2.89 (m, 9H), 2.83 (s, 1H), 2.39–2.33 (m, 2H), 2.00–1.93 (m, 2H), 1.90–1.87 (m, 3H), 1.85–1.78 (m, 1H), 1.61–1.52 (m, 2H), 1.48–1.21 (m, 7H), 1.21–0.55 (m, 31H), 0.11–−0.02 (m, 6H); ^{13}C NMR (151 MHz, $CDCl_3$) exists as rotational conformers: 172.4, 171.7, 171.6, 170.8, 170.8, 169.5, 168.1, 166.7, 156.4, 144.1, 143.9, 143.6, 143.4, 141.4, 141.3, 136.5, 129.3, 128.3, 127.9, 127.9, 127.7, 127.2, 127.1, 124.8, 120.1, 76.1, 76.1, 75.9, 71.7, 67.8, 66.7, 56.6, 56.4, 56.3, 54.3, 54.1, 53.8, 53.7, 52.7, 52.2, 47.2, 46.8, 45.0, 42.6, 38.6, 37.8, 37.7, 37.6, 37.5, 36.7, 36.5, 35.2, 35.1, 33.4, 32.5, 31.9, 30.6, 30.4, 30.2, 29.7, 29.7, 29.4, 26.1, 25.8, 24.9, 18.5, 18.0, 17.3, 17.2, 15.3, 14.9, 14.1, 14.1, 13.9, 12.8, 11.7, 11.6, 11.5, 10.4, −4.2, −4.7. HRMS (ESI-TOF) *m*/*z*: $C_{79}H_{105}N_5NaO_{13}Si^+$ $[M + Na]^+$: calcd: 1382.7370; found: 1382.7390.

3.13. Synthesis of Compound **31**

To a solution of compound **14** (28 mg, 36 µmol) in anhydrous CH_3CN (2.0 mL), diethylamine (Et_2NH) (1.0 mL) was added, and the mixture was stirred for 2 h at room temperature. The reaction mixture was then concentrated under reduced pressure, and the residue was dissolved in ethyl acetate (50.0 mL) and washed with 1 M HCl (aq.) (3.0 mL × 2) and brine. The organic phase was then dried over anhydrous Na_2SO_4, filtered, and concentrated to afford crude **29**, which was used in the next step without further purification. To a solution of compound **26** (16 mg, 20 µmol) in anhydrous CH_3CN (2.0 mL), diethylamine (Et_2NH) (1.0 mL) was added, and the mixture was stirred for 2 h at room temperature. The mixture was then concentrated under reduced pressure to afford crude **30**, which was used in the next step without further purification. The above crude acid **29** and amine **30** were dissolved in anhydrous THF (3.0 mL), and DEPBT (13 mg, 45 μmol) and DIPEA (7.8 μL, 45 μmol) were added successively at room temperature. The mixture was then stirred overnight. The reaction mixture was quenched with saturated NH_4Cl (5.0 mL), and the organic phase was extracted with ethyl acetate (30.0 mL × 3). The combined organic layers were washed with brine, dried over anhydrous Na_2SO_4, filtered, and concentrated. The resulting residue was purified by flash chromatography on silica gel (PE/EA = 2:3), yielding compound **31** (11.5 mg, 53%) as a colorless oil. $[\alpha]_D^{20.0} = -16.4$ (*c* 0.5, MeOH); ^{1}H NMR (600 MHz, $CDCl_3$) exists as rotational conformers: δ 7.39–7.13 (m, 5H), 7.13–7.03 (m, 1H), 7.02–6.91 (m, 1H), 6.81–6.66 (m, 1H), 5.98–5.87 (m, 1H), 5.78–5.68 (m, 1H), 5.67–5.59 (m, 1H), 5.38–5.30 (m, 1H), 5.30–5.22 (m, 1H), 5.13–5.07 (m, 1H), 5.07–4.96 (m, 1H), 4.96–4.82 (m, 1H), 4.71–4.61 (m, 2H), 4.59–4.36 (m, 2H), 4.34–4.26 (m, 1H), 3.94–3.84 (m, 1H), 3.84–3.72 (m, 1H), 3.32–3.11 (m, 2H), 3.11–2.80 (m, 8H), 2.42–2.27 (m, 2H), 2.10–2.01 (m, 1H), 1.97–1.80 (m, 4H), 1.79–1.38 (m, 18H), 1.38–1.06 (m, 15H), 1.04–0.82 (m, 18H), 0.09–−0.02 (m, 6H); ^{13}C NMR (151 MHz, $CDCl_3$) exists as rotational conformers: δ 173.1, 172.0, 171.3, 170.9, 170.7, 169.8, 167.9, 167.5, 155.3, 140.8, 136.5, 131.8, 129.9, 129.4, 128.4, 128.3, 126.8, 118.6, 79.4, 76.1, 74.9, 71.8, 65.5, 54.2, 53.2, 52.2, 51.9, 46.6, 42.8, 37.6, 36.8, 36.4, 35.3, 33.4, 32.4, 31.9, 31.3, 30.4, 29.7, 29.7, 29.4, 28.3, 28.3, 26.1, 25.8, 24.0, 22.7, 18.7, 18.0, 17.7, 15.5, 14.5, 14.5, 14.1, 14.1, 12.6, 11.7, 11.2, 10.4, −4.3, −4.7, −4.7; HRMS (ESI-TOF) *m*/*z*: $C_{58}H_{97}N_5NaO_{13}Si^+$ $[M + Na]^+$: calcd: 1122.6744; found: 1122.6726.

3.14. Synthesis of Lagunamide D (1)

To a solution of compound **31** (26 mg, 24 μmol) and $Pd(PPh_3)_4$ (2.7 mg, 2.4 μmol) in anhydrous THF (2.0 mL), PhNHMe (5.2 μL, 48 μmol) was added. The resulting mixture was stirred at room temperature for 1 h. The reaction was quenched with TFA (10 μL, 144 μmol), diluted with ethyl acetate (30.0 mL), and washed sequentially with 1 M HCl (aq.) (3.0 mL × 2). The organic phase was washed with brine, dried over anhydrous Na_2SO_4, filtered, and concentrated to afford the crude acid **32**, which was used in the next step without further purification. To a solution of the crude acid in anhydrous CH_2Cl_2 (2.5 mL), TFA (0.50 mL) was added, and the mixture was stirred at room temperature for 2 h. The mixture was concentrated under reduced pressure, the residue was dissolved in DMF (12.0 mL), and HOAt (16 mg, 0.12 mmol), 2,4,6-collidine (94 μL, 0.72 mmol), and HATU (90 mg, 0.24 mmol) were added successively. The mixture was stirred for 48 h and then concentrated under reduced pressure. The residue was dissolved in ethyl acetate and washed with 1 M HCl (aq.), water, and brine. The organic phase was then dried over anhydrous Na_2SO_4, filtered, and concentrated. The resulting residue was purified by flash chromatography on silica gel (PE/EA = 2:3 to pure EA), yielding lagunamide D (13 mg, 67%) as a colorless foam. $[\alpha]_D^{20.0} = -57.1$ (*c* 0.07, MeOH); ^{1}H NMR (600 MHz, DMSO-d_6) exists as rotational conformers: δ 8.49 (d, *J* = 6.4 Hz, 0.3H), 8.34 (d, *J* = 8.3 Hz, 0.1H), 7.23–7.05 (m, 5.1H), 6.92–6.74 (m, 0.2H), 6.74–6.54 (m, 0.2H), 5.81–5.67 (m, 0.2H), 5.28 (dd, *J* = 10.2, 5.3 Hz, 0.6H), 5.23–4.99 (m, 0.6H), 4.92 (d, *J* = 7.6 Hz, 0.6H), 4.90–4.81 (m, 1.0H), 4.81–4.72 (m, 0.7H), 4.72–4.44 (m, 0.9H), 4.31 (dq, *J* = 6.3, 6.3 Hz, 0.6H), 4.25–4.07 (m, 0.8H), 3.98 (d, *J* = −18.4 Hz, 0.5H), 3.92 (q, *J* = 6.6 Hz, 0.6H), 3.87–3.72 (m, 0.3H), 3.72–3.38 (m, 0.7H), 3.21 (s, 2.4H), 3.16–3.06 (m, 0.6H), 3.06–2.88 (m, 1.9H), 2.85 (s, 2.7H), 2.80–2.76 (m, 0.8H), 2.73 (s, 2.2H), 2.64 (s, 1.2H), 2.45–2.18 (m, 1.2H), 2.10 (ddd, *J* = −14.0, 9.8, 9.8 Hz, 0.9H), 1.95–1.85 (m, 1.2H), 1.85–1.64 (m, 4.9H), 1.62–1.08 (m, 11.0H), 1.06–0.41 (m, 21.0H); ^{13}C NMR (151 MHz, DMSO-d_6) δ 172.45, 170.80, 170.14, 170.11, 169.52, 168.23, 168.01, 144.45, 137.17, 129.18, 127.48, 126.83, 125.84, 75.36, 74.62, 69.30, 58.07, 52.45, 51.1, 50.40, 44.65, 40.89, 37.29, 37.10, 36.27, 35.79, 34.42, 33.86, 29.60, 29.36, 25.83, 23.19, 17.05, 14.89, 14.69, 14.06, 13.92, 12.93, 11.98, 11.40, 10.27, 9.60; HRMS (ESI-TOF) *m*/*z*: $C_{44}H_{69}N_5NaO_{10}^+$ $[M + Na]^+$: calcd: 850.4937; found: 850.4909.

4. Conclusions

In summary, we have accomplished the total synthesis of lagunamide D and confirmed its absolute stereochemical configuration. Key features of the synthesis include Ghosh's $TiCl_4$-promoted anti-aldol reaction to establish the C38 and C39 chiral centers, a CBS reduction to construct the C37 chiral hydroxyl group, and a cross-metathesis reaction followed by a Pinnick oxidation to build the unsaturated carboxylic acid moiety. This synthetic strategy was completed in a 14-step longest linear sequence, starting from the known intermediate **17**, with an overall yield of 4.6%, which demonstrated an efficient route for access to the structurally unique 26-membered cytotoxic cyclic depsipeptide.

Supplementary Materials: The following supporting information can be downloaded at https://www.mdpi.com/article/10.3390/md23030099/s1: Figure S1: Comparison of ^{1}H NMR (600 MHz) for Natural and Synthetic Lagunamide D in DMSO-*d6*; Table S1: Comparison of ^{13}C NMR (600 MHz) for Natural and Synthetic Lagunamide D in DMSO-*d6*.; NMR and spectra of compounds **1**, **2**, **4**, **10**, **12**, **14**, **18**, **20–22**, **26**, **27**, **31** and **S1–S3**.

Author Contributions: Conceptualization, J.L., J.-L.Y., T.Y. and J.-B.P.; investigation, J.-B.P., H.N., X.-E.L., J.H., H.X. and M.-J.C.; writing—original draft preparation, H.N., X.-E.L., J.H., H.X. and M.-J.C.; writing—review and editing, J.L., T.Y., J.-L.Y. and J.-B.P. All authors have read and agreed to the published version of the manuscript.

Funding: This research was funded by the Department of Education of Guangdong Province (2021ZDJS097), the Technology and Innovation Bureau of Longgang District (RCTDPT-2019-008), the Guangdong Basic and Applied Basic Research Foundation (2022A1515110592, 2023A1515012715, and 2024A1515010958), the Natural Science Foundation of Guangdong Province (2021A1515010344), the National Natural Science Foundation of China (Grant no. 82473801), and the Jiangmen Basic and Applied Basic Research Project (202301003003140).

Institutional Review Board Statement: Not applicable.

Data Availability Statement: Data are contained within the article or Supplementary Materials.

Conflicts of Interest: Author Tao Ye was employed by the company Qian Yan (Shenzhen) Pharmatech. Ltd. The remaining authors declare that the research was conducted in the absence of any commercial or financial relationships that could be construed as a potential conflict of interest.

References

1. Newman, D.J.; Cragg, G.M. Natural Products as Sources of New Drugs over the Nearly Four Decades from 01/1981 to 09/2019. *J. Nat. Prod.* **2020**, *83*, 770–803. [CrossRef]
2. Antunes, E.M.; Beukes, D.R.; Caro-Diaz, E.J.E.; Narchi, N.E.; Tan, L.T.; Gerwick, W.H. Chapter 5—Medicines from the sea. In *Oceans and Human Health*, 2nd ed.; Fleming, L.E., Alcantara Creencia, L.B., Gerwick, W.H., Goh, H.C., Gribble, M.O., Maycock, B., Solo-Gabriele, H., Eds.; Academic Press: San Diego, CA, USA, 2023; pp. 103–148.
3. Banday, A.H.; ul Azha, N.; Farooq, R.; Sheikh, S.A.; Ganie, M.A.; Parray, M.N.; Mushtaq, H.; Hameed, I.; Lone, M.A. Exploring the potential of marine natural products in drug development: A comprehensive review. *Phytochem. Lett.* **2024**, *59*, 124–135. [CrossRef]
4. Luesch, H.; Ellis, E.K.; Chen, Q.-Y.; Ratnayake, R. Progress in the discovery and development of anticancer agents from marine cyanobacteria. *Nat. Prod. Rep.* **2025**, *42*, 208–256. [CrossRef] [PubMed]
5. Jimenez, P.C.; Wilke, D.V.; Branco, P.C.; Bauermeister, A.; Rezende-Teixeira, P.; Gaudêncio, S.P.; Costa-Lotufo, L.V. Enriching cancer pharmacology with drugs of marine origin. *Br. J. Pharmacol.* **2020**, *177*, 3–27. [CrossRef] [PubMed]
6. Haque, N.; Parveen, S.; Tang, T.; Wei, J.; Huang, Z. Marine Natural Products in Clinical Use. *Mar. Drugs* **2022**, *20*, 528. [CrossRef]
7. Ghareeb, M.A.; Tammam, M.A.; El-Demerdash, A.; Atanasov, A.G. Insights about clinically approved and Preclinically investigated marine natural products. *Curr. Res. Biotechnol.* **2020**, *2*, 88–102. [CrossRef]
8. Papon, N.; Copp, B.R.; Courdavault, V. Marine drugs: Biology, pipelines, current and future prospects for production. *Biotechnol. Adv.* **2022**, *54*, 107871. [CrossRef] [PubMed]
9. Jiménez, C. Marine Natural Products in Medicinal Chemistry. *ACS Med. Chem. Lett.* **2018**, *9*, 959–961. [CrossRef] [PubMed]
10. Luo, D.; Putra, M.Y.; Ye, T.; Paul, V.J.; Luesch, H. Isolation, Structure Elucidation and Biological Evaluation of Lagunamide D: A New Cytotoxic Macrocyclic Depsipeptide from Marine Cyanobacteria. *Mar. Drugs* **2019**, *17*, 83. [CrossRef]

11. Tripathi, A.; Puddick, J.; Prinsep, M.R.; Rottmann, M.; Chan, K.P.; Chen, D.Y.-K.; Tan, L.T. Lagunamide C, a cytotoxic cyclodepsipeptide from the marine cyanobacterium *Lyngbya majuscula*. *Phytochemistry* **2011**, *72*, 2369–2375. [CrossRef] [PubMed]
12. Tripathi, A.; Puddick, J.; Prinsep, M.R.; Rottmann, M.; Tan, L.T. Lagunamides A and B: Cytotoxic and Antimalarial Cyclodepsipeptides from the Marine Cyanobacterium *Lyngbya majuscula*. *J. Nat. Prod.* **2010**, *73*, 1810–1814. [CrossRef] [PubMed]
13. Kobayashi, Y.; Tan, C.H.; Kishi, Y. Toward creation of a universal NMR database for stereochemical assignment: The case of 1,3,5-trisubstituted acyclic systems. *Helv. Chim. Acta* **2000**, *83*, 2562–2571. [CrossRef]
14. Kobayashi, Y.; Tan, C.-H.; Kishi, Y. Toward creation of a universal NMR database for stereochemical assignment: Complete structure of the desertomycin/oasomycin class of natural products structural properties of fatty acids and related compounds are inherent to the specfic stereochemical. *J. Am. Chem. Soc.* **2001**, *123*, 2076–2078. [CrossRef] [PubMed]
15. Luo, D.; Ratnayake, R.; Atanasova, K.R.; Paul, V.J.; Luesch, H. Targeted and functional genomics approaches to the mechanism of action of lagunamide D, a mitochondrial cytotoxin from marine cyanobacteria. *Biochem. Pharmacol.* **2023**, *213*, 115608. [CrossRef]
16. Dai, L.; Chen, B.; Lei, H.; Wang, Z.; Liu, Y.; Xu, Z.; Ye, T. Total synthesis and stereochemical revision of lagunamide A. *Chem. Commun.* **2012**, *48*, 8697–8699. [CrossRef]
17. Huang, W.; Ren, R.-G.; Dong, H.-Q.; Wei, B.-G.; Lin, G.-Q. Diverse Synthesis of Marine Cyclic Depsipeptide Lagunamide A and Its Analogues. *J. Org. Chem.* **2013**, *78*, 10747–10762. [CrossRef]
18. Gorges, J.; Kazmaier, U. Matteson Homologation-Based Total Synthesis of Lagunamide A. *Org. Lett.* **2018**, *20*, 2033–2036. [CrossRef]
19. Hagimoto, K.; Tojo, S.; Teruya, T.; Yoshida, M.; Kigoshi, H. Structure revision of lagunamide C to odoamide by total synthesis and biological evaluation. *Tetrahedron* **2024**, *154*, 133871. [CrossRef]
20. Kaneda, M.; Sueyoshi, K.; Teruya, T.; Ohno, H.; Fujii, N.; Oishi, S. Total synthesis of odoamide, a novel cyclic depsipeptide, from an Okinawan marine cyanobacterium. *Org. Biomol. Chem.* **2016**, *14*, 9093–9104. [CrossRef] [PubMed]
21. Grubbs, R.H. Olefin-Metathesis Catalysts for the Preparation of Molecules and Materials (Nobel Lecture). *Angew. Chem. Int. Ed.* **2006**, *45*, 3760–3765. [CrossRef] [PubMed]
22. Delaude, L.; Noels, A.F. Metathesis. In *Kirk-Othmer Encyclopedia of Chemical Technology*; John Wiley & Sons, Inc.: New York, NY, USA, 2005.
23. Ghosh, A.K.; Onishi, M. Synthesis of Enantiomerically Pure Anti-Aldols: A Highly Stereoselective Ester-Derived Titanium Enolate Aldol Reaction. *J. Am. Chem. Soc.* **1996**, *118*, 2527–2528. [CrossRef]
24. Ghosh, A.K.; Xu, C.-X. A Convergent Synthesis of the Proposed Structure of Antitumor Depsipeptide Stereocalpin A. *Org. Lett.* **2009**, *11*, 1963–1966. [CrossRef]
25. Liu, J.; Chen, Y.; Luesch, H.; Ye, T. Total Synthesis of des-Thiomethyllooekeyolide A. *Org. Lett.* **2022**, *24*, 7260–7264. [CrossRef] [PubMed]
26. Corey, E.J.; Bakshi, R.K.; Shibata, S. Highly enantioselective borane reduction of ketones catalyzed by chiral oxazaborolidines. Mechanism and synthetic implications. *J. Am. Chem. Soc.* **1987**, *109*, 5551–5553. [CrossRef]
27. Liu, J.; Wang, L.; Zhang, J.; Xu, Z.; Ye, T. The total synthesis and stereochemical assignment of scytonemin A. *Chem. Commun.* **2016**, *52*, 1002–1005. [CrossRef] [PubMed]
28. Rychnovsky, S.D.; Rogers, B.; Yang, G. Analysis of two carbon-13 NMR correlations for determining the stereochemistry of 1,3-diol acetonides. *J. Org. Chem.* **1993**, *58*, 3511–3515. [CrossRef]
29. Inanaga, J.; Hirata, K.; Saeki, H.; Katsuki, T.; Yamaguchi, M. A Rapid Esterification by Means of Mixed Anhydride and Its Application to Large-ring Lactonization. *Bull. Chem. Soc. Jpn.* **1979**, *52*, 1989–1993. [CrossRef]
30. Boden, E.P.; Keck, G.E. Proton-transfer steps in Steglich esterification: A very practical new method for macrolactonization. *J. Org. Chem.* **1985**, *50*, 2394–2395. [CrossRef]
31. Shiina, I.; Ibuka, R.; Kubota, M. A New Condensation Reaction for the Synthesis of Carboxylic Esters from Nearly Equimolar Amounts of Carboxylic Acids and Alcohols Using 2-Methyl-6-nitrobenzoic Anhydride. *Chem. Lett.* **2002**, *31*, 286–287. [CrossRef]
32. Devos, A.; Remion, J.; Frisque-Hesbain, A.-M.; Colens, A.; Ghosez, L. Synthesis of acyl halides under very mild conditions. *J. Chem. Soc. Chem. Commun.* **1979**, *24*, 1180–1181. [CrossRef]
33. Ye, Y.-h.; Li, H.; Jiang, X. DEPBT as an efficient coupling reagent for amide bond formation with remarkable resistance to racemization. *Pept. Sci.* **2005**, *80*, 172–178. [CrossRef] [PubMed]
34. Li, H.; Jiang, X.; Ye, Y.-h.; Fan, C.; Romoff, T.; Goodman, M. 3-(Diethoxyphosphoryloxy)-1,2,3-benzotriazin-4(3H)-one (DEPBT): A New Coupling Reagent with Remarkable Resistance to Racemization. *Org. Lett.* **1999**, *1*, 91–94. [CrossRef]
35. Umehara, M.; Takada, Y.; Nakao, Y.; Kimura, J. Intramolecular ester exchange of potent cytotoxic kulokekahilide-2. *Tetrahedron Lett.* **2009**, *50*, 840–843. [CrossRef]
36. Kaneda, M.; Kawaguchi, S.; Fujii, N.; Ohno, H.; Oishi, S. Structure–Activity Relationship Study on Odoamide: Insights into the Bioactivities of Aurilide-Family Hybrid Peptide–Polyketides. *ACS Med. Chem. Lett.* **2018**, *9*, 365–369. [CrossRef] [PubMed]

marine drugs

MDPI

Article

Synthesis and Biological Activity of Glycosyl Thiazolyl Disulfides Based on Thiacarpine, an Analogue of the Cytotoxic Alkaloid Polycarpine from the Ascidian *Polycarpa aurata*

Dmitry N. Pelageev [1,*], Yuri E. Sabutski [1], Svetlana M. Kovach [2], Nadezhda N. Balaneva [1], Ekaterina S. Menchinskaya [1], Ekaterina A. Chingizova [1], Anna L. Burylova [1,3] and Victor Ph. Anufriev [1]

1 G. B. Elyakov Pacific Institute of Bioorganic Chemistry, Russian Academy of Sciences, Prospect 100 let Vladivostoku 159, Vladivostok 690022, Russia; alixar2006@yandex.ru (Y.E.S.); balaneva@piboc.dvo.ru (N.N.B.); ekaterinamenchinskaya@gmail.com (E.S.M.); martyyas@mail.ru (E.A.C.); anaburylova1@gmail.com (A.L.B.); anufriev@piboc.dvo.ru (V.P.A.)

2 Institute of High Technologies and Advanced Materials, Far Eastern Federal University, Ajax Bay 10, Russky Island, Vladivostok 690922, Russia; svetakovach596403@gmail.com

3 Institute of the World Ocean, Far Eastern Federal University, Ajax Bay 10, Russky Island, Vladivostok 690922, Russia

* Correspondence: pelageev@mail.ru

Abstract: Polycarpine, a diimidazolyl disulfan alkaloid isolated from the ascidian *Polycarpa aurata*, showed high cytotoxic activity in vitro. However, in vivo experiments have shown that polycarpine has a high acute toxicity. At the same time, its synthetic thiazolyl analog, thiacarpine, showed less acute toxicity and had a greater therapeutic index, which makes its derivatives promising for further drug development. We assume that due to the presence of a disulfide bond in the molecules of polycarpine and thiacarpine and the possibility of its reduction in a living cell, the mercapto derivatives formed are responsible for the high activity of the original compounds. Based on this assumption, and to increase the selectivity of action, glycosyl disulfide conjugates of thiacarpine derivatives with thioglucose and thioxylose were synthesized and screened for their cytotoxic and antimicrobial activities. The target compounds did not show hemolytic activity at concentrations of up to 25 μM. Some of them exhibited moderate cytotoxic activity, blocked colony growth and migration of HeLa tumor cells, high antimicrobial activity, and inhibited biofilm formation comparable to or higher than that of a standard antibiotic (gentamicin) and antimycotic (nitrofungin).

Keywords: polycarpine; thiacarpine; bis(2-amino-4-phenyl-5-thiazolyl)disulfide; thioglycosides; *Polycarpa aurata*; cytotoxic activity; antimicrobial activity; biofilm formation; hemolysis

1. Introduction

Polycarpine, a diimidazolyl disulfane alkaloid isolated from the ascidia of the genus *Polycarpa*, is the first representative of a new structural type of alkaloids containing 2-aminoimidazole rings linked by a disulfide bridge (Figure 1) [1–4]. In vitro experiments showed that polycarpine exhibited high cytotoxic and antitumor activity. However, in vivo experiments showed that it had acute toxicity. At the same time, its synthetic thiazolyl analog, thiacarpine, also exhibited a marked antitumor effect on both solid and ascites tumors. When injected intraperitoneally, it effectively inhibited the development of solid tumors such as LLC and melanoma B-16. However, unlike polycarpine, which was usually effective at high therapeutic doses, thiacarpine had a higher therapeutic index [5].

This makes its derivatives promising for further drug development. Moreover, having a wide pharmacological spectrum, 2-aminothiazole derivatives are important substances in medicinal chemistry and drug development [6,7]. Thus, 2-aminothiazole derivatives exhibit antitumor [8–10], antiviral [11], antimicrobial [12–14], anticonvulsant [15], antidiabetic [16], antiprion [17], and other properties [18]. For example, in vitro studies on the antitumor activity of various 2-aminothiazole derivatives have demonstrated their potent and selective inhibitory activity against a wide range of human cancer cell lines, such as breast, leukemia, lung, colon, central nervous system (CNS), melanoma, ovarian, kidney, and prostate [19–21].

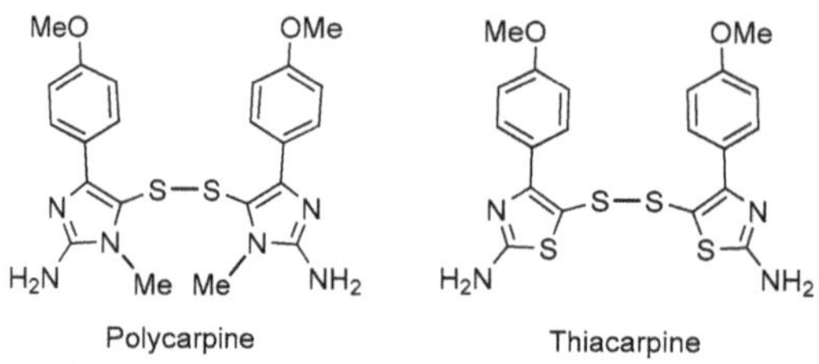

Figure 1. Structures of polycarpine and its synthetic analogue thiacarpine.

The combination of different fragments in one hybrid molecule leads to a significant change in biological properties. Thus, the introduction of nonpolar fragments increases lipophilicity and, as a rule, increases cytotoxicity by facilitating diffusion through cell membranes. The introduction of polar fragments can increase the water solubility and bioavailability. One promising means of conjugation is the formation of disulfide bonds. They are of great importance in biological processes. Disulfide bonds are involved in the formation of the tertiary structure of proteins as well as in thiol-disulfide exchange with the participation of glutathione. Disulfides have also been reported to exhibit various biological activities. For example, some unsymmetrical aryl-alkyl disulfides inhibited the growth of methicillin-resistant *Staphylococcus aureus* and *Bacillus anthracis* [22]. Yoon and co-workers reported that some unsymmetrical disulfide compounds were inhibitors of *Mycobacterium tuberculosis* and *Haemophilus influenzae*, by interfering with acetohydroxyacid synthase (AHAS), a key enzyme in the biosynthesis pathway of branched-chain amino acids [23,24].

Unsymmetrical monoterpenyl-hetaryl disulfides based on heterocyclic disulfides and monoterpene thiols had good indicators of antioxidant, antimicrobial, and antiviral activities [25]. Some aromatic disulfides were reported to exhibit antiviral activity [26–29]. Moreover, glycosyl disulfides have attracted significant attention as glycomimetics with wide biological applications [30]. For example, they can be used as prodrugs that are activated in living cells by reducing disulfide bonds [31].

Glycoconjugation, that is, the binding of a drug with different sugars, is a promising approach that may increase the cellular uptake of the therapeutic compound. So, the idea of conjugating anticancer drugs to glucose residue is based on the Warburg effect. This effect describes the ability of cancer tissues to consume larger amounts of glucose than normal tissues. Overexpression of glycolytic enzymes and glucose transporters GLUTs mediates this effect and has been recognized as a hallmark of cancer development. The use of the Warburg effect as an anticancer strategy has attracted much attention, and the idea of using sugar-conjugated anticancer drugs to enhance the selectivity of their uptake has developed significantly over the past decade. Several compounds using the Warburg effect are undergoing advanced clinical trials, while many others are in preclinical development [32–34].

A similar effect on microorganisms can be expected for xylose. Many bacteria, including *E. coli*, tend to use active transport for D-xylose. In yeasts and fungi, transportation can occur by facilitated diffusion or active transport, and is highly dependent on species and whether it can be utilized to sustain growth. Yeast, such as *Pichia*, *Candida*, and *Debaryomyces*, have been reported to have xylose-proton symporters that are substrate-specific, have a high affinity, and are reliant upon induction by xylose for some species [35].

We assume that because of the presence of the disulfide bond in polycarpine and thiacarpine molecules and the possibility of its reduction in living cells, the mercapto derivatives formed as a result of this reduction are responsible for the high activity of the parent compounds. Based on this assumption, in order to study antimicrobial and cytotoxic activity in this work, we obtained thiazole-glucose and thiazole-xylose conjugates based on thiacarpine and its derivatives, in which the thiazole and carbohydrate fragments are connected through two sulfur atoms. The target compounds are expected to have high water solubility and bioavailability, and may also exhibit selectivity on tumor cells or pathogenic microorganisms.

2. Results and Discussion

2.1. Synthesis of Glycosyl Disulfides

Despite the development of numerous methods for the synthesis of asymmetric disulfides [30], it is challenging to find the most effective method for the substrates under consideration. Bis(2-amino-4-phenyl-5-thiazolyl)disulfides **1a–e**, thiacarpine and its analogues, were the starting compounds in our work because of the instability of mercapto derivatives **2a–e** during purification. These mercapto derivatives **2a–e** can be obtained by the reduction with sodium dithionite but they are readily oxidized back to the starting disulfides **1a–e** in air. Oxidation of a mixture of mercapto derivatives **2a–e** and **3a,b** with iodine gave the target acetylated asymmetric disulfides **4a–e** in satisfactory yields (Scheme 1) [36]. The chosen method was found to be easy to perform and, considering the recovery of the starting disulfide (approximately 40%), the yields could be considered good.

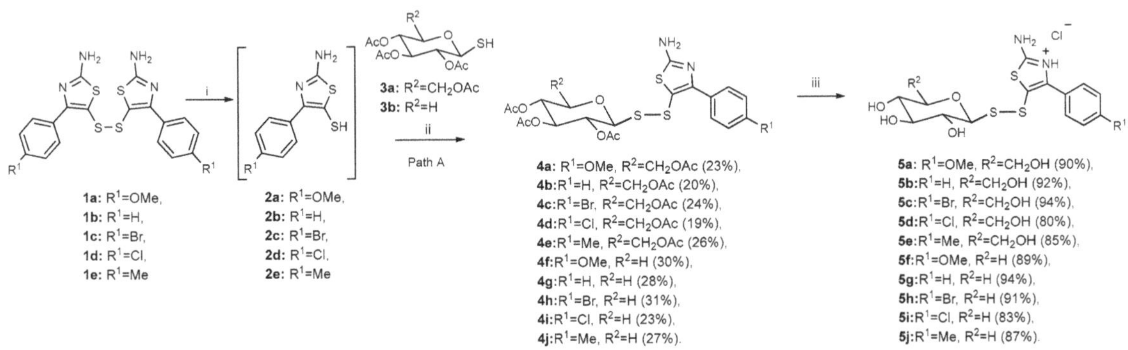

Scheme 1. Reagents and conditions: i, $Na_2S_2O_4$, acetone–H_2O (1:2 v/v), room temperature, 15 min; ii, EtOH, I_2, room temperature, 15 min; iii, MeOH/HCl, room temperature, 15 h.

The experiments with bis(2-amino-4-phenyl-5-thiazolyl)disulfide **1b** to test the typically effective alternative methods described in [37,38] showed that the use of sulfenyl halides **2b′** and **3b′** was ineffective (yield of about 15–19% for paths B and C compared to 28% for path A) and more difficult to perform, as required anhydrous solvents and had lower solubility of the starting disulfide (Scheme 2).

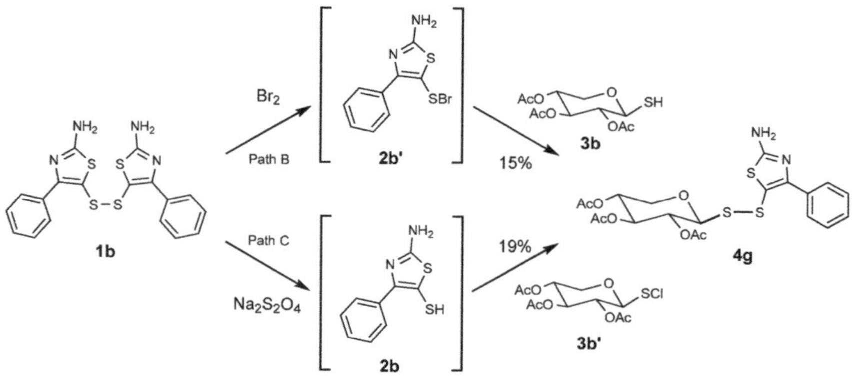

Scheme 2. The alternative methods of the disulfide synthesis.

Deacetylation of **4a–j** derivatives under the action of HCl in methanol gave glycosyl disulfides **5a–j** as hydrochlorides in excellent yields (Scheme 1).

2.2. Biological Activity of the Compounds

2.2.1. Cytotoxic Activity

The cytotoxic activities of the synthesized compounds were studied in tumor and normal human cells: HeLa (cervical cancer), Hep G2 (hepatocellular carcinoma), MDA-MB-231 (triple-negative breast cancer), MCF-7 (adenocarcinoma of the mammary gland ducts), PC-3 (prostate cancer), and BEAS-2B (bronchial epithelium). All compounds were also tested for their ability to destroy erythrocyte membranes. The experiments revealed that the studied compounds did not have hemolytic activity in the concentration range of up to 25 μM. The most stable cell lines were PC-3 and MCF-7, as none of the substances showed cytotoxic activity up to 25 μM during incubation for 24 h. As expected, acetylated derivatives **4a–j**, which are less polar substances, generally had higher toxicity than deacetylated derivatives **5a–j** and starting disulfides **1a–e**. Deacetylation mainly resulted in a marked decrease in cytotoxicity. The highest activity was observed for compounds with –OMe, –Me, and–Br substituents (Table 1). There was no pronounced effect of sugar backbone type on the cytotoxicity of the conjugates. It is worth noting that compound **4e** bearing an acetylated glucose moiety and a methyl substituent in the aromatic moiety showed the greatest cytotoxic effect on cancer HeLa cells (EC_{50} = 18.53 μM) and TNBC cells of the MDA-MB-231 line (EC_{50} = 14.95 μM). In addition, conjugate **4e** showed no cytotoxicity against normal cell culture BEAS-2B (up to 25 μM). Compounds **4c, 4f,** and **4h** exhibited similar cytotoxic activity against HeLa and MDA-MB-231 tumor cells and were selected for further investigation.

Table 1. Cytotoxicity (EC_{50}) of compounds on cancer and non-cancer cell lines (μM) *.

Compound	Cell Lines, EC_{50}, μM			
	HeLa	Hep G_2	MDA-MB-231 (TNBC)	BEAS 2B
1a	>25	>25	21.4	>25
4a	>25	>25	>25	19.9
4b	>25	>25	24.1	19.0
4c	19.4	24.3	21.7	15.5
4d	>25	>25	22.9	14.1

Table 1. *Cont.*

Compound	Cell Lines, EC_{50}, μM			
	HeLa	Hep G_2	MDA-MB-231 (TNBC)	BEAS 2B
4e	18.5	>25	15.0	>25
4f	20.4	22.6	22.9	23.5
4h	21.3	24.6	21.1	19.9
4j	>25	>25	23.7	>25
5a	>25	>25	24.9	>25
5b	>25	>25	>25	20.8
5e	>25	>25	23.5	22.6
5g	>25	>25	>25	22.0
5h	>25	>25	>25	23.5
cisplatin	10.2	14.8	81.5	63.3

* The cytotoxic activity of compounds **1b–1e**, **4 g**, **4i**, **5c**, **5d**, **5f**, **5i**, and **5j** on all cell lines was higher than 25 μM. The cytotoxic activity of all compounds on cell lines PC-3, MCF-7, and erythrocytes was higher than 25 μM.

2.2.2. HeLa Cell Migration

Cell migration is an important process in cancer metastasis; therefore, the search for drugs that will help prevent this process remains relevant. The effects of these compounds on cell migration were evaluated using an in vitro wound scratch migration assay. In the control group, HeLa cells migrated to completely close the wound area after 24 h (Figure 2). However, in the treatment groups, cell migration into the wound areas was significantly reduced at 24 h in a dose-dependent manner. All selected compounds **4c**, **4e**, **4f**, **4h** showed similar migration inhibition effects. The maximum migration inhibition effect was observed for compounds **4e** and **4h** at a concentration of 10 μM, and was approximately 43% for both.

2.2.3. Compounds Reduced the Number of Colonies Forming of HeLa Cells

To observe the long-term effects of the test compounds on HeLa cells, a colony formation assay was performed. The cells were treated with concentrations below the EC_{50} for 14 days. Colony formation was significantly reduced by all test compounds at the studied concentrations (Figure 3). The maximum inhibitory effect was observed at 10 μM, amounting to 76% for **4c** and 78% for **4f**. Compound **4f**, at a concentration of 5 μM, had less of an effect on colony formation. Thus, colony growth inhibition was approximately 16% of that of the control.

2.2.4. Antimicrobial Activity

The antimicrobial activity of the synthesized series of disulfides was studied against the Gram-positive bacteria *Staphylococcus aureus*, Gram-negative bacteria *Escherichia coli*, and yeast-like fungi *Candida albicans* using a double dilution method in liquid nutrient media. The antimicrobial activity was assessed by changing the optical density of the medium using a plate spectrophotometer. There was no general pattern in the change in activity between the acetylated and deacetylated derivatives. This can be explained by the interaction of these hybrid structures with different targets in the living cells. These interactions can cause effects with different contributions and directions (increase or decrease toxicity). As a rule, deacetylation led to a decrease in activity; however, in the case of halogen derivatives **4c**, **4d**, and **4h**, the activity of the deacetylated products **5c**, **5d**, and **5h** was higher. Bromine (**4c**, **4h**, **5c**, and **5h**) and chlorine (**4d**, **4i**, **5d**, and **5i**) derivatives of the synthesized series of disulfide conjugates showed the highest antimicrobial activity against the test strains of microorganisms (Table 2). In addition, bromine derivatives were found to be more selective for growth inhibition of Gram-positive bacteria and yeast (Figure 4). There was no clear effect of the carbohydrate fragment on the activity of the studied compounds, but among the most active, the xyloside derivative **5h** had the strongest growth inhibitory activity, with MIC_{50} of 1.15 (*S. aureus*), 1.56 (*C. albicans*), and 3.08 (*E. coli*) μM.

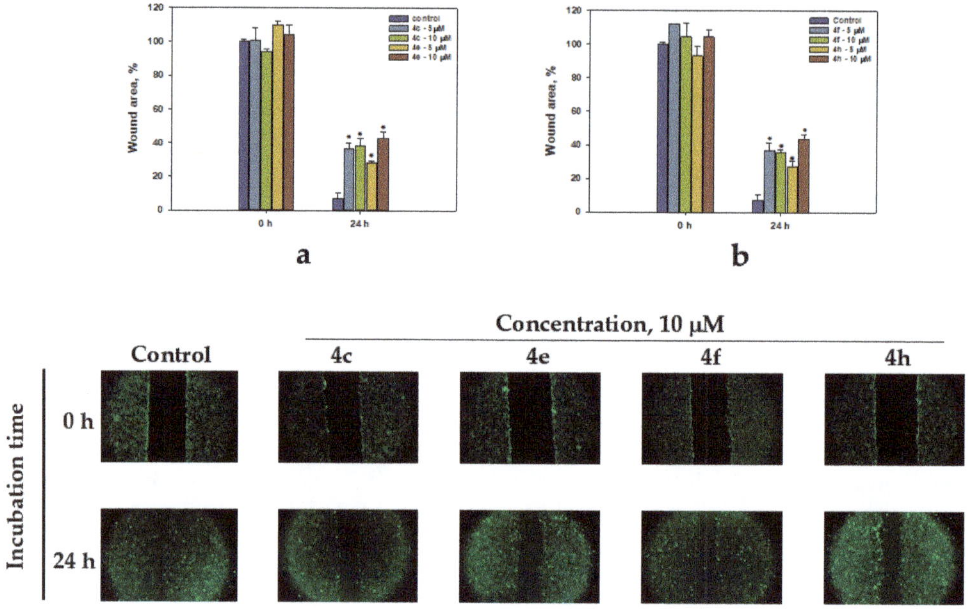

Figure 2. Cell migration into wound areas processed by Image J 1.52 software: (**a**) Compounds **4c** and **4e** at 5 and 10 μM concentrations; (**b**) Compounds **4f** and **4h** at 5 and 10 μM concentrations; (**c**) Migration of HeLa cells into wound areas observed with an MIB-2-FL fluorescence microscope of ten-fold magnification, studied compounds at 10 μM concentration. Data are presented as means ± SEM. * p-value ≤ 0.05 is considered significant.

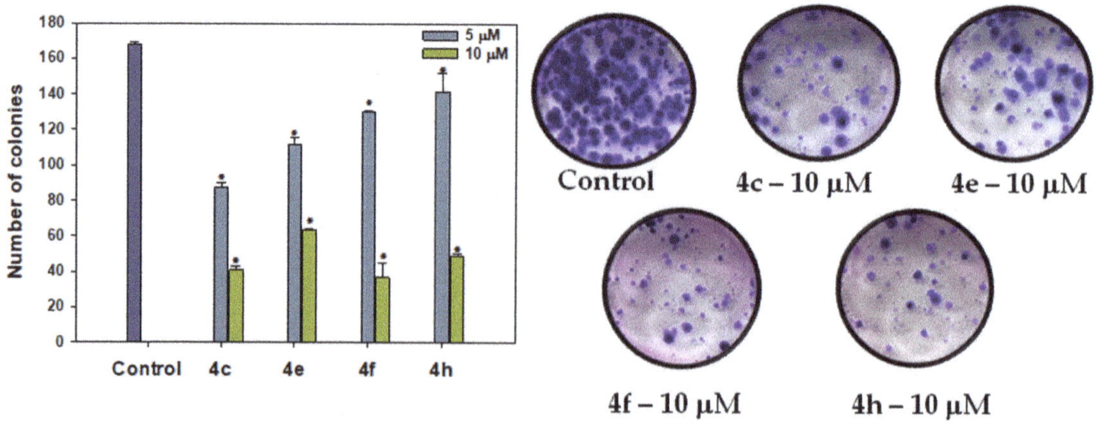

Figure 3. Number of HeLa cell colonies after treatment with different concentrations of the studied compounds. Data are presented as means ± SEM. * p-value ≤ 0.05 considered significant.

Table 2. Antimicrobial activity and inhibition of biofilm formation of disulfides (**4a–5j**) against *S. aureus*, *E. coli*, and *C. albicans* are presented in MIC_{50}, μM (gentamicin/nitrofungin are positive controls) *.

Compound	Inhibition of Microbial Growth MIC_{50}, μM			Inhibition of Biofilm Formation MIC_{50}, μM		
	S. aureus	*E. coli*	*C. albicans*	*S. aureus*	*E. coli*	*C. albicans*
1a	10.3 ± 1.1	>50	38.2 ± 3.2	34.5 ± 3.7	>50	35.3 ± 3.4
1b	5.2 ± 0.5	13.9 ± 1.3	6.2 ± 0.6	17.3 ± 1.1	5.9 ± 0.5	11.5 ± 1.1
1c	3.4 ± 0.4	15.7 ± 2.3	3.1 ± 0.4	>50	>50	12.4 ± 2.5
1d	2.8 ± 0.2	30.9 ± 3.0	5.0 ± 0.4	>50	>50	25.1 ± 3.1
1e	30.7 ± 2.1	33.9 ± 3.9	19.5 ± 2.0	34.0 ± 3.1	31.6 ± 3.6	23.4 ± 2.6
4a	32.5 ± 3.2	>50	31.5 ± 3.1	36.2 ± 3.1	>50	22.1 ± 2.4
4b	28.4 ± 3.1	31.2 ± 2.0	20.5 ± 2.7	27.4 ± 1.5	34.3 ± 3.4	15.9 ± 1.0
4c	2.3 ± 0.3	6.9 ± 0.5	7.1 ± 0.7	7.9 ± 0.5	8.0 ± 0.8	14.1 ± 1.3
4d	19.2 ± 2.0	16.1 ± 1.7	6.9 ± 0.9	16.7 ± 1.1	17.0 ± 1.2	7.0 ± 0.3
4e	>50	>50	17.7 ± 0.3	25.1 ± 2.3	27.1 ± 2.1	18.3 ± 1.5
4f	32.1 ± 3.7	39.5 ± 4.0	34.1 ± 2.1	35.4 ± 2.1	23.2 ± 2.0	22.1 ± 2.1
4g	34.0 ± 1.6	42.1 ± 4.1	35.7 ± 3.0	36.0 ± 3.1	38.1 ± 3.0	37.5 ± 4.0
4h	2.4 ± 0.2	5.8 ± 0.4	4.3 ± 0.5	6.3 ± 0.5	10.0 ± 0.9	7.1 ± 0.4
4i	3.1 ± 0.3	8.7 ± 0.9	2.8 ± 0.3	6.3 ± 0.4	13.5 ± 1.2	4.1 ± 0.1
4j	25.0 ± 1.4	25.5 ± 2.0	18.1 ± 1.0	19.4 ± 1.3	14.2 ± 1.0	13.5 ± 1.6
5c	3.0 ± 0.2	5.0 ± 0.5	1.6 ± 0.2	10.7 ± 1.1	12.4 ± 1.1	8.7 ± 0.7
5d	2.5 ± 0.2	6.6 ± 0.5	3.1 ± 2.3	18.6 ± 1.3	6.0 ± 0.6	10.9 ± 1.0
5e	>50	>50	38.5 ± 3.4	>50	>50	17.3 ± 0.4
5f	>50	>50	36.2 ± 2.1	>50	>50	16.1 ± 0.4
5g	>50	24.9 ± 2.2	25.3 ± 1.0	>50	42.1 ± 3.5	38.1 ± 3.0
5h	1.2 ± 0.1	3.1 ± 0.3	1.6 ± 0.1	11.4 ± 1.0	8.9 ± 0.7	3.2 ± 0.3
5i	13.7 ± 1.1	21.0 ± 3.0	13.8 ± 1.2	20.1 ± 2.0	12.1 ± 1.1	25.0 ± 2.0
5j	34.5 ± 3.0	38.0 ± 3.0	15.9 ± 1.1	38.0 ± 3.6	5.6 ± 0.6	24.1 ± 2.1
Gentamicin	4.3 ± 0.8	5.1 ± 0.7	–	4.6 ± 0.5	5.0 ± 0.5	–
Nitrofungin	–	–	4.1 ± 0.5	–	–	4.3 ± 0.4

* The activity of compounds **5a** and **5b** against all microorganism strains was higher than 50 μM.

The synthesized disulfides were also tested for their ability to inhibit biofilm formation by test strains of microorganisms using the modified method of Walencka [39], and the data are presented in Table 2. It was shown that the studied series of synthesized disulfides (**4a–5j**) had less pronounced inhibition of biofilm formation compared to the inhibition of planktonic forms of microorganisms. This is most likely due to the fact that the compounds inhibit the growth of microorganisms and they do not have time to form a biofilm under the action of tested compounds. Bromine and chlorine derivatives of disulfides had the most pronounced inhibitory effect on biofilms of the test strains of microorganisms (Figure 4). The most pronounced inhibitory effect on biofilm formation of the yeast-like fungi *C. albicans* was demonstrated by bromine derivative **5h** and chlorine derivative **4i**, with MIC_{50} of 3.21 and 4.08 μM. Bromine derivatives **4h** and **5c** inhibited biofilm formation by *C. albicans* with MIC_{50} 7.11 and 8.69 μM, and chlorine derivative **4d** with MIC_{50} 7.03 μM.

The studied series of synthetic disulfides had a more pronounced effect on the biofilm formation of the yeast-like fungi *C. albicans* in comparison with bacteria.

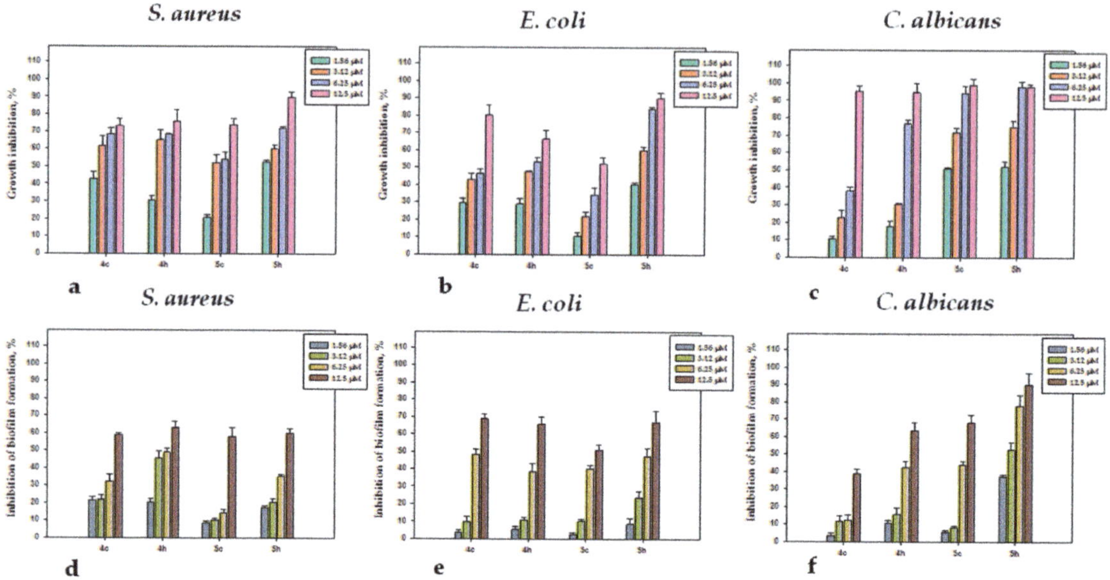

Figure 4. The influence of brominated disulfides **4c**, **4h**, **5c**, **5h** on growth *S. aureus* (**a**), *E. coli* (**b**), *C. albicans* (**c**) and inhibited biofilm formation *S. aureus* (**d**), *E. coli* (**e**), *C. albicans* (**f**). All experiments were performed in triplicate. Data are presented as mean ± SEM.

Among the studied disulfides, the most significant activity inhibiting the biofilm formation of Gram-negative bacteria *E. coli* was demonstrated by compounds **5j**, **5d**, **4c**, and **5h** with MIC_{50} of 5.62, 6.00, 8.04, and 8.92 μM, respectively (Table 2). The greatest activity in relation to the inhibition of biofilm formation by the Gram-positive bacterium *S. aureus* was shown by bromine derivatives **4h** and **4c**, with MIC_{50} of 6.32 and 7.94 μM and chlorine derivative **4i** with MIC_{50} of 6.25 μM.

3. Materials and Methods

3.1. General Information

All reagents and solvents were obtained from commercial suppliers and used without further purification. The starting bis(2-amino-4-phenyl-5-thiazolyl) disulfides **1a–e** [8,12], tetra-O-acetyl-1-thio-β-D-glucopyranose **3a**, and tri-O-acetyl-1-thio-β-D-xylopyranose **3b** [40] were obtained according to previously reported procedures. Melting points were determined using a Boetius apparatus and uncorrected. IR spectra in $CHCl_3$ and KBr were obtained using a Bruker Vector-22 FT-IR spectrophotometer. ^{1}H and ^{13}C NMR spectra were recorded on Bruker Avance DPX-300 spectrometer. $CDCl_3$ and DMSO-d_6 were used as solvents, with $SiMe_4$ ($\delta = 0$ ppm) or the signal of the residual solvent ($CHCl_3$: $\delta_H = 7.26$, $\delta_c = 77.16$, DMSO: $\delta_H = 2.50$, $\delta_c = 39.52$ ppm) as the internal reference. HRESIMS spectra were measured using an Agilent 6510 Q-TOF LC mass spectrometer. The reaction course was monitored by TLC. The copies of ^{1}H NMR and ^{13}C NMR spectra for synthesized compounds **4a–j**, **5a–j** can be found in Supplementary Materials.

3.1.1. General Procedure for the Synthesis of Acetylated Conjugates **4a–j**

Reduction of thiazole disulfides **1a–e**.

Sodium dithionite (85%, 8.2 g, 40 mmol, 20 eq) was added to a stirring suspension of the corresponding disulfide **1a–e** (2 mmol) in an acetone-water mixture (90 mL, 1:2 *v*/*v*) at 10 °C. The reaction mixture was stirred for 15 min at room temperature until a yellowish solution was formed. The mixture was diluted with cold water (100 mL) and cooled to 5 °C for 1 h. The precipitate of mercaptothiazole **2a–e** was filtered and washed with cold water (5 mL). The filtrate was extracted with chloroform (3 × 50 mL) and the extract was evaporated under reduced pressure at 40 °C. The yellowish residue containing compounds **2a–e** was combined with the filtered precipitate and immediately used in the next synthesis stage.

Oxidation of mercaptanes with I_2.

To a mixture of acetylated mercaptosugar **3a** or **3b** (4 mmol) and corresponding freshly prepared mercaptothiazole **2a–e** in 70 mL of EtOH (mixture can be warmed to 40 °C for better solubility), a solution of I_2 (0.8 M in 95% ethanol) was slowly added until a persistent yellow-brown color was observed. The reaction mixture was stirred for 15 min at room temperature, and the excess iodine was quenched with a sodium thiosulfate solution (5% in H_2O) until a light yellow solution was formed. Sodium hydrogen carbonate (0.5 g) was added to neutralize the formed HI and the reaction mixture was stirred for 20 min. Inorganic salts were filtered off, the obtained solution was evaporated, and the residue was subjected to column chromatography (elution with a hexane-benzene-acetone mixture, 2:1:1 *v*/*v*) to obtain the corresponding conjugate **4a–j**.

5-[(2,3,4,6-Tetra-O-acetyl-β-D-glucopyranosyl)disulfanyl]-2-amino-4-(4-methoxyphenyl) thiazole (**4a**); yield 553 mg (23%, recovery of the starting disulfide **1a** 43%), white solid, mp 82–83 °C. ^{1}H NMR (300 MHz, $CDCl_3$) δ: 7.80 (d, *J* = 8.8 Hz, 2H, 2×Ar-H), 6.97 (d, *J* = 8.8 Hz, 2H, 2×Ar-H), 5.32 (s, 2H, -NH_2), 5.04–5.16 (m, 2H, H^3, H^4), 5.01 (t, *J* = 9.4 Hz, 1H, H^2), 4.48 (d, *J* = 9.4 Hz, 1H, H^1), 4.26 (dd, *J* = 12.4, 4.8 Hz, 1H, H^{6a}), 4.14 (dd, *J* = 12.4, 2.3 Hz, 1H, H^{6b}), 3.86 (s, 3H, -OCH_3), 3.49–3.54 (m, 1H, H^5), 2.09 (s, 3H, -$COCH_3$), 2.02 (s, 3H, -$COCH_3$), 2.00 (s, 6H, 2×-$COCH_3$). ^{13}C NMR (75 MHz, $CDCl_3$) δ: 171.1, 170.3, 169.4, 169.3 (×2), 160.1, 157.6, 131.1 (×2), 126.2, 113.7 (×2), 111.9, 87.4, 76.3, 73.9, 69.7, 68.3, 62.0, 55.4, 21.1, 20.7 (×3). IR ($CHCl_3$, ν, cm^{-1}): 3498, 3396, 3092, 3003, 2963, 2840, 1755, 1603, 1524, 1504, 1465, 1441, 1417, 1369, 1331, 1250, 1211, 1178, 1089, 1057, 1037. HRMS (ESI): *m/z* $[M - H]^-$ calcd for $C_{24}H_{27}N_2O_{10}S_3$: 599.0833; found: 599.0831.

5-[(2,3,4,6-Tetra-O-acetyl-β-D-glucopyranosyl)disulfanyl]-2-amino-4-phenylthiazole (**4b**); yield 456 mg (20%, recovery of the starting disulfide **1b** 45%), white solid, mp 114–115 °C. ^{1}H NMR (300 MHz, $CDCl_3$) δ: 7.78–7.82 (m, 2H, 2×Ar-H), 7.36–7.47 (m, 3H, 3×Ar-H), 5.36 (s, 2H, -NH_2), 5.05–5.15 (m, 2H, H^3, H^4), 5.02 (t, *J* = 9.4 Hz, 1H, H^2), 4.46 (d, *J* = 9.4 Hz, 1H, H^1), 4.27 (dd, *J* = 12.4, 4.7 Hz, 1H, H^{6a}), 4.12 (dd, *J* = 12.4, 2.1 Hz, 1H, H^{6b}), 3.44–3.49 (m, 1H, H^5), 2.10 (s, 3H, -$COCH_3$), 2.03 (s, 3H, -$COCH_3$), 2.00 (s, 6H, 2× -$COCH_3$). ^{13}C NMR (75 MHz, $CDCl_3$) δ: 171.1, 170.3, 169.4, 169.3 (×2), 157.9, 133.8, 129.8 (×2), 128.9, 128.4 (×2), 113.6, 87.4, 76.3, 73.9, 69.7, 68.2, 62.0, 21.1, 20.7 (×3). IR ($CHCl_3$, ν, cm^{-1}): 3498, 3396, 3064, 3003, 1755, 1603, 1505, 1468, 1439, 1369, 1333, 1241, 1228, 1206, 1194, 1090, 1058. HRMS (ESI): *m/z* $[M - H]^-$ calcd for $C_{23}H_{25}N_2O_9S_3$: 569.0727; found: 569.0723.

5-[(2,3,4,6-Tetra-O-acetyl-β-D-glucopyranosyl)disulfanyl]-2-amino-4-(4-bromophenyl) thiazole (**4c**); yield 623 mg (24%, recovery of the starting disulfide **1c** 38%), white solid, mp 98–100 °C. ^{1}H NMR (300 MHz, $CDCl_3$) δ: 7.71 (d, *J* = 8.4 Hz, 2H, 2×Ar-H), 7.57 (d, *J* = 8.4 Hz, 2H, 2×Ar-H), 5.29 (s, 2H, -NH_2), 5.08–5.20 (m, 2H, H^3, H^4), 5.04 (t, *J* = 9.4 Hz, 1H, H^2), 4.50 (d, *J* = 9.4 Hz, 1H, H^1), 4.31 (dd, *J* = 12.4, 4.9 Hz, 1H, H^{6a}), 4.17 (dd, *J* = 12.4, 2.2 Hz, 1H, H^{6b}), 3.55–3.60 (m, 1H, H^5), 2.10 (s, 3H, -$COCH_3$), 2.04 (s, 3H, -$COCH_3$), 2.01 (s, 3H, -$COCH_3$), 2.00 (s, 3H, -$COCH_3$). ^{13}C NMR (75 MHz, $CDCl_3$) δ: 171.0, 170.3, 169.4, 169.3 (×2), 156.6, 132.8, 131.5 (×2), 131.3 (×2), 123.1, 114.2, 87.1, 76.5, 73.9, 69.7, 68.4, 62.1,

21.1, 20.7 (×3). IR ($CHCl_3$, ν, cm^{-1}): 3498, 3396, 3053, 2982, 2361, 1756, 1603, 1506, 1457, 1395, 1369, 1328, 1241, 1230, 1203, 1193, 1163, 1058, 1011. HRMS (ESI): *m/z* $[M - H]^-$ calcd for $C_{23}H_{24}BrN_2O_9S_3$: 646.9833; found: 646.9834.

5-[(2,3,4,6-Tetra-O-acetyl-β-D-glucopyranosyl)disulfanyl]-2-amino-4-(4-chlorophenyl) thiazole (**4d**); yield 460 mg (19%, recovery of the starting disulfide **1d** 47%), white solid, mp 116–118 °C. ^{1}H NMR (300 MHz, $CDCl_3$) δ: 7.76 (d, *J* = 8.6 Hz, 2H, 2×Ar-H), 7.41 (d, *J* = 8.6 Hz, 2H, 2×Ar-H), 5.39 (s, 2H, -NH_2), 5.09–5.20 (m, 2H, H^3, H^4), 5.04 (t, *J* = 9.5 Hz, 1H, H^2), 4.51 (d, *J* = 9.5 Hz, 1H, H^1), 4.31 (dd, *J* = 12.5, 4.9 Hz, 1H, H^{6a}), 4.17 (dd, *J* = 12.5, 2.2 Hz, 1H, H^{6b}), 3.56–3.62 (m, 1H, H^5), 2.10 (s, 3H, -$COCH_3$), 2.04 (s, 3H, -$COCH_3$), 2.01 (s, 6H, 2× -$COCH_3$). ^{13}C NMR (75 MHz, $CDCl_3$) δ: 171.1, 170.3, 169.5, 169.4, 169.3, 156.6, 134.8, 132.2, 131.0 (×2), 128.6 (×2), 113.9, 86.9, 76.4, 73.8, 69.5, 68.3, 62.1, 21.1, 20.8 (×3). IR ($CHCl_3$, ν, cm^{-1}): 3498, 3396, 3020, 2959, 1753, 1603, 1506, 1459, 1432, 1400, 1369, 1328, 1247, 1193, 1164, 1092, 1058. HRMS (ESI): *m/z* $[M - H]^-$ calcd for $C_{23}H_{24}ClN_2O_9S_3$: 603.0338; found: 603.0333.

5-[(2,3,4,6-Tetra-O-acetyl-β-D-glucopyranosyl)disulfanyl]-2-amino-4-(p-tolyl)thiazole (**4e**); yield 608 mg (26%, recovery of the starting disulfide **1e** 37%), white solid, mp 90–92 °C. ^{1}H NMR (300 MHz, $CDCl_3$) δ: 7.67 (d, *J* = 8.1 Hz, 2H, 2×Ar-H), 7.25 (d, *J* = 8.4 Hz, 2H, 2×Ar-H), 5.74 (s, 2H, -NH_2), 5.01–5.11 (m, 2H, H^3, H^4), 4.98 (t, *J* = 9.4 Hz, 1H, H^2), 4.40 (d, *J* = 9.4 Hz, 1H, H^1), 4.23 (dd, *J* = 12.4, 4.7 Hz, 1H, H^{6a}), 4.10 (dd, *J* = 12.4, 2.0 Hz, 1H, H^{6b}), 3.39–3.44 (m, 1H, H^5), 2.39 (s, 3H, -CH_3), 2.08 (s, 3H, -$COCH_3$), 2.02 (s, 3H, -$COCH_3$), 1.99 (s, 3H, -$COCH_3$), 1.98 (s, 3H, -$COCH_3$). ^{13}C NMR (75 MHz, $CDCl_3$) δ: 171.0, 170.3, 169.7, 169.4 (×2), 158.0, 138.9, 130.9, 129.6 (×2), 129.1 (×2), 112.5, 87.4, 76.2, 73.8, 69.6, 68.2, 62.0, 21.4, 21.0, 20.7 (×3). IR ($CHCl_3$, ν, cm^{-1}): 3499, 3396, 3061, 2959, 2361, 2342, 2361, 2342, 1755, 1603, 1504, 1469, 1369, 1329, 1306, 1242, 1230, 1214, 1193, 1090, 1057. HRMS (ESI): *m/z* $[M - H]^-$ calcd for $C_{24}H_{27}N_2O_9S_3$: 583.0884; found: 583.0879.

5-[(2,3,4-Tri-O-acetyl-β-D-xylopyranosyl)disulfanyl]-2-amino-4-(4-methoxyphenyl) thiazole (**4f**); yield 634 mg (30%, recovery of the starting disulfide **1a** 35%), white solid, mp 85–86 °C. ^{1}H NMR (300 MHz, $CDCl_3$) δ: 7.75 (d, *J* = 8.8 Hz, 2H, 2×Ar-H), 6.97 (d, *J* = 8.8 Hz, 2H, 2×Ar-H), 5.80 (s, 2H, -NH_2), 5.06 (t, *J* = 8.5 Hz, 1H, H^3), 4.97 (t, *J* = 8.6 Hz, 1H, H^2), 4.68–4.76 (m, 1H, H^4), 4.48 (d, *J* = 8.6 Hz, 1H, H^1), 4.03 (dd, *J* = 11.6, 5.3 Hz, 1H, H^{5a}), 3.85 (s, 3H, -OCH_3), 3.13 (dd, *J* = 11.6, 9.6 Hz, 1H, H^{5b}), 2.02 (s, 6H, 2×-$COCH_3$), 2.00 (s, 3H, -$COCH_3$). ^{13}C NMR (75 MHz, $CDCl_3$) δ: 170.1, 169.8, 169.5, 169.4, 160.1, 157.5, 131.0 (×2), 126.3, 113.7 (×2), 111.7, 87.9, 72.4, 69.5, 68.5, 65.9, 55.4, 20.8 (×3). IR ($CHCl_3$, ν, cm^{-1}): 3499, 3396, 2976, 2840, 1755, 1603, 1524, 1504, 1465, 1441, 1417, 1369, 1331, 1249, 1178, 1037. HRMS (ESI): *m/z* $[M - H]^-$ calcd for $C_{21}H_{23}N_2O_8S_3$: 527.0622; found: 527.0614.

5-[(2,3,4-Tri-O-acetyl-β-D-xylopyranosyl)disulfanyl]-2-amino-4-phenylthiazole (**4g**); yield 558 mg (28%, recovery of the starting disulfide **1b** 34%), white solid, mp 204–206 °C. ^{1}H NMR (300 MHz, $CDCl_3$) δ: 7.79–7.82 (m, 2H, 2×Ar-H), 7.38–7.48 (m, 3H, 3×Ar-H), 5.33 (s, 2H, -NH_2), 5.05 (t, *J* = 8.5 Hz, 1H, H^3), 4.97 (t, *J* = 8.5 Hz, 1H, H^2), 4.67–4.74 (m, 1H, H^4), 4.47 (d, *J* = 8.6 Hz, 1H, H^1), 4.00 (dd, *J* = 11.6, 5.3 Hz, 1H, H^{5a}), 3.09 (dd, *J* = 11.6, 9.6 Hz, 1H, H^{5b}), 2.03 (s, 3H, -$COCH_3$), 2.02 (s, 3H, -$COCH_3$), 2.01 (s, 3H, -$COCH_3$). ^{13}C NMR (75 MHz, $CDCl_3$) δ: 170.1, 169.8, 169.4, 169.2, 158.2, 133.9, 129.7 (×2), 128.9, 128.3 (×2), 113.8, 87.9, 72.4, 69.5, 68.5, 66.0, 20.9, 20.8 (×2). IR ($CHCl_3$, ν, cm^{-1}): 3501, 3398, 3106, 2985, 2869, 1754, 1603, 1507, 1460, 1371, 1328, 1245, 1193, 1164, 1122, 1092, 1069, 1035. HRMS (ESI): *m/z* $[M - H]^-$ calcd for $C_{20}H_{21}N_2O_7S_3$: 497.0516; found: 497.0512.

5-[(2,3,4-Tri-O-acetyl-β-D-xylopyranosyl)disulfanyl]-2-amino-4-(4-bromophenyl)thiazole (**4h**); yield 808 mg (31%, recovery of the starting disulfide **1c** 46%), white solid, mp 171–173 °C. ^{1}H NMR (300 MHz, $CDCl_3$) δ: 7.73 (d, *J* = 8.6 Hz, 2H, 2×Ar-H), 7.58 (d, *J* = 8.6 Hz, 2H, 2×Ar-H), 5.24 (s, 2H, -NH_2), 5.09 (t, *J* = 8.5 Hz, 1H, H^3), 5.00 (t, *J* = 8.6 Hz, 1H, H^2), 4.66–4.74 (m, 1H, H^4), 4.53 (d, *J* = 8.6 Hz, 1H, H^1), 4.06 (dd, *J* = 11.6, 5.2 Hz, 1H,

H^{5a}), 3.15 (dd, *J* = 11.6, 9.4 Hz, 1H, H^{5b}), 2.04 (s, 6H, 2× -$COCH_3$), 2.01 (s, 3H, -$COCH_3$). ^{13}C NMR (75 MHz, $CDCl_3$) δ: 170.1, 169.9, 169.4 (×2), 156.7, 132.8, 131.6 (×2), 131.2 (×2), 123.1, 114.1, 87.8, 72.2, 69.5, 68.5, 65.9, 20.8 (×3). IR ($CHCl_3$, ν, cm^{-1}): 3502, 3398, 3056, 2978, 2415, 2361, 1755, 1603, 1505, 1459, 1395, 1371, 1327, 1245, 1232, 1224, 1214, 1188, 1071, 1035, 1011. HRMS (ESI): *m/z* $[M-H]^-$ calcd for $C_{20}H_{20}BrN_2O_7S_3$: 574.9621; found: 574.9615.

5-[(2,3,4-Tri-O-acetyl-β-D-xylopyranosyl)disulfanyl]-2-amino-4-(4-chlorophenyl)thiazole (**4i**); yield 490 mg (23%, recovery of the starting disulfide **1d** 48%), white solid, mp 196–197 °C. ^{1}H NMR (300 MHz, $CDCl_3$) δ: 7.78 (d, *J* = 8.5 Hz, 2H, 2×Ar-H), 7.42 (d, *J* = 8.5 Hz, 2H, 2×Ar-H), 5.36 (s, 2H, -NH_2), 5.10 (t, *J* = 8.5 Hz, 1H, H^3), 5.01 (t, *J* = 8.5 Hz, 1H, H^2), 4.66–4.74 (m, 1H, H^4), 4.53 (d, *J* = 8.6 Hz, 1H, H^1), 4.06 (dd, *J* = 11.6, 5.2 Hz, 1H, H^{5a}), 3.16 (dd, *J* = 11.6, 9.4 Hz, 1H, H^{5b}), 2.04 (s, 3H, -$COCH_3$), 2.01 (s, 6H, 2× -$COCH_3$). ^{13}C NMR (75 MHz, $CDCl_3$) δ: 170.1, 169.9, 169.4, 169.2, 156.7, 134.8, 132.4, 130.9 (×2), 128.6 (×2), 114.1, 87.7, 72.2, 69.4, 68.5, 65.9, 20.9 (×2), 20.8. IR ($CHCl_3$, ν, cm^{-1}): 3501, 3398, 3106, 2985, 2869, 1754, 1603, 1507, 1460, 1371, 1328, 1245, 1193, 1164, 1122, 1092, 1069, 1035. HRMS (ESI): *m/z* $[M-H]^-$ calcd for $C_{20}H_{20}ClN_2O_7S_3$: 531.0126; found: 531.0125.

5-[(2,3,4-Tri-O-acetyl-β-D-xylopyranosyl)disulfanyl]-2-amino-4-(p-tolyl)thiazole (**4j**); yield 543 mg (27%, recovery of the starting disulfide **1e** 44%), white solid, mp 199–200 °C. ^{1}H NMR (300 MHz, $CDCl_3$) δ: 7.69 (d, *J* = 8.1 Hz, 2H, 2×Ar-H), 7.26 (d, *J* = 8.1 Hz, 2H, 2×Ar-H), 5.50 (s, 2H, -NH_2), 5.05 (t, *J* = 8.5 Hz, 1H, H^3), 4.96 (t, *J* = 8.6 Hz, 1H, H^2), 4.67–4.74 (m, 1H, H^4), 4.45 (d, *J* = 8.6 Hz, 1H, H^1), 4.01 (dd, *J* = 11.6, 5.3 Hz, 1H, H^{5a}), 3.09 (dd, *J* = 11.6, 9.5 Hz, 1H, H^{5b}), 2.39 (s, 3H, -CH_3), 2.03 (s, 3H, -$COCH_3$), 2.02 (s, 3H, -$COCH_3$), 2.00 (s, 3H, -$COCH_3$). ^{13}C NMR (75 MHz, $CDCl_3$) δ: 170.1, 169.8, 169.4, 169.3, 158.3, 138.9, 131.2, 129.6 (×2), 129.1 (×2), 112.9, 88.1, 72.5, 69.6, 68.6, 66.0, 21.5, 20.8 (×3). IR ($CHCl_3$, ν, cm^{-1}): 3501, 3397, 3114, 3019, 2983, 2869, 1755, 1602, 1505, 1470, 1432, 1371, 1329, 1306, 1248, 1193, 1118, 1068, 1035. HRMS (ESI): *m/z* $[M-H]^-$ calcd for $C_{21}H_{23}N_2O_7S_3$: 511.0673; found: 511.0669.

3.1.2. General Procedure for the Synthesis of Deacetylated Derivatives 5a–j

The corresponding acetylated disulfide **4a–j** (0.5 mmol) was added to the solution of HCl in absolute MeOH (7 mL, ~1.6 M) and stirred for 15 h at room temperature. The solvent was removed under reduced pressure, and the residue was recrystallized from a mixture of MeOH-acetone (2:3 *v*/*v*, 5 mL) to give the hydrochloride of deacetylated product **5a–j**.

5-[(β-D-glucopyranosyl)disulfanyl]-2-amino-4-(4-methoxyphenyl)thiazole hydrochloride (5a); yield 211 mg (90%), white solid, mp 169–170 °C. ^{1}H NMR (300 MHz, DMSO-d_6) δ: 8.83 (br s, 1H, -N^+H), 7.70 (d, J = 8.8 Hz, 2H, 2×Ar-H), 7.06 (d, J = 8.8 Hz, 2H, 2×Ar-H), 5.23 (br.s, 6H, 4× -OH, -NH_2), 4.35 (d, J = 8.8 Hz, 1H, H^1), 3.81 (s, 3H, -OCH_3), 3.68 (dd, J = 11.8, 1.5 Hz, 1H, H^{6a}), 3.52 (dd, J = 11.8, 5.0 Hz, 1H, H^{6b}), 3.07–3.18 (m, 3H, H^2, H^3, H^4), 3.00–3.04 (m, 1H, H^5). ^{13}C NMR (75 MHz, DMSO-d_6) δ: 169.6, 160.1, 147.5, 130.6 (×2), 122.3, 113.9 (×2), 110.6, 88.5, 81.5, 77.9, 72.1, 69.5, 60.5, 55.4. IR (KBr, ν, cm^{-1}): 3392, 3271, 3048, 2361, 2342, 1172, 1717, 1699, 1636, 1619, 1570, 1541, 1507, 1405, 1385, 1313, 1279, 1256, 1211, 1181, 1112, 1054, 1024, 883, 832, 736, 720. HRMS (ESI): m/z $[M-H]^-$ calcd for $C_{16}H_{20}ClN_2O_6S_3$: 467.0177; found: 467.0175.

5-[(β-D-glucopyranosyl)disulfanyl]-2-amino-4-phenylthiazole hydrochloride (**5b**); yield 202 mg (92%), white solid, mp 178–180 °C. ^{1}H NMR (300 MHz, DMSO-d_6) δ: 8.65 (br.s, 1H, -N^+H), 7.72–7.75 (m, 2H, 2×Ar-H), 7.46–7.53 (m, 3H, 3×Ar-H), 5.95 (br s, 6H, 4× -OH, -NH_2), 4.35 (d, *J* = 8.7 Hz, 1H, H^1), 3.67 (dd, *J* = 11.8, 1.5 Hz, 1H, H^{6a}), 3.50 (dd, *J* = 11.8, 5.0 Hz, 1H, H^{6b}), 3.05–3.15 (m, 3H, H^2, H^3, H^4), 2.99–3.03 (m, 1H, H^5). ^{13}C NMR (75 MHz, DMSO-d_6) δ: 169.8, 148.2, 133.3, 129.5, 129.2 (×2), 128.4 (×2), 112.3, 88.6, 81.6, 77.9, 72.0, 69.5, 60.6. IR (KBr, ν, cm^{-1}): 3375, 3275, 2932, 2892, 2360, 1628, 1587, 1570, 1543, 1488, 1448,

1425, 1385, 1323, 1278, 1207, 1183, 1091, 1061, 1016, 985, 919, 870, 788, 765, 732. HRMS (ESI): *m/z* $[M - H]^-$ calcd for $C_{15}H_{18}ClN_2O_5S_3$: 437.0072; found: 437.0070.

5-[(β-D-glucopyranosyl)disulfanyl]-2-amino-4-(4-bromophenyl)thiazole hydrochloride (**5c**); yield 243 mg (94%), white solid, mp 145–147 °C. ^{1}H NMR (300 MHz, DMSO-d_6) δ: 8.28 (br s, 1H, -N$^+$H), 7.72 (d, *J* = 8.8 Hz, 2H, 2×Ar-H), 7.68 (d, *J* = 8.8 Hz, 2H, 2×Ar-H), 5.46 (br s, 6H, 4× -OH, -NH$_2$), 4.33 (d, *J* = 8.7 Hz, 1H, H^1), 3.65 (dd, *J* = 11.7, 1.5 Hz, 1H, H^{6a}), 3.50 (dd, *J* = 11.7, 5.0 Hz, 1H, H^{6b}), 3.07–3.26 (m, 3H, H^2, H^3, H^4), 2.96–3.00 (m, 1H, H^5). ^{13}C NMR (75 MHz, DMSO-d_6) δ: 169.8, 148.6, 131.3 (×2), 131.1 (×2), 130.9, 122.6, 112.5, 88.5, 81.6, 78.0, 72.1, 69.4, 60.5. IR (KBr, ν, cm^{-1}): 3289, 2932, 2360, 2341, 1635, 1621, 1592, 1540, 1485, 1434, 1385, 1350, 1271, 1055, 1007, 915, 883, 824, 732, 712. HRMS (ESI): *m/z* $[M - H]^-$ calcd for $C_{15}H_{17}BrClN_2O_5S_3$: 514.9177; found: 514.9178.

5-[(β-D-glucopyranosyl)disulfanyl]-2-amino-4-(4-clorophenyl)thiazole hydrochloride (**5d**); yield 189 mg (80%), white solid, mp 149–150 °C. ^{1}H NMR (300 MHz, DMSO-d_6) δ: 8.40 (br s, 1H, -N$^+$H), 7.80 (d, *J* = 8.5 Hz, 2H, 2×Ar-H), 7.55 (d, *J* = 8.5 Hz, 2H, 2×Ar-H), 5.47 (br s, 6H, 4× -OH, -NH$_2$), 4.33 (d, *J* = 8.8 Hz, 1H, H^1), 3.65 (dd, *J* = 11.8, 1.5 Hz, 1H, H^{6a}), 3.50 (dd, *J* = 11.8, 5.0 Hz, 1H, H^{6b}), 3.06–3.16 (m, 3H, H^2, H^3, H^4), 2.95–3.00 (m, 1H, H^5). ^{13}C NMR (75 MHz, DMSO-d_6) δ: 169.8, 148.9, 133.8, 130.9 (×2), 130.1, 128.4 (×2), 112.3, 88.5, 81.6, 78.0, 72.1, 69.4, 60.5. IR (KBr, ν, cm^{-1}): 3372, 2362, 1637, 1621, 1560, 1385, 1349, 1271, 1095, 1054, 1016, 914, 882, 827, 732, 717. HRMS (ESI): *m/z* $[M - H]^-$ calcd for $C_{15}H_{17}Cl_2N_2O_5S_3$: 470.9682; found: 470.9684.

5-[(β-D-glucopyranosyl)disulfanyl]-2-amino-4-(p-tolyl)thiazole hydrochloride (**5e**); yield 193 mg (85%), white solid, mp 175–176 °C. ^{1}H NMR (300 MHz, DMSO-d_6) δ: 8.84 (br s, 1H, -N$^+$H), 7.62 (d, *J* = 8.0 Hz, 2H, 2×Ar-H), 7.32 (d, *J* = 8.0 Hz, 2H, 2×Ar-H), 5.82 (br s, 6H, 4× -OH, -NH$_2$), 4.34 (d, *J* = 8.7 Hz, 1H, H^1), 3.68 (dd, *J* = 11.8, 1.5 Hz, 1H, H^{6a}), 3.51 (dd, *J* = 11.8, 5.0 Hz, 1H, H^{6b}), 3.07–3.15 (m, 3H, H^2, H^3, H^4), 2.99–3.04 (m, 1H, H^5), 2.36 (s, 3H, -CH$_3$). ^{13}C NMR (75 MHz, DMSO-d_6) δ: 169.7, 147.1, 139.5, 129.1 (×2), 129.0 (×2), 126.9, 111.9, 88.5, 81.6, 77.9, 72.0, 69.5, 60.5, 21.0. IR (KBr, ν, cm^{-1}): 3277, 2907, 2361, 2343, 1717, 1699, 1628, 1586, 1566, 1542, 1504, 1435, 1385, 1346, 1320, 1273, 1209, 1186, 1115, 1086, 1057, 1021, 985, 870, 839, 817, 789, 734, 713. HRMS (ESI): *m/z* $[M - H]^-$ calcd for $C_{16}H_{20}ClN_2O_5S_3$: 451.0228; found: 451.0227.

5-[(β-D-xylopyranosyl)disulfanyl]-2-amino-4-(4-methoxyphenyl)thiazole hydrochloride (**5f**); yield 195 mg (89%), white solid, mp 149–150 °C. ^{1}H NMR (300 MHz, DMSO-d_6) δ: 8.73 (br s, 1H, -N$^+$H), 7.70 (d, *J* = 8.8 Hz, 2H, 2×Ar-H), 7.06 (d, *J* = 8.8 Hz, 2H, 2×Ar-H), 5.72 (br s, 5H, 3× -OH, -NH$_2$), 4.37 (d, *J* = 8.3 Hz, 1H, H^1), 3.81 (s, 3H, -OCH$_3$), 3.72 (dd, *J* = 11.1, 4.8 Hz, 1H, H^{5a}), 3.18–3.26 (m, 1H, H^3), 3.09–3.14 (m, 2H, H^2, H^4), 2.96 (t, *J* = 10.5 Hz, 1H, H^{5b}). ^{13}C NMR (75 MHz, DMSO-d_6) δ: 169.5, 159.9, 149.1, 130.4 (×2), 123.2, 113.7 (×2), 110.1, 89.6, 77.0, 71.9, 69.0, 68.9, 55.3. IR (KBr, ν, cm^{-1}): 3153, 3046, 2836, 2361, 2341, 1171, 1614, 1574, 1508, 1403, 1386, 1307, 1285, 1262, 1179, 1097, 1061, 1027, 968, 896, 831, 784, 740, 720. HRMS (ESI): *m/z* $[M - H]^-$ calcd for $C_{15}H_{18}ClN_2O_5S_3$: 437.0072; found: 437.0081.

5-[(β-D-xylopyranosyl)disulfanyl]-2-amino-4-phenylthiazole hydrochloride (**5g**); yield 192 mg (94%), white solid, mp 159–160 °C. ^{1}H NMR (300 MHz, DMSO-d_6) δ: 8.54 (br s, 1H, -N$^+$H), 7.71–7.74 (m, 2H, 2×Ar-H), 7.46–7.53 (m, 3H, 3×Ar-H), 5.72 (br s, 5H, 3× -OH, -NH$_2$), 4.35 (d, *J* = 8.3 Hz, 1H, H^1), 3.70 (dd, *J* = 11.1, 4.8 Hz, 1H, H^{5a}), 3.16–3.23 (m, 1H, H^3), 3.07–3.13 (m, 2H, H^2, H^4), 2.93 (t, *J* = 10.8 Hz, 1H, H^{5b}). ^{13}C NMR (75 MHz, DMSO-d_6) δ: 169.7, 148.7, 130.5, 129.5, 129.2 (×2), 128.4 (×2), 112.1, 89.6, 77.1, 71.9, 69.1 (×2). IR (KBr, ν, cm^{-1}): 3371, 3279, 2926, 2859, 2684, 1670, 1625, 1592, 1572, 1542, 1487, 1458, 1421, 1385, 1343, 1280, 1240, 1214, 1182, 1158, 1095, 1061, 998, 965, 895, 818, 768, 731. HRMS (ESI): *m/z* $[M - H]^-$ calcd for $C_{14}H_{16}ClN_2O_4S_3$: 406.9966; found: 406.9968.

5-[(β-D-xylopyranosyl)disulfanyl]-2-amino-4-(4-bromophenyl)thiazole hydrochloride (**5h**); yield 222 mg (91%), white solid, mp 144–146 °C. ^{1}H NMR (300 MHz, DMSO-d_6) δ: 8.16 (br s, 1H, -$N^{+}H$), 7.73 (d, J = 8.8 Hz, 2H, 2×Ar-H), 7.68 (d, J = 8.8 Hz, 2H, 2×Ar-H), 5.61 (br s, 5H, 3× -OH, -NH_2), 4.35 (d, J = 8.3 Hz, 1H, H^1), 3.71 (dd, J = 11.1, 5.0 Hz, 1H, H^{5a}), 3.20–3.27 (m, 1H, H^3), 3.08–3.16 (m, 2H, H^2, H^4), 2.93 (t, J = 10.3 Hz, 1H, H^{5b}). ^{13}C NMR (75 MHz, DMSO-d_6) δ: 169.8, 150.0, 131.2 (×2), 131.1 (×2), 130.9, 122.4, 112.0, 89.6, 77.1, 72.0, 69.1 (×2). IR (KBr, ν, cm^{-1}): 3367, 2361, 1626, 1566, 1542, 1508, 1487, 1458, 1435, 1385, 1292, 1211, 1184, 1088, 1053, 1007, 967, 897, 825, 712. HRMS (ESI): m/z $[M - H]^-$ calcd for $C_{14}H_{15}BrClN_2O_4S_3$: 484.9071; found: 484.9074.

5-[(β-D-xylopyranosyl)disulfanyl]-2-amino-4-(4-clorophenyl)thiazole hydrochloride (**5i**); yield 184 mg (83%), white solid, mp 135–137 °C. ^{1}H NMR (300 MHz, DMSO-d_6) δ: 8.07 (br s, 1H, -$N^{+}H$), 7.78 (d, J = 8.5 Hz, 2H, 2×Ar-H), 7.55 (d, J = 8.5 Hz, 2H, 2×Ar-H), 5.96 (br s, 5H, 3× -OH, -NH_2), 4.35 (d, J = 8.0 Hz, 1H, H^1), 3.70 (dd, J = 11.2, 4.8 Hz, 1H, H^{5a}), 3.18–3.25 (m, 1H, H^3), 3.07–3.15 (m, 2H, H^2, H^4), 2.92 (t, J = 10.4 Hz, 1H, H^{5b}). ^{13}C NMR (75 MHz, DMSO-d_6) δ: 169.8, 149.5, 133.8, 130.9 (×2), 130.4, 128.3 (×2), 112.1, 89.6, 77.1, 72.0, 69.1 (×2). IR (KBr, ν, cm^{-1}): 3372, 1699, 1619, 1566, 1542, 1487, 1458, 1429, 1385, 1354, 1292, 1236, 1093, 1049, 1010, 964, 897, 826, 779, 733, 718. HRMS (ESI): m/z $[M - H]^-$ calcd for $C_{14}H_{15}Cl_2N_2O_4S_3$: 440.9576; found: 440.9571.

5-[(β-D-xylopyranosyl)disulfanyl]-2-amino-4-(p-tolyl)thiazole hydrochloride (**5j**); yield 184 mg (87%), white solid, mp 134–136 °C. ^{1}H NMR (300 MHz, DMSO-d_6) δ: 8.64 (br s, 1H, -$N^{+}H$), 7.62 (d, J = 8.0 Hz, 2H, 2×Ar-H), 7.31 (d, J = 8.0 Hz, 2H, 2×Ar-H), 5.53 (br s, 5H, 3× -OH, -NH_2), 4.36 (d, J = 8.1 Hz, 1H, H^1), 3.72 (dd, J = 11.1, 4.8 Hz, 1H, H^{5a}), 3.18–3.26 (m, 1H, H^3), 3.08–3.17 (m, 2H, H^2, H^4), 2.96 (t, J = 10.4 Hz, 1H, H^{5b}), 2.36 (s, 3H, -CH_3). ^{13}C NMR (75 MHz, DMSO-d_6) δ: 169.6, 148.1, 139.3, 129.0 (×2), 128.9 (×2), 127.3, 111.5, 89.6, 77.1, 71.9, 69.1 (×2), 21.0. IR (KBr, ν, cm^{-1}): 3290, 2919, 2858, 1624, 1569, 1505, 1435, 1385, 1294, 1234, 1215, 1188, 1089, 1053, 1003, 957, 897, 818, 782, 733, 713. HRMS (ESI): m/z $[M - H]^-$ calcd for $C_{15}H_{18}ClN_2O_4S_3$: 421.0123; found: 421.0117.

3.2. Cell Lines

Human erythrocytes were purchased from the blood transfusion station Vladivostok. Human breast cancer cell lines MCF-7^{HTB-22}, and MDA-MB-231$^{CRM-HTB-26}$, liver hepatocellular carcinoma Hep G2$^{HB-8065}$, prostate adenocarcinoma PC-3$^{CRL-1435}$, cervical adenocarcinoma HeLa$^{CRM-CCL-2}$, and normal bronchial epithelial cells BEAS-2B $^{CRL-3588}$ were received from ATCC (Manassas, VA, USA).

DMEM medium (Biolot, Russia) with 1% penicillin/streptomycin and 10% fetal bovine serum (FBS) (Biolot, Russia) was used for cultivation of Hep G2, PC-3, HeLa, and Beas-2b. MEM medium (Biolot, Russia) with 1% penicillin/streptomycin sulfate (Biolot, Russia) and FBS (Biolot, Russia) to a final concentration of 10% for MCF-7 and MDA-MB-231 cells.

3.3. MTT Assay to Determine the Effect on Cell Viability

The effect of the studied compounds on the viability of human cancer and normal cells was determined using the MTT (3-[4,5-dimethylthiazol-2-yl]-2,5 diphenyl tetrazolium bromide) assay. Briefly, 6×10^3 cells per well were seeded into 96-well plates and incubated for 24 h for adhesion, followed by incubation for 24 h with different concentrations of the substances. After incubation, the medium containing the test substances was replaced with 100 μL of fresh medium. Then, 10 μL of MTT (Sigma-Aldrich, Madison, WI, USA) reagent (5 mg/mL MTT in PBS) was added into the cells and the plates for additional 4 h. Thereafter, 100 μL of SDS-HCl solution (1 g SDS/10 mL dH_2O/17 μL 6N HCl) was added to each well and incubated for 18 h. The absorbance of the converted formazan dye was measured using a Multiskan FC microplate photometer (Thermo Scientific, Waltham, MA,

USA) at a wavelength of 570 nm. All experiments were performed in triplicate. Cytotoxic activity was expressed as a percentage of the cell viability.

3.4. Wound Scratch Migration Assay

To analyze the effect of the tested compounds on the migration of HeLa tumor cells, special migration inserts (Culture-insert 2 Well 24, ibiTreat, Martinsried, Germany) were used, which left a gap of 500 ± 50 μm (according to the manufacturer's data) between the cells attached to the plate. HeLa cells at a concentration of 5×10^5 were added to each well of the migration insert for 24 h, the insert was removed, and the cells were washed twice with PBS to remove cell debris and floating cells and loaded with the fluorescent probe CFDA-SE (Lumiprobe, Moscow, Russia) at a concentration of 10 μM for 5 min. The cells were treated with different concentrations of the studied compounds for 0 and 24 h. Cells treated with culture medium alone were used as vehicle controls. Cell migration in the wound area was observed under a fluorescence microscope (MIB-2-FL, LOMO, St. Petersburg, Russia) with a 10× objective.

3.5. Colony Formation Assay to Determine the Effect on Cell Proliferation

The effect of the test compounds on HeLa cell proliferation was analyzed using a clonogenic assay. Briefly, HeLa cells were cultured in 6-well plates at a density of 1×10^2 cells per well, and compounds were added at concentrations of 5 or 10 μM. Untreated culture medium was used as a control. The cells were incubated for 14 days at 37 °C with 5% CO_2 until the cells in the control plates formed colonies that were visible to the eye and had a good size (at least 50 cells per colony). Before fixation and staining, the medium was removed and the cells were washed twice with PBS. The colonies were then fixed with methanol for 25 min and stained with 0.5% crystal violet for 25 min at room temperature. The plates were then washed with water and air-dried.

3.6. Antimicrobial Activity

The antimicrobial activity of the compounds was determined against Gram-positive bacteria *Staphylococcus aureus* (ATCC 21027), Gram-negative bacteria *Escherichia coli* (VKPM B-7935), and yeast-like fungi *Candida albicans* (KMM 455) (all test strains were obtained from the Collection of Marine Microorganisms KMM PIBOC FEB RAS) in liquid nutrient media. Test cultures of *S. aureus*, *E. coli*, and *C. albicans* were grown in Petri dishes on a solid nutrient medium (Mueller–Hinton broth with the addition of agar—16.0 g/L) at 37 °C for 24 h. The antimicrobial activity of the compounds was determined by the change in optical density and expressed as the percentage of bacterial inhibition at different concentrations of substances added to the well of the microorganism suspension, compared to the control [41]. The compounds were dissolved in dimethyl sulfoxide (DMSO) at a concentration of 10 mM and stored at −20 °C. Before the experiment, the solution of substances in DMSO was diluted with PBS at a concentration of 0.5–100.0 μM and added to the wells so that the concentration of DMSO in the culture medium was less than 1%. Antimicrobial activity was determined in 96-well microplates in a liquid Mueller–Hinton nutrient medium. For *S. aureus*, *E. coli*, and *C. albicans*, a bacterial suspension of 10^6 CFU in 1 mL of the media was used, 90 μL was added to each well of the microplates and then incubated in a thermostatted shaker at 37 °C for 18 h. Inhibition of microorganism growth was assessed by measuring the optical density at 620 nm using a microplate reader (Thermo Fisher Scientific, Waltham, MA, USA) after preliminary shaking of the plates for 10 min. All experiments were performed in triplicate. Gentamicin (*S. aureus* and *E. coli*) and nitrofungin (*C. albicans*) were used as positive controls, and 1% DMSO in PBS was used as a negative control.

3.7. Inhibition of Biofilm Formation

Biofilm formation was performed according to the method described by Walencka et al. [39], with minor modifications. The compounds were dissolved in dimethyl sulfoxide (DMSO) at a concentration of 10 mM and stored at −20 °C. Before the experiment, the solution of substances in DMSO was diluted with PBS at a concentration of 0.5–100.0 μM and added to the wells so that the concentration of DMSO in the culture medium was less than 1%. Biofilm formation was assessed in 96-well microplates in a liquid Mueller–Hinton nutrient medium. For *S. aureus*, *E. coli*, and *C. albicans*, a bacterial suspension of 10^6 CFU in 1 mL of medium was used, 90 μL was added to each well of the microplates and then incubated in a thermostatted shaker at 37 °C for 24 h. After incubation, the suspension of planktonic microorganisms was removed from the plate and washed with PBS. Next, 100 μL of PBS and 10 μL of MTT (3-(4,5-dimethylthiazol-2-yl)-2,5-diphenyltetrazolium bromide, MTT reagent, Sigma) stock solution (5 mg/mL) were added to the wells and incubated for 3 h at 37 °C. After incubation, all the solution was removed from the wells, 100 μL of DMSO was added, and the plate was shaken for 10 min until all formazan crystals had dissolved. The absorption was measured using a plate reader (Thermo Fisher Scientific, Waltham, MA, USA) at a wavelength of 570 nm. The activity of the substances was assessed by the change in optical density compared with that of the control. All experiments were performed in triplicate. Gentamicin (*S. aureus* and *E. coli*) and nitrofungin (*C. albicans*) were used as positive controls, and 1% DMSO in PBS was used as a negative control.

4. Conclusions

In this study, we developed a procedure for the synthesis of new carbohydrate-thiazole disulfides based on the alkaloid thiacarpine and its analogs **1a–e**. It was found that the type of sugar residue had a weaker influence on the activity of the synthesized compounds than the substituent type in the phenyl moiety of the thiazole ring. Acetylation of the sugar residue and the presence of –Me, –Br, and –OMe substituents of the aromatic part of the heterocyclic fragment are the most important factors for cytotoxic activity. The most promising compounds for the study of antitumor potential, **4c**, **4e**, **4f**, and **4h**, showed good migration inhibition and colony formation inhibition in cancer cell lines. The highest antimicrobial activity was observed for synthetic bromine **4c**, **4h**, **5c**, **5h**, and chlorine derivatives **4i** and **5d** which exhibited antimicrobial activity and inhibited biofilm formation by the Gram-positive bacteria *S. aureus*, Gram-negative bacteria *E. coli*, and yeast-like fungi *C. albicans*, comparable to the action of a standard antibiotic (gentamicin) and antimycotic (nitrofungin), but did not demonstrate hemolytic activity at concentrations up to 25 μM. The results also show that the introduction of carbohydrate fragments (glucose or xylose) into the molecule does not guarantee an increase in antimicrobial activity or selectivity of action on tumor cells, but in some cases, such a desired effect can be observed. Thus, of the studied substances, compound **5h** containing a xylose moiety, showed the most potent antimicrobial activity, on average twice as high as the starting symmetric disulfide **1c** and the comparison drugs.

Supplementary Materials: The following supporting information can be downloaded at: https://www.mdpi.com/article/10.3390/md23030117/s1. The copies of ^{1}H NMR and ^{13}C NMR spectra for compounds **4a–j**, **5a–j**.

Author Contributions: Conceptualization, V.P.A.; methodology, Y.E.S.; validation, Y.E.S., E.S.M. and E.A.C.; formal analysis, Y.E.S., E.S.M. and E.A.C.; investigation, D.N.P., Y.E.S., S.M.K., N.N.B., E.S.M., A.L.B. and E.A.C.; resources, D.N.P., Y.E.S., E.S.M. and E.A.C.; writing—original draft preparation, D.N.P., Y.E.S., E.S.M. and E.A.C.; writing—review and editing, D.N.P., Y.E.S., E.S.M. and E.A.C.; visualization, D.N.P., Y.E.S., E.S.M. and E.A.C.; supervision, D.N.P.; project administration,

D.N.P.; funding acquisition, D.N.P. All authors have read and agreed to the published version of the manuscript.

Funding: This research was funded by Russian Science Foundation, grant number 23-23-00357.

Institutional Review Board Statement: Not applicable.

Informed Consent Statement: Not applicable.

Data Availability Statement: Data are contained within the article and Supplementary Materials.

Acknowledgments: We thank Artur R. Chingizov for assistance in studying antimicrobial activity, R. S. Popov for MS measurements, and V. P. Glazunov for recording IR spectra. The study was carried out using the equipment of the Collective Facilities Center "The Far Eastern Center for Structural Molecular Research (NMR/MS) PIBOC FEB RAS".

Conflicts of Interest: The authors declare no conflicts of interest.

References

1. Kang, H.; Fenical, W. Polycarpine dihydrochloride: A cytotoxic dimeric disulfide alkaloid from the Indian Ocean ascidian *Polycarpa clavate*. *Tetrahedron Lett.* **1996**, *37*, 2369–2372. [CrossRef]
2. Fedoreyev, S.A.; Radchenko, O.S.; Novikov, V.L.; Isakov, V.V.; Ilyin, S.G.; Popov, A.M.; Elyakov, G.B.; Murphy, P.T.; Willis, R.H.; Baker, J.T. Polycarpine, a novel cytotoxic sulfur-containing alkaloid from the marine ascidian *Polycarpa aurata* and related compounds. In Proceedings of the Eighth International Symposium on Marine Natural Products, Tenerife, Canary Islands, Spain, 10–15 September 1995; pp. 196–197.
3. Wang, W.; Oda, T.; Fujita, A.; Mangindaan, R.E.P.; Nakazawa, T.; Ukai, K.; Kobayashi, H.; Namikoshi, M. Three new sulfur-containing alkaloids, polycarpaurines A, B, and C, from an Indonesian ascidian *Polycarpa aurata*. *Tetrahedron* **2007**, *63*, 409–412. [CrossRef]
4. Abas, S.A.; Hossain, M.B.; Helm, D.; Schmitz, F.J.; Laney, M.; Cabuslay, R.; Schatzman, R.C. Alkaloids from the Tunicate *Polycarpa aurata* from Chuuk Atoll. *J. Org. Chem.* **1996**, *61*, 2709–2712. [CrossRef]
5. Popov, A.M.; Novikov, V.L.; Radchenko, O.S.; Elyakov, G.B. The cytotoxic and antitumor activities of the imidazole alkaloid polycarpin from the ascidian *Polycarpa aurata* and its synthetic analogues. *Dokl. Biochem. Biophys.* **2002**, *385*, 213–218. [CrossRef]
6. Das, D.; Sikdar, C.; Bairagi, M. Recent developments of 2-aminothiazoles in medicinal chemistry. *Eur. J. Med. Chem.* **2016**, *109*, 89–98. [CrossRef] [PubMed]
7. Elsadek, F.M.; Ahmed, M.B.; Farahat, F.M. An overview on synthetic 2-aminothiazole—Based compounds associated with four biological activities. *Molecules* **2021**, *26*, 1449. [CrossRef]
8. Radchenko, O.S.; Novikov, V.L.; Willis, R.H.; Murphy, P.T.; Elyakov, G.B. Synthesis of polycarpine, a cytotoxic sulfur-containing alkaloid from the ascidian *Polycarpa aurata* and related compounds. *Tetrahedron Lett.* **1997**, *38*, 3581–3584. [CrossRef]
9. Wan, Y.; Long, J.; Gao, H.; Tang, Z. 2-Aminothiazole: A privileged scaffold for the discovery of anti-cancer agents. *Eur. J. Med. Chem.* **2021**, *210*, 112953. [CrossRef] [PubMed]
10. Alizadeh, S.R.; Hashemi, S.M. Development and therapeutic potential of 2-aminothiazole derivatives in anticancer drug discovery. *Med. Chem. Res.* **2021**, *30*, 771–806. [CrossRef]
11. Minickaite, R.; Grybaite, B.; Vaickelioniene, R.; Kavaliauskas, P.; Petraitis, V.; Petraitiene, R.; Tumosiene, I.; Jonuskiene, I.; Mickevicius, V. Synthesis of novel aminothiazole derivatives as promising antiviral, antioxidant and antibacterial candidates. *Int. J. Mol. Sci.* **2022**, *23*, 7688. [CrossRef]
12. Siddiqui, H.L.; Zia-Ur-Rehman, M.; Ahmad, N.; Weaver, G.W.; Lucas, P.D. Synthesis and antibacterial activity of bis [2-amino-4-phenyl-5-thiazolyl] disulfides. *Chem. Pharm. Bull.* **2007**, *55*, 1014–1017. [CrossRef]
13. Cascioferro, S.; Parrino, B.; Carbone, D.; Schillaci, D.; Giovannetti, E.; Cirrincione, G.; Diana, P. Thiazoles, their benzofused systems, and thiazolidinone derivatives: Versatile and promising tools to combat antibiotic resistance. *J. Med. Chem.* **2020**, *63*, 7923. [CrossRef] [PubMed]
14. Lemilemu, F.; Bitew, M.; Demissie, T.B.; Eswaramoorthy, R.; Endale, M. Synthesis, antibacterial and antioxidant activities of thiazole-based schiff base derivatives: A combined experimental and computational study. *BMC Chem.* **2021**, *15*, 67. [CrossRef]
15. Siddiqui, N.; Ahsan, W. Synthesis, anticonvulsant and toxicity screening of thiazolyl–thiadiazole derivatives. *Med. Chem. Res.* **2011**, *20*, 261–268. [CrossRef]
16. Grewal, A.S.; Kharb, R.; Prasad, D.N.; Dua, J.S.; Lather, V. Design synthesis and evaluation of novel 3,5-disubstituted benzamide derivatives as allosteric glucokinase activators. *BMC Chem.* **2019**, *13*, 2. [CrossRef] [PubMed]
17. Gallardo-Godoy, A.; Gever, J.; Fife, K.L.; Silber, B.M.; Prusiner, S.B.; Renslo, A.R. 2-Aminothiazoles as therapeutic leads for prion diseases. *J. Med. Chem.* **2011**, *54*, 1010–1021. [CrossRef] [PubMed]

18. Patel, P.J.; Patel, S.G.; Upadhyay, D.B.; Ravi, L.; Dhanasekaran, A.; Patel, H.M. An efficient, catalyst-free and aqueous ethanol-mediated synthesis of 5-((2-aminothiazol-5-yl)(phenyl)methyl)-6-hydroxypyrimidine-2,4(1*H*,3*H*)-dione derivatives and their antioxidant activity. *RSC Adv.* **2023**, *13*, 24466. [CrossRef]
19. Kayagil, I.; Demirayak, S. Synthesis and anticancer activities of some thiazole derivatives. *Phosphorus Sulfur Silicon* **2009**, *184*, 2197–2207. [CrossRef]
20. Lee, Y.-S.E.; Chuang, S.-H.; Huang, L.Y.L.; Lai, C.-L.; Lin, Y.-H.; Yang, J.-Y.; Liu, C.-W.; Yang, S.-C.; Lin, H.-S.; Chang, C.-C.; et al. Discovery of 4-aryl-N-arylcarbonyl-2-aminothiazoles as Hec1/Nek2 inhibitors. Part I: Optimization of in vitro potencies and pharmacokinetic properties. *J. Med. Chem.* **2014**, *57*, 4098–4110. [CrossRef]
21. Liao, M.; Huang, D.; Cheng, Y.-X. 2-Amino-4-(aminomethyl)thiazole-based derivatives as potential antitumor agents: Design, synthesis, cytotoxicity and apoptosis inducing activities. *Mendeleev Commun.* **2023**, *33*, 73–76. [CrossRef]
22. Turos, E.; Revell, K.D.; Ramaraju, P.; Gergeres, D.A.; Greenhalgh, K.; Young, A.; Sathyanarayan, N.; Dickey, S.; Lim, D.; Alhamadsheh, M.M.; et al. Unsymmetric aryl-alkyl disulfide growth inhibitors of methicillin-resistant *Staphylococcus aureus* and *Bacillus anthracis*. *Bioorg. Med. Chem.* **2008**, *16*, 6501–6508. [CrossRef]
23. Choi, K.J.; Yu, Y.G.; Hahn, H.G.; Choi, J.D.; Yoon, M.Y. Characterization of acetohydroxyacid synthase from *Mycobacterium tuberculosis* and the identification of its new inhibitor from the screening of a chemical library. *FEBS Lett.* **2005**, *579*, 4903–4910. [CrossRef] [PubMed]
24. Choi, K.J.; Noh, K.M.; Kim, D.E.; Ha, B.H.; Kim, E.E.; Yoon, M.Y. Identification of the catalytic subunit of acetohydroxyacid synthase in *Haemophilus influenzae* and its potent inhibitors. *Arch. Biochem. Biophys.* **2007**, *466*, 24–30. [CrossRef]
25. Sudarikov, D.V.; Gyrdymova, Y.V.; Borisov, A.V.; Lukiyanova, J.M.; Rumyantcev, R.V.; Shevchenko, O.G.; Baidamshina, D.R.; Zakarova, N.D.; Kayumov, A.R.; Sinegubova, E.O.; et al. Synthesis and Biological Activity of Unsymmetrical Monoterpenylhetaryl Disulfides. *Molecules* **2022**, *27*, 5101. [CrossRef]
26. Sepúlveda, C.S.; García, C.C.; Levingston Macleod, J.M.; López, N.; Damonte, E.B. Targeting of arenavirus RNA synthesis by a carboxamide-derivatized aromatic disulfide with virucidal activity. *PLoS ONE* **2013**, *8*, e81251. [CrossRef]
27. Lara, H.H.; Ixtepan-Turrent, L.; Garza-Treviño, E.N.; Flores-Teviño, S.M.; Borkow, G.; Rodriguez-Padilla, C. Antiviral propierties of 5, 5′-dithiobis-2-nitrobenzoic acid and bacitracin against T-tropic human immunodeficiency virus type 1. *Virol. J.* **2011**, *8*, 137. [CrossRef]
28. García, C.C.; Topisirovic, I.; Djavani, M.; Borden, K.L.; Damonte, E.B.; Salvato, M.S. An antiviral disulfide compound blocks interaction between arenavirus Z protein and cellular promyelocytic leukemia protein. *Biochem. Biophys. Res. Commun.* **2010**, *393*, 625–630. [CrossRef] [PubMed]
29. Wang, L.; Bao, B.; Song, G.; Chen, C.; Zhang, X.; Lu, W.; Wang, Z.; Cai, Y.; Li, S.; Fu, S. Discovery of unsymmetrical aromatic disulfides as novel inhibitors of SARS-CoV main protease: Chemical synthesis, biological evaluation, molecular docking and 3D-QSAR study. *Eur. J. Med. Chem.* **2017**, *137*, 450–461. [CrossRef] [PubMed]
30. Morais, G.R.; Falconer, R.A. Glycosyl disulfides: Importance, synthesis and application to chemical and biological systems. *Org. Biomol. Chem.* **2021**, *19*, 82–100. [CrossRef]
31. Vrudhula, V.M.; MacMaster, J.F.; Li, Z.; Kerr, D.E.; Senter, P.D. Reductively activated disulfide prodrugs of paclitaxel. *Bioorg. Med. Chem. Lett.* **2002**, *12*, 3591–3594. [CrossRef]
32. Calvaresi, E.C.; Hergenrother, P.J. Glucose conjugation for the specific targeting and treatment of cancer. *Chem. Sci.* **2013**, *4*, 2319–2333. [CrossRef]
33. Shi, Y.; Liu, S.; Ahmad, S.; Gao, Q. Targeting key transporters in tumor glycolysis as a novel anticancer strategy. *Curr. Top. Med. Chem.* **2018**, *18*, 454–466. [CrossRef] [PubMed]
34. Fu, J.; Yang, J.; Seeberger, P.H.; Yin, J. Glycoconjugates for glucose transporter-mediated cancer-specific targeting and treatment. *Carbohydr. Res.* **2020**, *498*, 108195. [CrossRef] [PubMed]
35. McClintock, M.K.; Zhang, K. Chapter 8: Xylose Metabolism and Its Metabolic Engineering Applications. In *Engineering Microbial Metabolism for Chemical Synthesis. Reviews and Perspectives*; Yan, Y., Ed.; World Scientific: Singapore, 2018; pp. 209–235. [CrossRef]
36. Cheng, J.; Miller, C.J. Quantum interference effects in self-assembled asymmetric disulfide monolayers: Comparisons between experiment and ab initio/Monte Carlo theories. *J. Phys. Chem. B* **1997**, *101*, 1058–1062. [CrossRef]
37. Yang, F.; Wang, W.; Li, K.; Zhao, W.; Dong, X. Efficient one-pot construction of unsymmetrical disulfide bonds with TCCA. *Tetrhedron Lett.* **2017**, *58*, 218–222. [CrossRef]
38. Ishigeev, R.S.; Potapov, V.A.; Skurchenko, I.V.; Khabibulina, A.G.; Amosova, S.V. Synthesis of new polycyclic compounds via the reaction of quinoline-8-sulfenyl halides with cyclic alkenes. *Chem. Heterocycl. Comp.* **2021**, *57*, 314–319. [CrossRef]
39. Walencka, E.; Sadowska, B.; Rózalska, S.; Hryniewicz, W.; Rózalska, B. Lysostaphin as a potential therapeutic agent for staphylococcal biofilm eradication. *Pol. J. Microbiol.* **2005**, *54*, 191–200.

40. Fujihira, T.; Chida, M.; Kamijo, H.; Takido, T.; Seno, M. Novel synthesis of 1-thioglycopyranoses via thioiminium salts. *J. Carbohyd. Chem.* **2002**, *21*, 287–292. [CrossRef]
41. Zhuravleva, O.I.; Chingizova, E.A.; Oleinikova, G.K.; Starnovskaya, S.S.; Antonov, A.S.; Kirichuk, N.N.; Menshov, A.S.; Popov, R.S.; Kim, N.Y.; Berdyshev, D.V.; et al. Anthraquinone derivatives and other aromatic compounds from marine fungus *Asteromyces cruciatus* KMM 4696 and their effects against *Staphylococcus aureus*. *Mar. Drugs* **2023**, *21*, 431. [CrossRef]

marine drugs

MDPI

Article

Synthesis and Evaluation of Antitumor and Anti-Angiogenesis Activity of Pyrone- or Pyridone-Embedded Analogs of Cortistatin A

Yuri Fujimoto [1], Kanako Mizuno [2], Yuta Nakamura [1], Masayoshi Arai [2] and Naoyuki Kotoku [1,2,*]

[1] College of Pharmaceutical Sciences, Ritsumeikan University, 1-1-1 Noji-higashi, Kusatsu 525-8577, Shiga, Japan; ph0162fp@ed.ritsumei.ac.jp (Y.F.); ph0187si@ed.ritsumei.ac.jp (Y.N.)
[2] Graduate School of Pharmaceutical Sciences, Osaka University, 1-6 Yamadaoka, Suita 565-0871, Osaka, Japan; m.kombbbbb@gmail.com (K.M.); araim@phs.osaka-u.ac.jp (M.A.)
* Correspondence: kotoku@fc.ritsumei.ac.jp; Tel.: +81-77-561-4920

Abstract: Simplified analogs of cortistatin A were synthesized and biologically evaluated to develop novel antitumor substances that target angiogenesis. To analyze the effect of substituents at positions corresponding to C-2 and/or C-4 of the A-ring, various pyrone- or pyridone-embedded analogs were designed and synthesized. Among the prepared analogs, the pyridone analog **19** bearing a methyl group at C-2 and a hydroxyl group at C-4 showed potent and selective growth inhibitory activity against human umbilical vein endothelial cells (HUVECs, IC_{50} = 0.001 μM, selective index over that against human epidermoid carcinoma KB3-1 cells = 6400), exceeding those of natural products. The analog **19** of oral administration exhibited excellent in vivo antitumor activity in mice subcutaneously inoculated with sarcoma S180 cells.

Keywords: Cortistatin A; simplified analog; antitumor effect; anti-angiogenic substance

1. Introduction

Marine natural products have garnered considerable attention as rich and promising sources of drug candidates, particularly in the field of anticancer drug discovery [1,2]. Generally, novel bioactive compounds are identified through bioassay-guided separation using simple phenotype screening. Phenotypic screening is a promising method for the discovery of first-in-class drug candidates with a novel mode of action, and the mechanistic study of these compounds might reveal an unknown signaling pathway as a target for drug discovery [3].

However, only small amounts of bioactive compounds can be isolated from the extracts of marine organisms such as sponges and tunicates, and the sustainable supply of active compounds has been a challenge for further evaluation and drug development. Chemical synthesis of bioactive natural products and their analogs can overcome this drawback. In contrast, natural products often exhibit diverse bioactivities by binding to multiple target molecules (proteins) because of their complex chemical structures containing various functional groups. Successful examples indicate that the truncation of its partial structure or several moieties is effective, in some cases, for extracting the essential scaffold of the natural product, resulting in a reduction in the number of target proteins without losing specific bioactivity. In addition, structural simplification leads to the supply of a substantial amount of the compound for further studies such as in vivo activity evaluation and mechanistic analysis. Furthermore, the Absorption, Distribution, Metabolism, Excretion, and Toxicity (ADMET) profiles of the compounds can be improved by reducing the

 https://doi.org/10.3390/md23040179

molecular weight [4–6]. Therefore, the syntheses of truncated natural products based on structure–activity relationship (SAR) studies are expected to develop more accessible and promising drug leads with optimized activity or chemical stability.

Angiogenesis is a critical phenomenon in tumor growth and metastasis. A growing tumor must form new blood capillaries that provide nutrients and oxygen. New blood vessels are also used as a way for tumor cells to enter the circulation, resulting in cancer metastasis to other organs. Therefore, substances that inhibit angiogenesis have considerable potential as novel therapeutic agents for cancer treatment [7]. Previously, our research group focused on identifying anti-angiogenic substances as novel anti-cancer drug seeds from marine organisms and isolated cortistatins, a family of novel *abeo*-9(10-19)-androstane-type steroidal alkaloids, from the Indonesian marine sponge *Corticium simplex* [8–10]. Cortistatin A (**1**, Figure 1), a major constituent of *C. simplex*, shows potent and highly selective antiproliferative activity against human umbilical vein endothelial cells (HUVECs). Compound **1** also exhibited potent in vitro anti-angiogenic activity and inhibited the migration and tubular formation of HUVECs induced by vascular endothelial growth factor (VEGF) or basic fibroblast growth factor (bFGF). In addition, mechanistic study implied that the selective growth inhibitory activity of **1** against HUVECs is independent on the VEGF signal pathway, one of the main pathways of angiogenesis and thus the target of most existing anti-angiogenesis drugs [11].

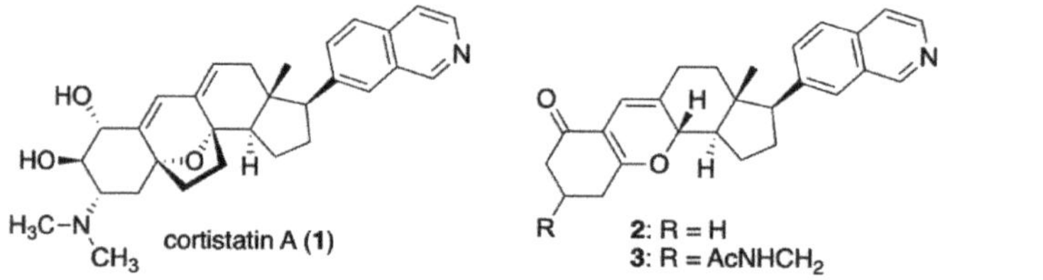

Figure 1. The chemical structure of cortistatin A (**1**) and its simplified analogs (**2**,**3**).

Because of their unique chemical and biological properties, cortistatins are promising novel anti-angiogenic drug leads. However, the supply of cortistatins from natural sources to validate the feasibility of their use as potential drug leads is impractical. Although many synthetic studies on cortistatins [12–14] including six total syntheses [15–20] have been reported, the overall yields were insufficient in most cases. Therefore, we focused on developing structurally simplified analogs and identified a useful compound, **2** (Figure 1). Analog **2** exhibited good antiproliferative activity in HUVECs with significant selectivity and potent in vivo anti-tumor activity following oral administration [21]. Since then, we have focused on developing a more promising anticancer drug lead through structural optimization of analog **2** as a scaffold and establishing a more practical synthetic method [22]. This resulted in the generation of a novel analog with potent activity and selectivity exceeding those of natural cortistatin A (**1**), as well as significant in vivo anti-angiogenic activity, the detailed results of which are presented in this report.

2. Results and Discussions

2.1. Design of Pyrone- or Pyridone-Embedded Analogs

As shown in Figure 1, the anthracene-like planar ABC-ring system of simplified analogs **2** and **3** developed by our group mimics the core structure of **1**, an *abeo*-9(10-19)-androstane-type rearranged steroidal backbone with an oxa-bridge between the 5- and 8-position. The tricyclic structure was prepared by Knoevenagel condensation of aldehyde **4** and cyclohexane-1,3-dione derivatives (Figure 2A). Considering the σ-symmetry of cyclohexane-1,3-dione, regioselective functionalization of the A-ring was possible only at the C-3 position of the natural product using 5-substituted cyclohexane-1,3-diones. As the analog **3**, with a acetamide moiety at C-3, exhibited potent growth inhibitory activity against HUVECs (IC_{50} = 0.0026 μM) and high selectivity over KB3-1 cells (IC_{50} = 8.2 μM, selective index (S.I.) = 3150), synthesis and evaluation of the analogs with C-2 and/or C-4-substitutents are highly desirable.

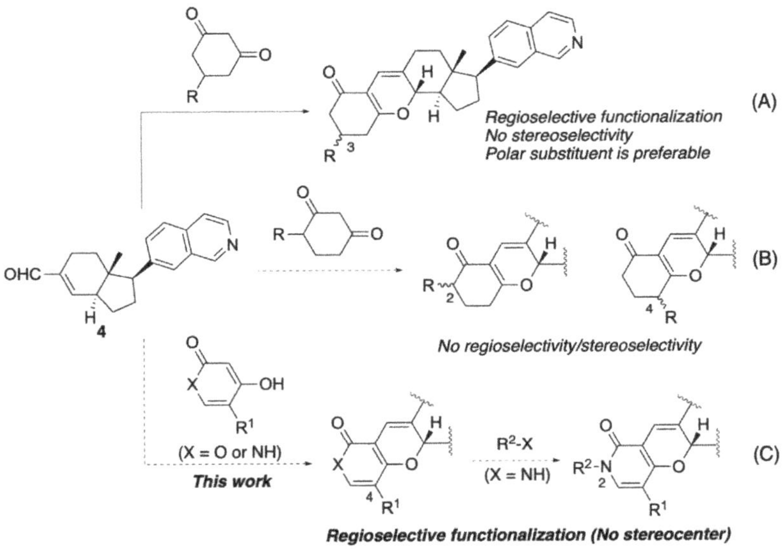

Figure 2. (**A**) General synthetic strategy of cortistatin A analog with a substituent at C-3. (**B**) Synthetic strategy of analogs with C-2 or C-4 substituent. (**C**) Synthetic strategy of novel analogs with substituents at C-2 or C-4 in this work using 4-hydroxy-2-pyrone or pyridone.

However, the above strategy might not be effective for preparing C-2- or C-4-substituted analogs because the Knoevenagel condensation between aldehyde **4** and 4-substituted cyclohexane-1,3-dione derivatives provides a mixture of two regioisomers in an uncontrolled manner (Figure 2B). Furthermore, no stereocontrol of the newly formed asymmetric center was achieved in either case.

Subsequently, we designed novel type of analogs in this work, as shown in Figure 2C. 4-Hydroxy-2-pyrone possesses a cyclic β-keto ester structure that may function as a surrogate for the cyclohexane-1,3-dione derivative in the synthesis of the analogs. The asymmetric nature of the 4-hydroxy-2-pyrone system gives the desired cyclized product with a unified structure, and the substituent at C-5 of the pyrone (R^1 in Figure 2C) leads to 2-oxa analogs with a substituent at C-4. The resulting AB-ring system, the 2*H*,5*H*-pyrano[4,3-*b*]pyran-5-one structure, has been observed in some meroterpenoid natural products, and successful total synthesis of the compounds was achieved through the formal [3 + 3] cycloaddition method [23,24].

Another promising alternative to the A-ring unit is 4-hydroxy-2-pyridone with a cyclic β-keto amide structure, and condensation-electrocyclization with aldehyde **4** would afford aza-analogs. Similarly, the synthesis of 2,6-dihydro-5*H*-pyrano[3,2-*c*]pyridin-5-one derivatives leads to natural products or bioactive compounds have been reported [25–29]. The nitrogen atom of pyridone corresponds to C-2 of the natural product and can be used as a base for another substituent R^2 to analyze the effect of verification at this position (Figure 2C).

2.2. *Synthesis of Pyrone- or Pyridone-Embedded Analogs of Cortistatin A*

2.2.1. Synthesis of Pyrone-Embedded Analogs

Based on the above strategy, the synthesis of pyrone-embedded analogs was performed first, as shown in Scheme 1. Aldehyde **4**, the common precursor of all the analogs in this work, was prepared from (+)-Hajos-Parrish ketone (**5**) through a procedure developed by our group [22]. Commercially available 4-hydroxy-6-methyl-2*H*-pyran-2-one (**6**) was reacted with **4** to afford the desired pyrone-embedded analog **7** in moderate yield. The use of piperidine as a base gave a better reaction yield than ethylenediamine, which was the optimized base in our previous work using cyclohexane-1,3-dione derivatives as A-ring parts [21]. Another analog, **11**, with a hydroxymethyl moiety at C-4, was obtained in a similar manner using the corresponding pyrone derivative **10**. According to literature [30], ethyl acetoacetate (**8**) reacts with malonyl chloride to give compound **9** in good yield. Subsequent reduction of the ester moiety of **9** with BH_3 [31] and condensation cyclization of the resulting compound **10** with aldehyde **4** afforded the analog **11** in good yield.

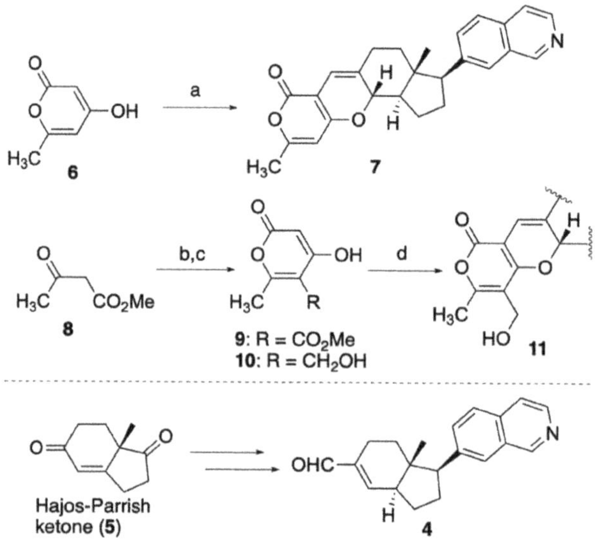

Scheme 1. Synthesis of pyrone-embedded analogs **7** and **11**. Reagents and conditions: (a) **4**, piperidine, 1,4-dioxane, 54%; (b) malonyl chloride, CH_2Cl_2, 74%; (c) $BH_3 \cdot S(CH_3)_2$, CH_2Cl_2/THF, 78%; (d) **4**, piperidine, 1,4-dioxane, 76%.

2.2.2. Synthesis of Pyridone-Embedded Analogs

Next, the synthesis of the pyridone-embedded analogs was attempted. Analog **13**, which has the simplest A-ring structure, was obtained by condensation of commercially available pyridine-2,4-diol (**12**) and aldehyde **4** (Scheme 2). Ethylenediamine diacetate was effective instead of piperidine in this case, although the reaction yield was not very high. *N*-Methyl analog **15** was obtained in the same manner using 4-hydroxy-1-methylpyridin-2(1*H*)-one (**14**), which was prepared from **12** [32].

Tracking the condensation reaction revealed that compound **iv**, the geometrical isomer of the desired Knoevenagel condensation product **iii** giving the electrocyclization product, was the main byproduct (Scheme 3). This means that the reaction is not in equilibrium, and the yield of the analog depends on the ratio of **iii** and **iv**. Indeed, no reaction was observed after the ethylenediamine treatment of isolated compound **iv**.

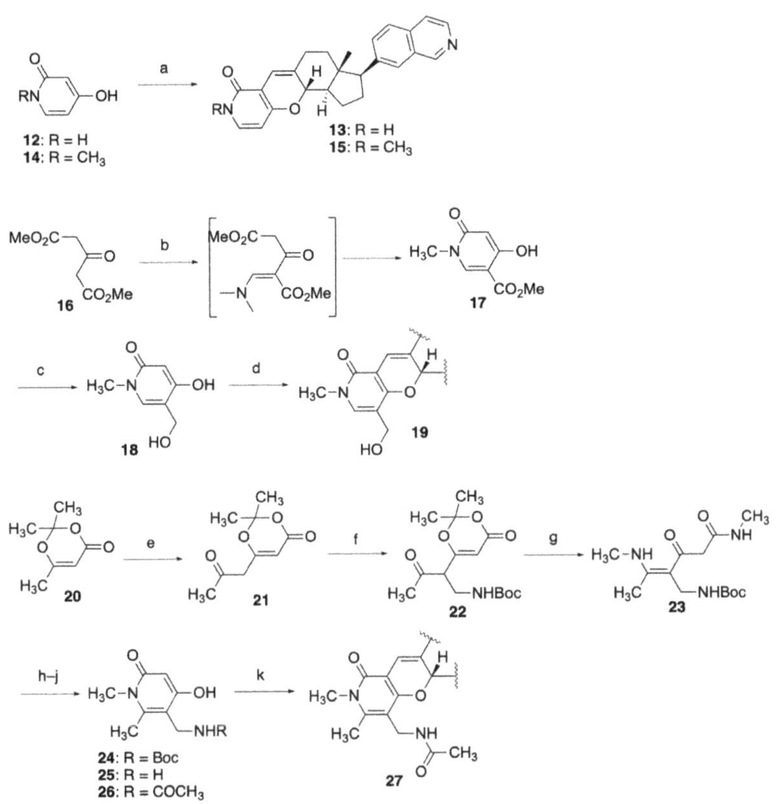

Scheme 2. Synthesis of pyridone-embedded analogs. Reagents and conditions: (a) ethylenediamine diacetate, DMF, 27% for **13**; 57% for **15**; (b) *N*,*N*-dimethylformamide dimethyl acetal, CH_3NH_2, MeOH, 37%; (c) DIBAL, toluene, −78 °C, 39%; (d) ethylenediamine diacetate, DMF, 45%; (e) LHMDS, AcCl, THF, 50%; (f) *N*-Boc(tosyl)methylamine, NaH, THF, 55%; (g) CH_3NH_2, toluene, 75 °C, 50%; (h) CH_3CO_2H, toluene; (i) TFA, CH_2Cl_2; (j) Ac_2O, K_2CO_3, DMF, 34% (3 steps); (k) ethylenediamine diacetate, DMF, 30%.

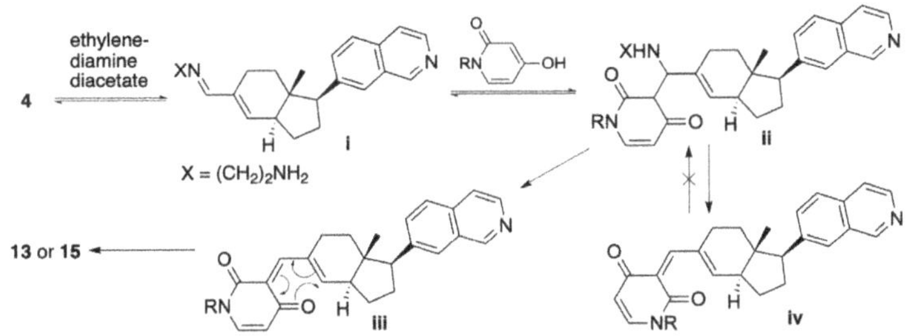

Scheme 3. Knoevenagel condensation-electrocyclization of aldehyde **4** and pyridone derivatives.

The pyridone-embedded analogs with polar substituents at C-4 were synthesized as follows: According to the literature [33], dimethyl acetone-1,3-dicarboxylate (**16**) was reacted with *N*,*N*-dimethylformamide dimethyl acetal to provide an enaminoketone, and subsequent cyclization occurred to give compound **17** by the treatment with methylamine. The ester moiety of **17** was then converted into a primary hydroxyl group via DIBAL reduction, yielding compound **18**. Finally, condensation with aldehyde **4** afforded the desired analog **19**.

Furthermore, analog **27** with an acetamide moiety at C-4 was prepared through a separate reaction because the substitution of the hydroxyl group of **19** with a nitrogen-based functionality under various conditions did not give satisfactory results. The acetylation of commercially available 2,2,6-trimethyl-4*H*-1,3-dioxine-4-one (**20**) afforded compound **21** [34]. The dienolate ion derived from **21** was then reacted with *N*-Boc(tosyl)methylamine to give compound **22** with a nitrogen-containing side chain in moderate yield [35]. Subsequent treatment with an excess amount of methylamine provided enamine-amide **23**, which was annulated in the presence of acetic acid by heating to give pyridone derivative **24**. The one-pot transformation of **22** to **24**, methylamine treatment, and subsequent heating did not yield satisfactory results. Removal of the Boc group of **24** using trifluoroacetic acid (TFA) and subsequent treatment of amine **25** with acetic anhydride under basic conditions provided compound **26**, the target A-ring fragment with an acetamidomethyl moiety at the C-4 position. Finally, condensation cyclization with aldehyde **4**, catalyzed by ethylenediamine diacetate, afforded desired analog **27**.

2.3. Biological Evaluation of Pyrone- or Pyridone-Embedded Analogs

2.3.1. Antiproliferative Activities of the Analogs Against Endothelial or Cancer Cells

The antiproliferative activities of the synthetic analogs against HUVECs and human epidermoid carcinoma KB3-1 cells were evaluated and the results are summarized in Table 1. It revealed that pyrone-embedded analogs **7** and **11** exhibited moderate or good antiproliferative activity against HUVEC (IC_{50} = 0.09 and 0.02 μM, respectively). Similar to the C-3 substitution described in our previous study (**2** vs. **3**) [22], the polar substituent introduced at C-4 was found to have a positive effect. In contrast, analog **7** showed weakened cytotoxicity against KB3-1 cells (IC_{50} = 62.8 μM). Compound **13** showed 9-fold higher potency than **7**, indicating that pyridone might be a more suitable A-ring structure than pyrone. The additional 3.3-fold potency of analog **15** over **13** clearly shows that *N*-methylation has a positive effect. Surprisingly, the introduction of a nonpolar substituent at that position increased bioactivity because cortistatin A (**1**) has a hydroxyl group at C-2. The introduction of a polar substituent at C-4 further enhanced the antiproliferative activity against HUVECs (analog **19** over **15**), the IC_{50} value of which exceeded that of the natural product without losing cell selectivity (6400 selective index value (IC_{50} against KB3-1 cells/IC_{50} against HUVECs)). Analog **27**, with an acetamide moiety at C-4, showed weaker activity against HUVECs (IC_{50} = 0.01 μM), whereas the same substituent at C-3 exhibited greater enhancing effect in the case of the analog **3** [22].

Table 1. Antiproliferative activities of cortistatin A analogs.

Compound	IC_{50} (μM)		S.I. [a]
	HUVECs	KB3-1	
1	0.0018 [b]	7.0 [b]	3900 [b]
2	0.035 [c]	10.5 [c]	300 [c]
3	0.0026 [c]	8.2 [c]	3150 [c]
7	0.09	62.8	700
11	0.02	10	500
13	0.01	11	1100
15	0.003	8.6	2870
19	0.001	6.4	6400
27	0.01	13.4	1340
28	0.56	4.8	8.6

[a] S.I. = selective index: IC_{50} against KB3-1 cells/IC_{50} against HUVECs. [b] Reported IC_{50} values in ref. [8]. [c] Reported IC_{50} values in Ref. [21].

In 2015, Shair et al. reported that cortistatin A (**1**) exhibited potent antiproliferative activity against some types of acute myeloid leukemia (AML) cells through the inhibition of cyclin-dependent kinase 8 (CDK8). They also showed that most solid tumor cell lines were not affected by treatment with **1**, although the effect of the compound on endothelial cells was not tested [36]. Subsequently, simplified steroidal analogs of **1** were found to exhibit similar potent inhibitory activity against CDK8 by Gray et al. in 2018. They also developed a proteolysis-targeting chimera (PROTAC) derived from a steroidal analog as an effective CDK8 [37].

To analyze the role of CDK8 in the proliferation of HUVECs, we prepared compound **28** (Figure 3), a steroidal analog, as a potent inhibitor of CDK8 (IC_{50} = 24 nM) [37] and evaluated its antiproliferative activities against HUVECs and KB3-1 cells. The analog **28** showed weak antiproliferative activity against HUVECs (IC_{50} = 0.56 μM) and low selectivity over KB3-1 cells (Table 1). This result implies that CDK8 contributes less to the proliferation of HUVECs at this time, although it is unclear whether the difference in activity between CDK8 inhibition and HUVECs growth inhibition is caused by the presence of another molecule responsible for the proliferation of HUVECs or by the low cell membrane permeability of **28**.

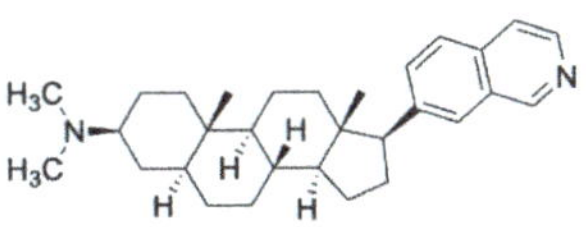

Figure 3. The chemical structure of a steroidal analog (**28**).

2.3.2. In Vivo Activity Evaluation of Analog 19

We evaluated in vivo activity of compound **19**, the most potent analog tested in this study, on the formation of new blood vessels, by Matrigel plug assay [21] in mice. As shown in Figure 4, oral administration of compound **19** prevented the formation of new blood capillaries in the Matrigel plug induced by bFGF. Compound **19** significantly decreased the hemoglobin content in the plug even after administration of 0.1 mg/kg administration, and the 1 mg/kg dose of **19** reduced the hemoglobin content to the same level as the negative control. These results indicate that analog **19** effectively inhibited in vivo angiogenesis.

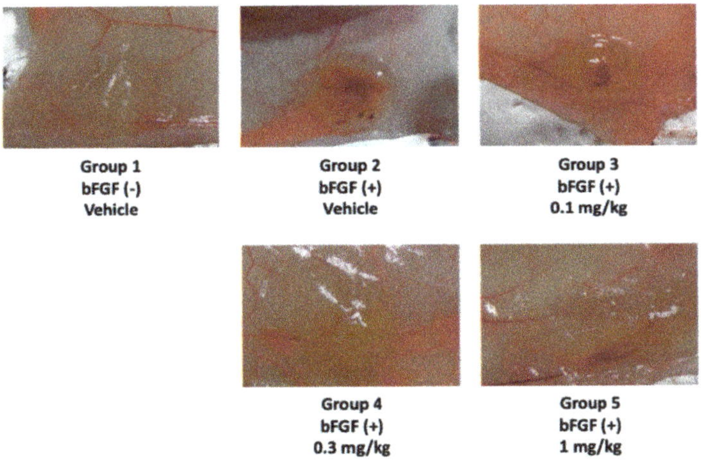

Figure 4. Pictures of the representative implanted Matrigel of the control and the treated group with the indicated amount of analog **19**.

During the assay, the mean body weights of mice in both the control and compound-treated groups were measured to determine the acute toxicity of the analogs. As shown in Table 2, no body weight loss was observed in any group even after day 9 of the treated group of 1 mg/kg administration. In addition, the hepatic toxicity of the compound was evaluated by measuring the activities of aspartate aminotransferase (AST) and alanine aminotransferase (ALT) in mouse serum on day 9. No significant changes in those enzyme activities were observed between the 1 mg/kg treatment group (AST: 57.8 ± 4.5 IU/L, ALT: 48.4 ± 3.3 IU/L) and control group (AST: 59.6 ± 3.1 IU/L, ALT: 43.6 ± 4.7 IU/L). These results indicated that analog **19** exhibited potent antiangiogenic activity in vivo without severe toxicity.

Table 2. In vivo anti-angiogenic effect, body weight measurement, and hepatotoxicity evaluation of analog **19**.

		19	Body Weight (g) [a]		Hb Content	AST	ALT
	bFGF	(mg/kg)	Day 1	Day 9	(μg/mg) [b]	(IU/L)	(IU/L)
1	–	–	26.03 ± 0.30	26.33 ± 0.33	0.65 ± 0.10	–	–
2	+	–	25.62 ± 0.52	25.98 ± 0.48	8.12 ± 1.25	59.6 ± 3.1	43.6 ± 4.7
3	+	0.1	25.70 ± 0.58	26.12 ± 0.58	3.27 ± 0.83	–	–
4	+	0.3	25.60 ± 0.64	26.14 ± 0.62	2.42 ± 0.79	–	–
5	+	1.0	26.30 ± 0.41	26.64 ± 0.39	0.79 ± 0.24	57.8 ± 4.5	48.4 ± 3.3

[a] The mean body weight of five mice in each group (mean ± SD). [b] Hemoglobin content (μg)/isolated Matrigel (mg) (mean ± SD).

We further examined the in vivo antitumor effects of analog **19**. Orally administered compound **19** of only 0.1 mg/kg exhibited significant tumor growth inhibition, with ~75% reduction compared to the control group, and more than 85% tumor weight reduction was observed with 1 mg/kg administration (Figure 5). Similar to the Matrigel plug assay, body weight loss and diarrhea, which are typical signs of acute toxicity, were not observed. The results of these in vivo experiments indicated that the potent anti-tumor activity of analog **19** was caused by the strong inhibition of angiogenesis promoted by the implanted tumor.

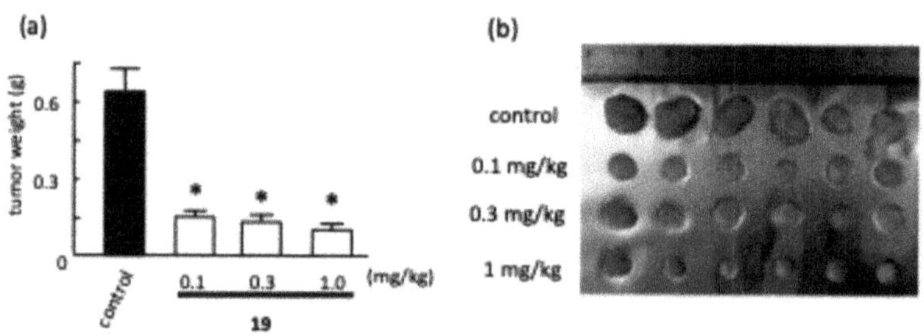

Figure 5. In vivo anti-tumor effect of analog **19**. (**a**) Tumor weight of each group (mean ± SD); *: $p < 0.01$. (**b**) Image of surged tumors after two weeks.

3. Materials and Methods

3.1. General

The following instruments were used to obtain physical data: a JASCO (Tokyo, Japan) DIP-370 digital polarimeter (L = 50 mm) for specific rotations; a JEOL (Tokyo, Japan) JNM-ECZ500R/S1 (^{1}H-NMR: 500 MHz, ^{13}C-NMR: 125 MHz) spectrometer or an Agilent (Santa Clara, CA, USA) NMR system (^{1}H-NMR: 600 MHz, ^{13}C-NMR: 151 MHz) for ^{1}H and ^{13}C NMR data, using tetramethylsilane or solvent residual peaks ($CDCl_3$: 7.26/77.0 ppm; DMSO-d_6: 2.49/39.5 ppm; CD_3OD: 3.31/49.0 ppm) as internal standards; Waters (Milford,

MA, USA) Q-Tof Ultima API or Xevo G2-XS Q-Tof mass spectrometer for ESI-TOF MS. Silica gel 60N (Kanto (Tokyo, Japan) 63–210 μm) and pre-coated thin layer chromatography (TLC) plates (Merck (Darmstadt, Germany) $60F_{254}$) were used for column chromatography and TLC, respectively. Spots on the TLC plates were detected by spraying with an acidic *p*-anisaldehyde solution (*p*-anisaldehyde: 25 mL, *c*-H_2SO_4: 25 mL, AcOH: 5 mL, EtOH: 425 mL) or with a phosphomolybdic acid solution (phosphomolybdic acid: 25 g, EtOH: 500 mL) with subsequent heating. Compounds **4** [22], **9** [30], **10** [31], **14** [32], **17** [33], and **21** [34] were prepared according to the literature. Other chemicals were purchased from Sigma-Aldrich (St. Louis, MO, USA), Nacalai Tesque, Inc. (Kyoto, Japan), Tokyo Chemical Industry Co., Ltd. (Tokyo, Japan), or FUJIFILM Wako Pure Chemical Co. (Osaka, Japan). Hard copies of ^1H and ^{13}C NMR spectra can be found as Supplementary Materials.

3.2. *Assay for Cytotoxicity of Compounds Against HUVECs*

HUVECs (5×10^5 cells/vial) were purchased from Kurabo Inc. and grown in HuMedia-EG2 medium with growth supplements (Kurabo, Osaka, Japan). HUVECs in the culture medium were plated into each well of 96-well plates (2×10^3 cells/well/100 μL). After 24 h, the serially diluted compounds as a 5% DMSO/EtOH or EtOH solution (1 μL) were added, and then the plates were incubated for an additional 72 h in a humidified atmosphere of 5% CO_2 at 37 °C. The cell proliferation was detected by WST-8 colorimetric reagent (Nacalai Tesque, Inc., Kyoto, Japan). The IC_{50} value was determined by linear interpolation from the growth inhibition curve, and the averaged IC_{50} values of the triplicate experiment are shown in Table 1.

3.3. *Antiproliferative Activity of the Compounds Against Cancer Cells*

KB3-1 cells were cultured in RPMI-1640 medium supplemented with 10% heat-inactivated fetal bovine serum and kanamycin (50 μg/mL). Cells were plated into 96-well microplates at 2×10^3 cells/100 μL assay medium/well, and various concentrations of test compounds were added to each well as a 5% DMSO/EtOH or EtOH solution (1 μL). The plates were incubated at 37 °C in a humidified atmosphere of 5% CO_2 for 72 h, and cell proliferation was determined by WST-8 colorimetric assay as above, and the averaged IC_{50} values of the triplicate experiment are shown in Table 1.

3.4. *In Vivo Matrigel Plug Assay and Toxicity Tests of Analog* **19**

All animal procedures were approved by the Committee on Animal Experimentation of Osaka University (Approval number: DouYaku 24-8-1). The measurements of in vivo angiogenesis using Matrigel plugs were performed as described previously [21]. An aliquot (250 μL) of Matrigel containing 200 ng/mL of bFGF and 100 U/mL of heparin was injected subcutaneously into the ventral side of female ddY mice (6 weeks old, $N = 4$, Japan SLC, Inc., Shizuoka, Japan). Then, analog **19** was orally administered on every other day (total 5 times: day 1, 3, 5, 7, and 9) as a suspension in 1% sodium carboxymethyl cellulose (CMC-Na). At day 10, the Matrigel plugs were photographed and removed. The levels of new vessels were quantified by measuring the hemoglobin of the Matrigel plug (μg hemoglobin/mg Matrigel) with the Drabkin reagent Kit.

The body weight of mice of the control group (bFGF (+) or (−)) and the groups treated with the testing compound (0.1, 0.3, and 1 mg/kg) at day 1 and day 9 were measured. The mean activities of aspartate aminotransferase (AST) and alanine aminotransferase (ALT) in mouse serum at day 10 of control group and the 1 mg/kg treated group were measured using the LabAssay™ AST or ALT kit (FUJIFILM Wako Pure Chemical Co., Osaka, Japan), respectively.

3.5. *In Vivo* Antitumor Effect of Analog **19**

Murine sarcoma S180 cells (1 × 10^6 cells/body) were implanted subcutaneously into the right ventral flank of female ddY mice (6 weeks old). After one week from implantation, analog **19** was orally administered on every other day for 14 days (total 7 times) as a suspension in 1% CMC-Na. Then, the tumor was isolated and weighed to calculate the inhibition ratio. The control group and the group treated with the testing compound consisted of six mice each in this study.

3.6. *Synthesis*

3.6.1. (3*S*,3a*R*,11a*S*,11b*R*)-3-(Isoquinolin-7-yl)-3a,9-dimethyl-1,2,3,3a,4,5,11a,11b-octahydro-7*H*-cyclopenta[h]pyrano[4,3-b]chromen-7-one (**7**)

4-Hydroxy-6-methyl-2-pyrone (**6**, 25.0 mg, 0.20 mmol) and piperidine (9.8 µL, 0.10 mmol) were added to a solution of **4** (19.3 mg, 0.07 mmol) in 1,4-dioxane (0.8 mL) and the whole mixture was stirred for 18 h. H_2O was added to the mixture and the whole mixture was extracted with $CHCl_3$. The organic layer was dried over Na_2SO_4 and was concentrated in vacuo. The crude material was purified by column chromatography (SiO_2; $CHCl_3$/MeOH/H_2O = 100:3:1, lower phase) to afford **7** (14.3 mg, 54%).

$[\alpha]^{24}_D$ +15.5° (*c* = 1.24 in $CHCl_3$). ^{1}H-NMR (500 MHz, $CDCl_3$) δ: 9.22 (s, 1H), 8.49 (s, 1H), 7.78 (s, 1H), 7.75 (d, *J* = 8.6 Hz, 1H), 7.62 (d, *J* = 5.7 Hz, 1H), 7.55 (d, *J* = 8.6 Hz, 1H), 6.16 (s, 1H), 5.76 (s, 1H), 5.00 (d, *J* = 10.9 Hz, 1H), 3.03 (t, *J* = 9.5 Hz, 1H), 2.44–2.34 (m, 3H), 2.20 (s, 3H), 2.17–2.13 (m, 3H), 1.76–1.72 (m, 1H), 1.61 (dd, *J* = 12.1, 3.5 Hz, 1H), 1.51 (td, *J* = 12.6, 6.3 Hz, 1H), 0.62 (s, 3H). ^{13}C-NMR (125 MHz, $CDCl_3$) δ: 163.8, 162.4, 161.6, 152.3, 142.6, 139.0, 134.7, 132.1, 131.4, 128.2, 126.3, 125.9, 120.1, 111.2, 99.7, 98.1, 80.8, 56.6, 55.4, 46.7, 36.8, 29.5, 26.3, 23.8, 20.1, 12.4. ESI MS: *m/z* 400 (M + H)$^+$. HR-ESI MS: *m/z* 400.1907, calcd for $C_{26}H_{26}NO_3$. Found: 400.1902.

3.6.2. (3*S*,3a*R*,11a*S*,11b*R*)-10-(Hydroxymethyl)-3-(isoquinolin-7-yl)-3a,9-dimethyl-1,2,3,3a,4,5,11a,11b-octahydro-7*H*-cyclopenta[h]pyrano[4,3-b]chromen-7-one (**11**)

Compound **10** (27.3 mg, 0.18 mmol) and piperidine (8.7 µL, 0.09 mmol) were added to a solution of **4** (12.9 mg, 0.04 mmol) in 1,4-dioxane (0.8 mL) and the whole mixture was stirred for 22 h. H_2O was added to the mixture and the whole mixture was extracted with $CHCl_3$. The organic layer was dried over Na_2SO_4 and was concentrated in vacuo. The crude material was purified by column chromatography (SiO_2; $CHCl_3$/MeOH/H_2O = 100:3:1, lower phase) to afford **11** (14.3 mg, 76%).

$[\alpha]^{22}_D$ +22.4° (*c* = 0.93 in $CHCl_3$). ^{1}H-NMR (500 MHz, $CDCl_3$) δ: 9.22 (s, 1H), 8.48 (d, *J* = 5.7 Hz, 1H), 7.78–7.76 (m, 2H), 7.64 (d, *J* = 5.7 Hz, 1H), 7.55 (d, *J* = 8.6 Hz, 1H), 6.16 (s, 1H), 5.05 (d, *J* = 10.9 Hz, 1H), 4.46 (s, 2H), 3.02 (t, *J* = 9.5 Hz, 1H), 2.46–2.34 (m, 3H), 2.32 (s, 3H) 2.23–2.12 (m, 4H), 1.81–1.76 (m, 1H), 1.62 (dd, *J* = 12.1, 5.2 Hz, 1H), 1.51 (td, *J* = 12.1, 5.2 Hz, 1H), 0.62 (s, 3H). ^{13}C-NMR (125 MHz, $CDCl_3$) δ: 162.5, 161.6, 160.7, 152.2, 142.4, 138.9, 134.8, 132.1, 131.4, 128.5, 126.3, 125.9, 120.2, 111.2, 110.4, 98.7, 81.2, 56.6, 55.5, 55.4, 46.8, 36.8, 29.4, 26.2, 23.8, 17.3, 12.3. ESI MS: *m/z* 430 (M + H)$^+$. HR-ESI MS: *m/z* 430.2013, calcd for $C_{27}H_{28}NO_4$. Found: 430.2025.

3.6.3. (3*S*,3a*R*,11a*S*,11b*R*)-3-(Isoquinolin-7-yl)-3a-methyl-2,3,3a,4,5,8,11a,11b-octahydrocyclopenta[7,8]chromeno[3,2-c]pyridin-7(1*H*)-one (**13**)

Pyridine-2,4-diol (**12**, 7.9 mg, 0.70 mmol) and ethylenediamine diacetate (1.3 mg, 0.007 mmol) were added to a solution of **4** (10.3 mg, 0.035 mmol) in DMF (0.35 mL) at 0 °C, and the whole mixture was stirred at 50 °C for 5 h. H_2O was added to the mixture and the whole mixture was extracted with $CHCl_3$. The organic layer was dried over Na_2SO_4 and was concentrated in vacuo. The crude material was purified by column chromatography (SiO_2; $CHCl_3$/MeOH/H_2O = 60:3:1, lower phase) to afford **13** (3.7 mg, 27%).

$[\alpha]^{20}{}_D$ +9.5° (c = 0.077 in $CHCl_3$). ^{1}H NMR (500 MHz, $CDCl_3$) δ: 11.05 (brs, 1H), 9.22 (s, 1H), 8.48 (d, J = 5.6 Hz, 1H), 7.79 (s, 1H), 7.75 (d, J = 8.3 Hz, 1H), 7.62 (d, J = 6.0 Hz, 1H), 7.56 (d, J = 8.5 Hz, 1H), 7.06 (d, J = 7.5 Hz, 1H), 6.36 (s, 1H), 5.89 (d, J = 7.2 Hz, 1H), 4.98 (d, J = 10.3 Hz, 1H), 3.03 (t, J = 9.5 Hz, 1H), 2.47 (dd, J = 15.8, 4.3 Hz, 1H), 2.41–2.34 (m, 2H), 2.22–2.15 (m, 3H), 1.80–1.72 (m, 1H), 1.63–1.49 (m, 2H), 0.62 (s, 3H). ^{13}C NMR (151 MHz, $CDCl_3$) δ: 162.7, 162.46, 152.3, 142.6, 139.2, 134.7, 133.2, 132.3, 132.2, 132.0, 126.3, 125.8, 120.1, 111.9, 100.4, 79.9, 56.7, 55.4, 46.6, 36.7, 29.7, 29.4, 26.4, 24.0, 12.4. ESI MS: m/z 385 (M + H)$^+$. HR-ESI MS: m/z 385.1911, calcd for $C_{25}H_{25}N_2O_2$. Found: 385.1935.

3.6.4. (3*S*,3a*R*,11a*S*,11b*R*)-3-(Isoquinolin-7-yl)-3a,8-dimethyl-2,3,3a,4,5,8,11a,11b-octahydrocyclopenta[7,8]chromeno[3,2-c]pyridin-7(1*H*)-one (**15**)

Compound **14** (30 mg, 0.24 mmol) and ethylenediamine diacetate (3.6 mg, 0.02 mmol) were added to a solution of **4** (36.0 mg, 0.12 mmol) in DMF (1.2 mL) at 0 °C, and the whole mixture was stirred at 50 °C for 5 h. H_2O was added to the mixture and the whole mixture was extracted with $CHCl_3$. The organic layer was dried over Na_2SO_4 and was concentrated in vacuo. The crude material was purified by column chromatography (SiO_2; $CHCl_3/MeOH/H_2O$ = 60:3:1, lower phase) to afford **15** (28 mg, 57%).

$[\alpha]^{20}{}_D$ +21.5° (c = 0.271 in $CHCl_3$). ^{1}H NMR (500 MHz, $CDCl_3$) δ 9.23 (s, 1H), 8.49 (s, 1H), 7.79 (s, 1H), 7.75 (d, J = 8.5 Hz, 1H), 7.63 (s, 1H), 7.56 (dd, J = 8.6, 1.9 Hz, 1H), 7.02 (d, J = 7.5 Hz, 1H), 6.42 (s, 1H), 5.82 (d, J = 7.5 Hz, 1H), 4.93 (d, J = 10.2 Hz, 1H), 3.47 (s, 3H), 3.03 (t, J = 8.8 Hz, 1H), 2.47 (dd, J = 15.2, 3.3 Hz, 1H), 2.40–2.32 (m, 2H), 2.22–2.14 (m, 3H), 1.78–1.72 (m, 1H), 1.62–1.58 (m, 1H), 1.51 (td, J = 13.1, 5.2 Hz, 1H), 0.61 (s, 3H). ^{13}C NMR (125 MHz, $CDCl_3$) δ: 160.85, 160.82, 152.5, 142.7, 139.4, 136.8, 136.7, 134.8, 132.3, 132.0, 126.4, 125.9, 120.3, 112.9, 107.5, 99.6, 79.8, 56.8, 55.4, 46.7, 37.3, 36.8, 29.5, 26.5, 24.2, 12.5. ESI MS: m/z 399 (M + H)$^+$. HR-ESI MS: m/z 399.2067, calcd for $C_{26}H_{27}N_2O_2$. Found: 399.2085.

3.6.5. 4-Hydroxy-5-(hydroxymethyl)-1-methylpyridin-2(1*H*)-one (**18**)

Diisobutylaluminium hydride (1.0 M in toluene, 1.2 mL, 1.2 mmol) was added to a solution of **17** (50 mg, 0.30 mmol) in toluene (2.4 mL) at –78 °C and the whole mixture was stirred at 0 °C for 7 h. Then, 5% HCl aq. was added to quench the reaction, and the whole mixture was concentrated in vacuo. The crude material was purified by column chromatography (SiO_2; $CHCl_3/MeOH/H_2O$ = 6:4:1) to afford **18** (16.6 mg, 39%).

^{1}H NMR (500 MHz, DMSO-d_6) δ: 10.63 (s, 1H), 7.43 (s, 1H), 5.62 (s, 1H), 4.88 (s, 1H), 4.22 (s, 2H), 3.37 (s, 3H). ^{13}C NMR (125 MHz, DMSO-d_6) δ: 165.0, 163.0, 137.7, 112.4, 97.7, 56.1, 35.8. ESI MS: m/z 156 (M + H)$^+$. HR-ESI MS: m/z 156.0655, calcd for $C_7H_9NO_3$. Found: 156.0660.

3.6.6. (3*S*,3a*R*,11a*S*,11b*R*)-10-(Hydroxymethyl)-3-(isoquinolin-7-yl)-3a,8-dimethyl-2,3,3a,4,5,8,11a,11b-octahydrocyclopenta[7,8]chromeno[3,2-c]pyridin-7(1*H*)-one (**19**)

Compound **18** (18.6 mg, 0.12 mmol) and ethylenediamine diacetate (2.2 mg, 0.01 mmol) were added to a solution of **4** (18.0 mg, 0.062 mmol) in DMF (0.6 mL) at 0 °C and the whole mixture was stirred at 50 °C for 5 h. H_2O was added to the mixture and the whole mixture was extracted with $CHCl_3$. The organic layer was dried over Na_2SO_4 and was concentrated in vacuo. The crude material was purified by column chromatography (SiO_2; $CHCl_3/MeOH/H_2O$ = 60:3:1, lower phase) to afford **19** (11.8 mg, 45%).

$[\alpha]^{20}{}_D$ +14.2° (c = 0.361 in $CHCl_3$). ^{1}H NMR (600 MHz, $CDCl_3$) δ: 9.21 (s, 1H), 8.48 (s, 1H), 7.78 (s, 1H), 7.75 (d, J = 8.5 Hz, 1H), 7.63 (d, J = 5.5 Hz, 1H), 7.55 (d, J = 8.3 Hz, 1H), 7.10 (s, 1H), 6.40 (s, 1H), 4.97 (d, J = 11.0 Hz, 1H), 4.44 (dd, J = 28.9, 12.9 Hz, 2H), 3.46 (s, 3H), 3.01 (t, J = 9.3 Hz, 1H), 2.90–2.60 (br, 1H), 2.47 (m, 1H), 2.41–2.31 (m, 2H), 2.23–2.11 (m, 3H), 1.81–1.72 (m, 1H), 1.61 (m, 1H), 1.51 (m, 1H), 0.61 (s, 3H). ^{13}C NMR (151 MHz, $CDCl_3$) δ: 160.5, 158.8, 152.2, 142.5, 139.1, 135.2, 134.7, 132.2, 132.1, 129.1, 126.3, 125.8, 120.1,

112.6, 111.6, 106.8, 79.9, 58.3, 56.6, 55.4, 46.6, 37.1, 36.8, 29.4, 26.3, 23.9, 12.4. ESI MS: m/z 429 $(M + H)^+$. HR-ESI MS: m/z 429.2173, calcd for $C_{27}H_{29}N_2O_3$. Found: 429.2199.

3.6.7. *tert*-Butyl (2-(2,2-Dimethyl-4-oxo-4*H*-1,3-dioxin-6-yl)-3-oxobutyl)carbamate (**22**)

Sodium hydride (335 mg, 8.38 mmol) was added to a solution of **21** (616 mg, 3.35 mmol) in THF (33.5 mL) at 0 °C, and the whole mixture was stirred at rt for 10 min. A solution of *tert*-butyl (tosylmethyl)carbamate (1.4 g, 5.0 mmol) in THF (10 mL) was added to the reaction mixture at 0 °C and the whole mixture was stirred for 1 h. Sat. NH_4Cl aq. was added to quench the reaction, and the whole mixture was extracted with Et_2O. The organic layer was dried over Na_2SO_4 and was concentrated in vacuo. The crude material was purified by column chromatography (SiO_2; *n*-hexane/AcOEt = 2:1) to afford **22** (581 mg, 55%).

^1H NMR (500 MHz, $CDCl_3$) δ: 5.36 (s, 1H), 4.96 (t, J = 6.4 Hz, 1H), 3.63 (t, J = 6.8 Hz, 1H), 3.52–3.47 (m, 1H), 3.42–3.37 (m, 1H), 2.20 (s, 3H), 1.64 (s, 6H), 1.46 (s, 9H). ^{13}C NMR (125 MHz, $CDCl_3$) δ: 202.6, 165.4, 160.1, 155.6, 107.1, 96.4, 79.8, 57.0, 38.7, 29.2, 28.2, 24.8, 24.7. ESI MS: m/z 336 $(M + Na)^+$. HR-ESI MS: m/z 336.1418, calcd for $C_{15}H_{23}NO_6Na$. Found: 336.1434.

3.6.8. *tert*-Butyl
(Z)-(5-(methylamino)-2-(1-(methylamino)ethylidene)-3,5-dioxopentyl)carbamate (**23**)

Methylamine (2.0 M in THF, 0.09 mL, 0.18 mmol) was added to a solution of **22** (28.4 mg, 0.09 mmol) in toluene (4.5 mL) and the whole mixture was stirred at 75 °C for 4 h. Concentration in vacuo gave the crude material, which was purified by column chromatography (SiO_2; $CHCl_3/MeOH/H_2O$ = 200:3:1, lower phase) to afford **23** (13.4 mg, 50%).

^1H NMR (500 MHz, $CDCl_3$) δ: 12.24 (brs, 1H), 6.94 (brs, 1H), 5.32 (brs, 1H), 3.99 (d, J = 5.0 Hz, 2H), 3.34 (s, 2H), 2.94 (d, J = 5.0 Hz, 3H), 2.76 (d, J = 5.0 Hz, 3H), 2.08 (s, 3H), 1.39 (s, 9H). ^{13}C NMR (125 MHz, $CDCl_3$) δ: 189.4, 168.9, 168.8, 155.6, 101.7, 78.9, 46.4, 39.4, 30.1, 28.3, 26.3, 15.1. ESI MS: m/z 322 $(M + Na)^+$. HR-ESI MS: m/z 322.1737, calcd for $C_{14}H_{25}N_3O_4Na$. Found: 322.1749.

3.6.9. *N*-((4-Hydroxy-1,2-dimethyl-6-oxo-1,6-dihydropyridin-3-yl)methyl)acetamide (**26**)

AcOH (14 μL, 0.48 mmol) was added to a solution of **23** (72 mg, 0.24 mmol) in toluene (2.4 mL) and the whole mixture was stirred at 110 °C for 8 h. Concentration in vacuo gave the crude material including compound **24**, which was dissolved in CH_2Cl_2 (1.2 mL). TFA (0.24 mL) was added to the solution and the whole mixture was stirred for 1 h. The reaction mixture was diluted with toluene (10 mL) and the whole mixture was concentrated in vacuo. The residue was dissolved in DMF (1.2 mL), and then K_2CO_3 (138 mg, 1.2 mmol) and Ac_2O (28 μL, 0.30 mmol) were successively added to the solution. The whole mixture was stirred for 2 h. MeOH (1.0 mL) was added to the reaction mixture, and the whole mixture was stirred for additional 2h. Concentration in vacuo gave the crude material, which was purified by column chromatography (SiO_2; $CHCl_3/MeOH/H_2O$ = 30:3:1, lower phase) to afford **26** (17.0 mg, 34% in 3 steps).

^1H NMR (500 MHz, $CD_3OD/CDCl_3$) δ: 5.81 (s, 1H), 4.25 (s, 2H), 3.49 (s, 3H), 2.43 (s, 3H), 1.91 (s, 3H). ^{13}C NMR (125 MHz, $CD_3OD/CDCl_3$) δ: 172.7, 167.1, 166.3, 148.3, 110.3, 97.3, 35.5, 31.8, 22.4, 17.0. ESI MS: m/z 233 $(M + Na)^+$. HR-ESI MS: m/z 233.0897, calcd for $C_{10}H_{14}N_2O_3$. Found: 233.0908.

3.6.10. *N*-(((3*S*,3a*R*,11a*S*,11b*R*)-3-(Isoquinolin-7-yl)-3a,8,9-trimethyl-7-oxo-1,2,3,3a,4,5,7,8,11a,11b-decahydrocyclopenta[7,8]chromeno[3,2-c]pyridin-10-yl)methyl)acetamide (**27**)

Compound **26** (15.3 mg, 0.068 mmol) and ethylenediamine diacetate (1.3 mg, 0.007 mmol) were added to a solution of **4** (10.0 mg, 0.034 mmol) in DMF (0.34 mL) at 0 °C and the whole mixture was stirred at 50 °C for 5 h. H_2O was added to the mixture and the whole mixture was extracted with $CHCl_3$. The organic layer was dried over Na_2SO_4 and was concentrated in vacuo. The crude material was purified by column chromatography (SiO_2; $CHCl_3$/MeOH/H_2O = 100:3:1, lower phase) to afford **27** (5.0 mg, 30%).

$[\alpha]^{20}{}_D$ −8.5° (*c* = 0.138 in $CHCl_3$). ^1H NMR (500 MHz, $CDCl_3$) δ: 9.25 (brs, 1H), 8.50 (brs, 1H), 7.81 (s, 1H), 7.78 (d, *J* = 8.5 Hz, 1H), 7.66 (brs, 1H), 7.58 (d, *J* = 8.6 Hz, 1H), 6.41 (s, 1H), 5.90 (brs, 1H), 4.95 (d, *J* = 10.8 Hz, 1H), 4.32 (dd, *J* = 14.1, 5.5 Hz, 1H), 4.23 (dd, *J* = 14.4, 5.2 Hz, 1H), 3.50 (s, 3H), 3.04 (t, *J* = 10.1 Hz, 1H), 2.49 (dd, *J* = 15.2, 5.2 Hz, 1H), 2.43–2.33 (m, 2H), 2.41 (s, 3H), 2.23–2.13 (m, 3H), 2.00 (s, 3H), 1.83–1.76 (m, 1H), 1.63 (dd, *J* = 12.6, 4.7 Hz, 1H), 1.52 (td, *J* = 12.8, 5.6 Hz, 1H), 0.63 (s, 3H). ^{13}C NMR (151 MHz, $CDCl_3$) δ 169.8, 160.5, 158.8, 152.3, 144.9, 142.6, 138.9, 134.7, 132.0, 131.3, 126.3, 125.8, 120.1, 113.0, 111.6, 107.0, 104.3, 80.0, 56.6, 55.40, 46.6, 36.8, 34.4, 31.5, 29.2, 26.3, 24.1, 23.2, 17.0, 12.3. ESI MS: *m*/*z* 484 $(M + H)^+$. HR-ESI MS: *m*/*z* 484.2595, calcd for $C_{30}H_{34}N_3O_3$. Found: 484.2623.

4. Conclusions

In summary, we developed a synthetic method for novel simplified analogs of cortistatin A (**1**) using 4-hydroxy-2-pyrone or 4-hydroxy-2-pyridone derivatives as A-ring fragments. Among those prepared in this work, the pyridone-embedded analog **19** is the most potent compound exhibiting significant in vivo anti-angiogenic and anti-tumor effect without acute toxicity and hepatotoxicity. Although some improvements in the reaction yield for the synthesis are needed, easy accessibility and more potent activity/selectivity than those of natural products are significant features of this compound, making it a promising candidate for anti-tumor drugs. Further studies to develop a more practical compound and elucidate its mechanism of action in angiogenesis are currently underway.

Supplementary Materials: The following supporting information can be downloaded at: https://www.mdpi.com/article/10.3390/md23040179/s1, Supplementary Data S1: NMR spectra of the new compounds.

Author Contributions: Conceptualization, N.K.; methodology, N.K., M.A., Y.F. and K.M.; validation, N.K.; formal analysis, N.K.; investigation, Y.F., K.M. and Y.N.; data curation, Y.F., K.M., and Y.N.; writing—original draft preparation, Y.F.; writing—review and editing, N.K. and M.A.; supervision, N.K.; project administration, N.K.; funding acquisition, N.K. and M.A. All authors have read and agreed to the published version of the manuscript.

Funding: This research was funded by the Hoansha Foundation and a Grant-in-Aid for Scientific Research C (Grant Nos. 18K05363 and 22K05339) from the Japan Society for the Promotion of Science (JSPS) to N.K. It was partially supported by the Research Support Project for Life Science and Drug Discovery (Basis for Supporting Innovative Drug Discovery and Life Science Research (BINDS)) from AMED under Grant Numbers JP24ama121054 and JP25ama121054, and a Grant-in-Aid for Scientific Research B (grant no. 21H02096) from JSPS to MA.

Institutional Review Board Statement: All animal procedures were approved by the Committee on Animal Experimentation of Osaka University (Approval number: DouYaku 24-8-1).

Data Availability Statement: The original data presented in the study are included in the article/Supplementary Material; further inquiries can be directed to the corresponding author.

Conflicts of Interest: The authors declare no conflicts of interest.

References

1. Carroll, A.R.; Copp, B.R.; Davis, R.A.; Keyzers, R.A.; Prinsep, M.R. Marine Natural Products. *Nat. Prod. Rep.* **2023**, *40*, 275–325. [CrossRef]
2. Molinski, T.F.; Dalisay, D.S.; Lievens, S.L.; Saludes, J.P. Drug development from marine natural products. *Nat. Rev. Drug Discov.* **2009**, *8*, 69–85. [CrossRef]
3. Swinney, D.C.; Anthony, J. How were new medicines discovered? *Nat. Rev. Drug Discov.* **2011**, *10*, 507–519. [CrossRef]
4. Wang, S.; Dong, G.; Sheng, C. Structural Simplification of Natural Products. *Chem. Rev.* **2019**, *119*, 4180–4220. [CrossRef]
5. Wach, J.-Y.; Gademann, K. Reduce to the Maximum: Truncated Natural Products as Powerful Modulators of Biological Processes. *Synlett* **2012**, *2012*, 163–170. [CrossRef]
6. Ueda, M. Chemical Biology of Natural Products on the Basis of Identification of Target Proteins. *Chem. Lett.* **2012**, *41*, 658–666. [CrossRef]
7. Carmeliet, P.; Jain, R.K. Angiogenesis in cancer and other diseases. *Nature* **2000**, *407*, 249–257. [CrossRef]
8. Aoki, S.; Watanabe, Y.; Sanagawa, M.; Setiawan, A.; Kotoku, N.; Kobayashi, M. Cortistatins A, B, C, and D, Anti-angiogenic Steroidal Alkaloids, from the Marine Sponge *Corticium simplex*. *J. Am. Chem. Soc.* **2006**, *128*, 3148–3149. [CrossRef]
9. Watanabe, Y.; Aoki, S.; Tanabe, D.; Setiawan, A.; Arai, M.; Kobayashi, M. Cortistatins E, F, G, and H, four novel steroidal alkaloids from marine sponge *Corticium simplex*. *Tetrahedron* **2007**, *63*, 4074–4079. [CrossRef]
10. Aoki, S.; Watanabe, Y.; Tanabe, D.; Setiawan, A.; Arai, M.; Kobayashi, M. Cortistatins J, K, L, novel abeo-9(10-19)-androstane-type steroidal alkaloids with isoquinoline unit, from marine sponge *Corticium simplex*. *Tetrahedron Lett.* **2007**, *48*, 4485–4488. [CrossRef]
11. Aoki, S.; Watanabe, Y.; Tanabe, D.; Arai, M.; Suna, H.; Miyamoto, K.; Tsujibo, H.; Tsujikawa, K.; Yamamoto, H.; Kobayashi, M. Structure–activity relationship and biological property of cortistatins, anti-angiogenic spongean steroidal alkaloids. *Bioorganic Med. Chem.* **2007**, *15*, 6758–6762. [CrossRef] [PubMed]
12. Narayan, A.R.H.; Simmons, E.M.; Sarpong, R. Synthetic Strategies Directed Towards the Cortistatin Family of Natural Products. *Eur. J. Org. Chem.* **2010**, *2010*, 3553–3567. [CrossRef]
13. Chen, D.Y.-K.; Tseng, C.-C. Chemistry of the cortistatins–a novel class of *anti*-angiogenic agents. *Org. Biomol. Chem.* **2010**, *8*, 2900–2911. [CrossRef] [PubMed]
14. Nising, C.F.; Bräse, S. Highlights in Steroid Chemistry: Total Synthesis versus Semisynthesis. *Angew. Chem. Int. Ed.* **2008**, *47*, 9389–9391. [CrossRef]
15. Shi, J.; Manolikakes, G.; Yeh, C.-H.; Guerrero, C.A.; Shenvi, R.A.; Shigehisa, H.; Baran, P.S. Scalable Synthesis of Cortistatin A and Related Structures. *J. Am. Chem. Soc.* **2011**, *133*, 8014–8027. [CrossRef]
16. Nicolaou, K.C.; Peng, X.-S.; Sun, Y.-P.; Polet, D.; Zou, B.; Lim, C.S.; Chen, D.Y.-K. Total Synthesis and Biological Evaluation of Cortistatins A and J and Analogues Thereof. *J. Am. Chem. Soc.* **2009**, *131*, 10587–10597. [CrossRef]
17. Lee, H.M.; Nieto-Oberhuber, C.; Shair, M.D. Enantioselective Synthesis of (+)-Cortistatin A, a Potent and Selective Inhibitor of Endothelial Cell Proliferation. *J. Am. Chem. Soc.* **2008**, *130*, 16864–16866. [CrossRef]
18. Flyer, A.N.; Si, C.; Myers, A.G. Synthesis of cortistatins A, J, K and L. *Nat. Chem.* **2010**, *2*, 886–892. [CrossRef]
19. Yamashita, S.; Iso, K.; Kitajima, K.; Himuro, M.; Hirama, M. Total Synthesis of Cortistatins A and J. *J. Org. Chem.* **2011**, *76*, 2408–2425. [CrossRef]
20. Nilson, M.G.; Funk, R.L. Total Synthesis of (±)-Cortistatin J from Furan. *J. Am. Chem. Soc.* **2011**, *133*, 12451–12453. [CrossRef]
21. Kotoku, N.; Sumii, Y.; Hayashi, T.; Tamura, S.; Kawachi, T.; Shiomura, S.; Arai, M.; Kobayashi, M. Creation of Readily Accessible and Orally Active Analogue of Cortistatin, A. *ACS Med. Chem. Lett.* **2012**, *3*, 673–677. [CrossRef] [PubMed]
22. Kotoku, N.; Ito, A.; Shibuya, S.; Mizuno, K.; Takeshima, A.; Nogata, M.; Kobayashi, M. Short-step Synthesis and Structure-activity Relationship of Cortistatin A Analogs. *Tetrahedron* **2017**, *73*, 1342–1349. [CrossRef]
23. Hsung, P.R.; Cole, P.K.; Zehnder, R.L.; Wang, J.; Wei, L.; Yang, X.; Coverdale, A.H. The total synthesis of (±)-arisugacin A. *Tetrahedron* **2003**, *59*, 311–324. [CrossRef]
24. Odani, A.; Ishihara, K.; Ohtawa, M.; Tomoda, H.; Omura, S. Total synthesis of pyripyropene A. *Tetrahedron* **2011**, *67*, 8195–8203. [CrossRef]
25. Fotiadou, A.D.; Zografos, A.L. Electrocyclization of Oxatrienes in the Construction of Structurally Complex Pyranopyridones. *Org. Lett.* **2012**, *14*, 5664–5667. [CrossRef]
26. Mihara, H.; Shibuguchi, T.; Kuramochi, A.; Ohshima, T.; Shibasaki, M. Short Synthesis of (+)-Cylindricine C and Formal Total Synthesis of (−)-Lepadiformine. *Heterocycles* **2007**, *72*, 421–438. [CrossRef]
27. Riveira, M.J.; Mischne, M.P. One-Pot Organocatalytic Tandem Aldol/Polycyclization Reactions between 1,3-Dicarbonyl Compounds and α,β,γ,δ-Unsaturated Aldehydes for the Straightforward Assembly of Cyclopenta[*b*]furan-Type Derivatives: New Insight into the Knoevenagel Reaction. *Chem. Eur. J.* **2012**, *18*, 2382–2388. [CrossRef]
28. Aabid, H.B.; Quiroga, G.N.; La-Venia, A.; Grover, H.K.; Riveira, M.J. Biomimetic Domino Knoevenagel/Cycloisomerization Strategy for the Synthesis of Citridone A and Derivatives. *J. Org. Chem.* **2021**, *86*, 12226–12236. [CrossRef]

29. Jacinto Demuner, A.; Moreira Valente, V.M.; Almeida Barbosa, L.C.; Rathi, A.; Donohoe, T.J.; Thompson, A.L. Synthesis and Phytotoxic Activity of New Pyridones Derived from 4-Hydroxy-6-Methylpyridin-2(1*H*)-one. *Molecules* **2009**, *14*, 4973–4986. [CrossRef]
30. Kurdyumov, A.V.; Muñoz, R.L.P.; Hsung, R.P. Total Syntheses of Daldiniapyrone, Annularin B, and (±)-Annularin F. *Synthesis* **2006**, *11*, 1787–1790. [CrossRef]
31. Shimizu, T.; Hiranuma, S.; Watanabe, T. Reduction of α-Pyrone Derivatives with Borane-Methyl Sulfide Complex. *Heterocycles* **1993**, *36*, 2445–2550. [CrossRef]
32. Robins, J.M.; Yang, H.; Miranda, K.; Peterson, A.M.; Clercq, D.E.; Balzarini, J. Synthesis and Biological Evaluation of 3,3-Difluoropyridine-2,4(1*H*,3*H*)-dione and 3-Deaza-3-fluorouracil Base and Nucleoside Derivatives. *J. Med. Chem.* **2009**, *52*, 3018–3027. [CrossRef] [PubMed]
33. Baškovč, J.; Dahmann, G.; Golobič, A.; Grošelj, U.; Kočar, D.; Stanovnik, B.; Svete, J. Diversity-Oriented Synthesis of 1-Substituted 4-Aryl-6-oxo-1,6-dihydropyridine-3-carboxamides. *ACS Comb. Sci.* **2012**, *14*, 513–519. [CrossRef] [PubMed]
34. Patel, H.B.; Mason, M.A.; Barret, M.G.A. Synthesis of 6-Substituted-4-Hydroxy-2-pyridinones via Intramolecular Ketene Trapping of Functionalized Enamine-Dioxinones. *Org. Lett.* **2011**, *13*, 5156–5159. [CrossRef]
35. Barrett, N.T.; Patel, H.B.; Barrett, M.G.A. Synthesis of *C*-5-substituted resorcylates and resorcinamides via formylation–aromatization of functionalized keto-dioxinones. *Tetrahedron* **2014**, *70*, 6894–6901. [CrossRef]
36. Pelish, H.E.; Liau, B.B.; Nitulescu, I.I.; Tangpeerachaikul, A.; Poss, Z.C.; da Silva, D.H.; Caruso, B.T.; Arefolov, A.; Fadeyi, O.; Christie, A.L.; et al. Mediator kinase inhibition further activates super-enhancer-associated genes in AML. *Nature* **2015**, *526*, 273–276. [CrossRef]
37. Hatcher, J.M.; Wang, E.S.; Johannessen, L.; Kwiatkowski, N.; Sim, T.; Gray, N.S. Development of Highly Potent and Selective Steroidal Inhibitors and Degraders of CDK8. *ACS. Med. Chem. Lett.* **2018**, *9*, 540–545. [CrossRef]

marine drugs

MDPI

Article

Precision-Engineered Dermatan Sulfate-Mimetic Glycopolymers for Multi-Targeted SARS-CoV-2 Inhibition †

Lihao Wang [1,‡], Lei Gao [1,‡], Chendong Yang [1], Mengfei Yin [1], Jiqin Sun [1], Luyao Yang [1], Chanjuan Liu [1], Simon F. R. Hinkley [2], Guangli Yu [1,3,*] and Chao Cai [1,3,*]

1 Key Laboratory of Marine Drugs of Ministry of Education, Shandong Key Laboratory of Glycoscience and Glycotherapeutics, School of Medicine and Pharmacy, Ocean University of China, Qingdao 266003, China; leowang@stu.ouc.edu.cn (L.W.); gaolei2@msu.edu (L.G.); sunzetao@hotmail.com (C.Y.); ymf@stu.ouc.edu.cn (M.Y.); 13262540703@163.com (J.S.); 2119083118@stu.ouc.edu.cn (L.Y.); liuchanjuan@ouc.edu.cn (C.L.)

2 The Ferrier Research Institute, Victoria University of Wellington, 69 Gracefield Road, Lower Hutt 5040, New Zealand; simon.hinkley@vuw.ac.nz

3 Laboratory for Marine Drugs and Bioproducts, Qingdao Marine Science and Technology Center, Qingdao 266003, China

* Correspondence: glyu@ouc.edu.cn (G.Y.); caic@ouc.edu.cn (C.C.)

† This article is dedicated to the memory of the late Prof. Robert J. Linhardt.

‡ These authors contributed equally to this work.

Abstract

The ongoing COVID-19 pandemic, caused by SARS-CoV-2, continues to pose major global health challenges despite extensive vaccination efforts. Variant escape, waning immunity, and reduced vaccine efficacy in immunocompromised populations underscore the urgent need for complementary antiviral therapeutics. Here, we report the design, synthesis, and biological evaluation of precision-engineered dermatan sulfate (DS)-mimetic glycopolymers as multi-targeted inhibitors of SARS-CoV-2. Guided by molecular docking and virtual screening, sulfation at the C2 and C4 positions of iduronic acid was identified as critical for binding to the viral spike protein and inhibiting host and viral enzymes, including heparanase (HPSE) and main protease (M^{pro}). Chemically synthesized DS disaccharides were covalently grafted onto polymer scaffolds via a post-modification strategy, yielding glycopolymers with well-defined assembly that form uniform nanoparticles under physiological conditions. Surface plasmon resonance and pseudovirus assays revealed strong binding to the viral spike protein ($K_D \approx 177$ nM), potent viral neutralization, and minimal cytotoxicity. Cellular uptake studies further demonstrated efficient internalization of nanoparticles and intracellular inhibition of HPSE and M^{pro}. These results establish a modular, non-anticoagulant, and glycosaminoglycan-mimetic platform for the development of broad-spectrum antiviral agents to complement vaccination and enhance preparedness against emerging coronavirus variants.

Keywords: dermatan sulfate; synthesis; disaccharide; glycopolymer; anti-SARS-CoV-2

1. Introduction

COVID-19, caused by severe acute respiratory syndrome-related coronavirus 2 (SARS-CoV-2), remains a persistent global health challenge. The World Health Organization reports over 7.1 million deaths worldwide [1–3], reflecting continued transmission and mortality despite extensive public health interventions. Successive viral mutations have sustained infection rates and complicated containment efforts [4–6]. Although approved vaccines have markedly reduced severe illness and mortality, their protection against infection and mild disease has diminished over time [7,8]. Antigenic drift among emerging variants further erodes vaccine efficacy, underscoring the limitations of vaccination alone for long-term viral control [9].

Similarly to the 2002 SARS-CoV strain, SARS-CoV-2 invades host cells through the binding of its surface spike protein to the angiotensin-converting enzyme 2 (ACE2) receptor [10–12]. In both viruses, the main protease (M^{pro}) is essential for viral replication. Beyond processing viral polyproteins, M^{pro} can also cleave host proteins, thereby creating conditions that favor infection and viral proliferation [13]. These parallels suggest a common therapeutic vulnerability. Targeting the spike protein–ACE2 interaction, together with the inhibition of M^{pro} activity, offers a promising strategy for developing broad-spectrum inhibitors capable of preventing future severe acute respiratory syndrome outbreaks [14–16].

Glycosaminoglycans (GAGs) are linear sulfated polysaccharides composed of repeating disaccharide units of hexosamine and uronic acid. Based on their disaccharide structures, GAGs are classified into heparan sulfate (HS), chondroitin sulfate (CS), heparin (HP), and keratan sulfate (KS), among others [17]. Since 2020, numerous studies have shown that HS contributes to SARS-CoV-2 infection. This effect is largely attributed to the ability of the spike receptor-binding domain (RBD) to bind HS in a manner that depends on both chain length and specific sequence features. HS appears to serve as an initial attachment site, enabling the virus to move through the glycocalyx via weak individual contacts that collectively produce strong overall binding. This positioning helps bring the virus to the cell surface, where it can subsequently engage ACE2 and initiate entry [18–21]. Building on this understanding, the Linhardt and Pomin groups jointly screened a series of marine-derived sulfated polysaccharides for their ability to inhibit infection by multiple SARS-CoV-2 variants in vitro [20,22,23]. Their results spurred a broader investigation into sulfated polysaccharides and their synthetic analogs as potential antiviral agents against COVID-19 [24]. Follow-up studies revealed that the selective desulfation of heparin alters its antiviral activity in distinct manners; specifically, *N*-desulfation markedly reduced antiviral activity against SARS-CoV compared to 6-*O*-desulfation. These findings underscore the critical role of sulfate patterning on cell-surface GAGs in determining their antiviral function [25].

While HS and HP have been extensively studied [26], dermatan sulfate (DS)—a structurally related glycosaminoglycan—remains comparatively underexplored. DS is composed of repeating GalNAc-β-(1→3)-IdoA-α-(1→4) disaccharide units and often occurs as copolymeric chains with chondroitin sulfate (CS). Variants of CS and DS were first identified in marine organisms, underscoring their structural diversity and potential biological significance [27,28]. Endogenous CS/DS contributes to cell proliferation, migration, neuronal differentiation, skeletal development, and immune regulation [29,30].

Beyond the spike protein and M^{pro}, heparanase (HPSE), an endo-β-*D*-glucuronidase [31], has also been implicated in SARS-CoV-2 infection [32]. HPSE commonly cleaves the heparan sulfate (HS) side chains of heparan sulfate proteoglycans (HSPGs), thereby diminishing viral adhesion to host cells and facilitating viral dissemination [33]. Notably, HPSE expression is markedly upregulated in cells infected with SARS-CoV-2. In contrast, HPSE-deficient macrophages show reduced viral load and inflammation, underscoring the enzyme's dual role in viral propagation and immune modulation [34]. Synthetic HPSE inhibitors that are structurally related to heparin, such as Roneparstat and PG545 (Pixatimod), have gained attention for their ability to target both the spike protein and HPSE, offering a promising multi-target antiviral strategy [35].

DS functions as a non-anticoagulant inhibitor of HPSE and offers lower side effects with improved safety, making it a promising candidate for anti–COVID-19 therapy. While HS plays a crucial role in mediating spike protein binding and viral entry, its interactions with a broad range of binding partners present a challenge. In designing biomimetic glycopolymers targeting HS, it is vital to focus on the selectivity of HS mimetics for specific binding proteins, particularly those like PF4 [36]. Non-selective binding to such proteins could result in undesirable side effects, such as thrombocytopenia. In contrast, the structural differences between DS and HS offer a potential advantage by reducing the likelihood of these side effects, making DS a safer alternative for targeting viral entry. However, natural DS suffers from inherent limitations, including heterogeneous molecular weights and impurities arising from variable site-specific sulfation patterns within chondroitin sulfate. To address these challenges, glycopolymer-based analogs inspired by natural polysaccharides have emerged as a promising alternative. The Hagg group demonstrated that negatively charged polysulfates can mimic natural HS and inhibit SARS-CoV-2 by interacting electrostatically with the spike protein [37]. Concurrently, the Nguyen group designed HS mimetics that have low affinity for heparin-binding proteins, such as PF4, thereby reducing potential side effects and enhancing the safety profile of antiviral glycopolymers [38]. Such synthetic glycopolymers enable precise control over structural features, yielding drug candidates with defined active motifs, enhanced uniformity, reduced toxicity, and improved efficacy [35]. Our laboratory previously developed a 'post-modification' strategy based on ring-opening metathesis polymerization (ROMP), enabling the covalent grafting of a synthetic regio-selectively sulphated galactosamine derivative onto a polymer backbone (Scheme 1) to generate multivalent glycopolymers with tunable bioactivity [39].

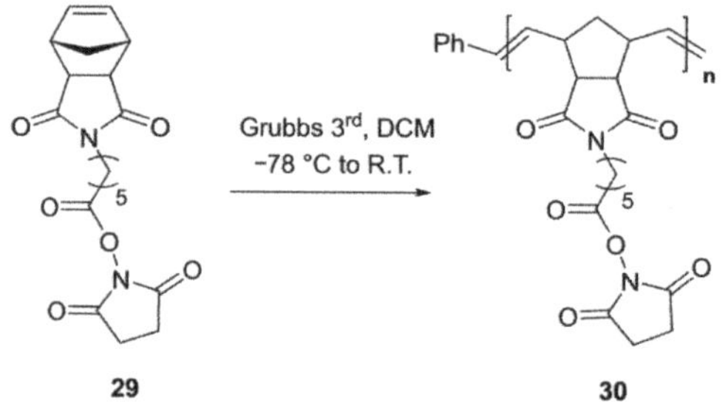

Scheme 1. Synthesis of polymer backbone **30**.

Here we report the design, synthesis, and in vitro antiviral evaluation of DS-mimetic glycopolymers. The functional disaccharide motifs were identified through molecular docking and virtual screening of selectively sulfated structures. Distinct sulfation patterns produced clear differences in binding affinity for the SARS-CoV-2 (2019-nCoV, Wuhan variant) spike protein and inhibitory activity toward M^{pro} and HPSE enzymes. These findings provide valuable insight for developing non-anticoagulant, glycosaminoglycan (GAG)-mimetic antivirals with broad therapeutic potential.

2. Results

2.1. Rational Screening, Design, and Synthesis of DS-Mimetic Disaccharide Modules

To evaluate the antiviral potential of GAG polysaccharides against SARS-CoV-2, we first performed molecular modeling and docking of representative GAG disaccharide units. Three-dimensional structures were generated using GLYCAM [40], and docking simulations were carried out with Vina-Carb [41]. The resulting scores are summarized in Table S1.

CS/DS were selected for further analysis due to their shared highly similar structural motifs to heparin and their comparatively lower incidence of reported side effects [42,43]. Docking results showed that disaccharides derived from CS and DS bind heparanase (HPSE) less strongly than those derived from heparan sulfate (HS). This weaker interaction suggests a reduced likelihood of off-target recognition by HS-binding proteins, thereby potentially minimizing unintended biological responses [28,38]. Within these two families, DS disaccharides present a clearer structure–activity trend [44]. Selective sulfation on DS units produced more distinct changes in predicted activity than comparable modifications on CS units, indicating that DS offers a more tunable platform for rational design. Moreover, the docking analysis of the six HS/HP disaccharide units (Table S1, entries 2–7) showed a clear trend: units containing IdoA (entries 5–7) had substantially higher binding scores across all three proteins than those glycopolymers containing GlcA (entries 2–4). This aligns with prior reports highlighting the key contribution of IdoA residues to GAG–protein interactions [45]. On this basis, we focused subsequent screening on DS disaccharides that incorporate IdoA units.

After visualizing the docking poses in 3D and evaluating the forces involved in a 2D diagram (Figures S1–S6), we observed that the addition of sulfate groups strengthens the DS disaccharide's binding within the RBD pocket. In particular, sulfation improves electrostatic attraction to the positively charged residue K403 and increases stabilizing contacts, including more hydrogen bonds (e.g., with K453 and K495) and additional hydrophobic interactions (e.g., with K505). The location of sulfation also mattered. Notably, sulfation at the C2 and C4 positions of iduronic acid in DS enhanced the predicted antiviral interactions more effectively than sulfation at the C4 and C6 positions of GalNAc. A plausible explanation is that IdoA-2/4S enables deeper insertion into the binding pocket, thereby positioning the GalNAc unit closer to the critical residue K449 [18]. Consistent with this interpretation, different sulfation patterns shifted the disaccharide's orientation in a manner that altered its contacts with K449. In **DM2**, GalNAc sulfation at C4 and C6 pulled the molecule away from K449, weakening or eliminating GalNAc–K449 interactions. In **DM3**, sulfation occurring exclusively on IdoA positioned GalNAc too close to K449 (approximately 1.42 Å), a distance potentially unfavorable for stable binding. In **DM4**, the more evenly distributed negative charge stabilized the disaccharide in the pocket and led to the strongest overall binding.

Guided by these results, we designed four DS-mimetic disaccharide models and conducted retrosynthetic analysis as shown in Scheme S1. Starting from *D*-glucose and *D*-galactosamine·HCl, the aldonic acid (IdoA) donor **6** (Schemes 2a and S2) [46] and the *N*-trichloroacetyl-galactosamine acceptor **9** (Scheme S3) [39] were prepared through multistep sequences. Glycosylation of these partners furnished the orthogonally protected disaccharide **11**. During the deprotection of **11**, an azide-bearing linker proved incompatible with the NH-TCA (2,2,2-trichloroacetyl) group, leading to incomplete deprotection (Scheme S4). We therefore replaced the reducing-end linker with alcohol **13**, protected by benzyl (Bn) and carbobenzyloxy (Cbz) groups, and revised the route to obtain the *N*-trichloroacetyl-galactosamine acceptor **15** (Schemes 2a and S5). The orthogonally protected disaccharide module **16** was synthesized with glycosylation between **6** and **15**, and DS disaccharide **17** was successfully achieved after reduction (Schemes 2a and S6).

Using disaccharide **17** as the core scaffold, four DS-mimetic disaccharides, including **DM1**, **DM2**, **DM3**, and **DM4**, were subsequently prepared through a combination of orthogonal deprotection and selective sulfation strategies (Schemes 2b and S7).

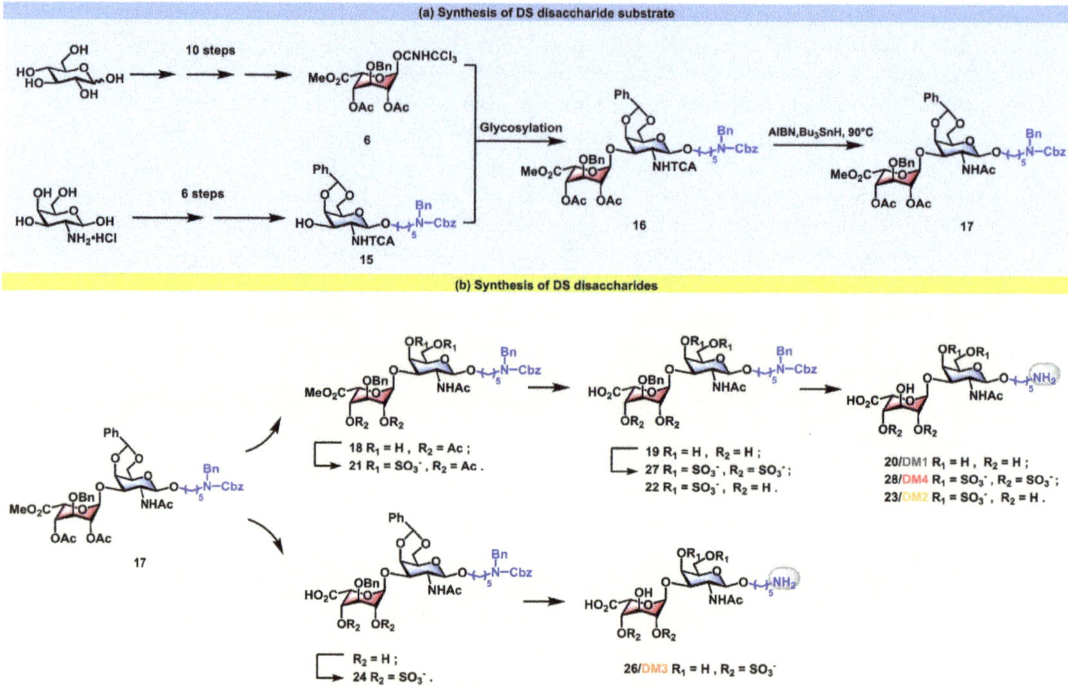

Scheme 2. (**a**) Synthetic route of DS disaccharide substrate. (**b**) Synthetic route of DS disaccharides.

2.2. Preparation, Characterization, and Protein-Binding Assessment of Diverse DS-Mimetic Glycopolymers

Following the successful synthesis of four distinct DS-mimetic disaccharides, a polymer scaffold featuring *N*-hydroxysuccinimide (NHS) ester functionalities (degree of polymerization = 62) was prepared using established methods (Figure 1a) [39]. These disaccharide units were subsequently grafted onto the scaffold in a methanol/water system, yielding four novel glycopolymers (Figure 1a and Scheme S8). The successful grafting and precise degree of sugar substitution (DSS) for each glycopolymer were verified by NMR spectroscopy (Figure 1b and Table 1).

Table 1. Composition and physicochemical characteristics of obtained DS-mimetic glycopolymers.

Glycopolymer	Sugar units	M_w (NMR) [a]	R_h (nm) [b]	R_m (nm) [c]	Zeta-potential [b]	DSS [d]
DMP1	**DM1** (0S)	33 kDa	348.20	27.98	−18.4	82%
DMP2	**DM2** (G4/6S)	36 kDa	327.30	21.09	−21.8	88%
DMP3	**DM3** (I2/4S)	31 kDa	246.60	12.52	−24.2	83%
DMP4	**DM4** (I2/4S, G4/6S)	33 kDa	269.45	15.83	−23.3	86%
MMP [e]	**GalNAc** (3/4/6S)	34 kDa	231.35	21.99	−12.0	84%

[a] Molecular weight (Mw) was determined by ^{1}H-NMR integration. [b] R_h and zeta potential were measured with Zetasizer Nano ZS90 instrument. [c] R_m were measured with TEM and processed with Nano Measurer 1.2. [d] DS = Degree of sugar substitution. [e] The compound was obtained using an established synthetic protocol [39].

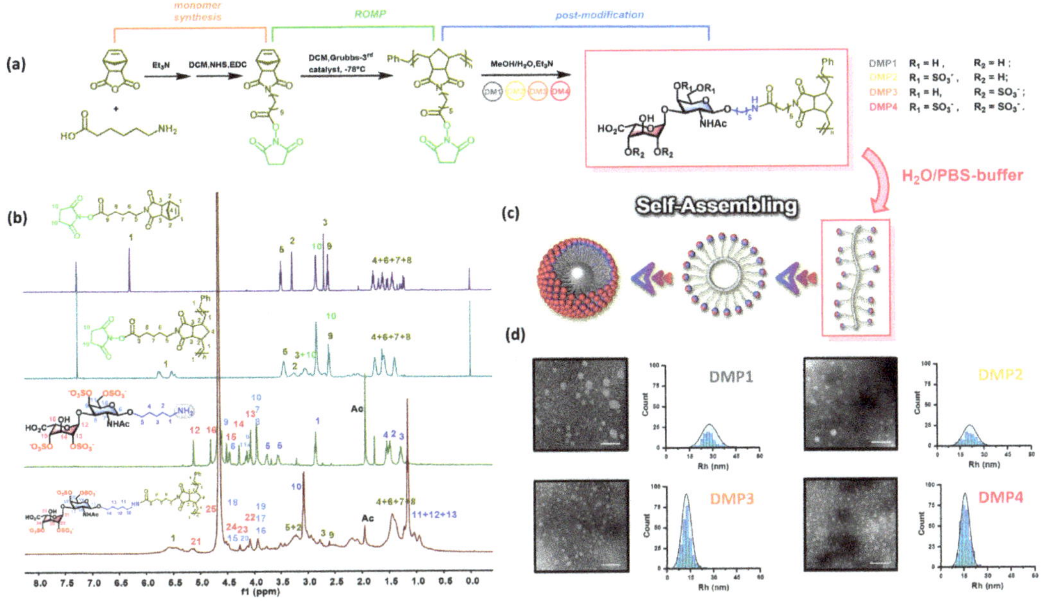

Figure 1. (**a**) Synthetic route of DS-mimetic glycopolymers. (**b**) Overlayed ^{1}H NMR spectra of the polymer backbone (**31**) in $CDCl_3$, DS-mimetic disaccharide **28** (**DM4**), and the relative glycopolymer (**DMP4**) in D_2O. (**c**) A schematic illustration of aqueous self-assembly of the glycopolymers into nanoparticles. (**d**) A TEM image of the resulting DS-mimetic glycopolymer nanoparticles (scale bar, 100 nm).

Consistent with our previous reports, these glycopolymers were observed to self-assemble into stable nanoparticles in aqueous solution, driven by the amphiphilic balance between the hydrophilic sugar side chains and the hydrophobic polymer backbone (Figure 1c). The particle size and uniformity of the resulting nanoparticles were characterized by transmission electron microscopy (TEM) and dynamic light scattering (DLS) (Figure 1d and Table 1). The glycopolymers self-assembled into nanoparticles with an average diameter of approximately 20 nm under physiological conditions (Figure 1d). Glycopolymers bearing sulfate modifications exhibited a more uniform size distribution and enhanced structural stability. Notably, glycopolymers **DMP3** and **DMP4**, which bear sulfate modifications at the C2 and C4 positions of IdoA within their disaccharide units, consistently formed smaller and more uniform nanoparticles (Table 1).

It is worth noting that the particle sizes measured by DLS were approximately 10–15 times larger than those observed by TEM. This discrepancy likely arises because during TEM analysis, the nanoparticles are well dispersed on the copper grid after solvent evaporation, whereas in DLS, strong interparticle interaction and the hydration layer around micelles increase the apparent hydrodynamic diameter (Z-average, R_h) [47].

Relative to **DMP2**, both **DMP3** and **DMP4** exhibit more negative (higher-magnitude) ζ-potentials (Table 1). Notably, **DMP3** outperforms **DMP2** despite carrying the same number of anionic groups (sulfate and carboxylate). This is attributed to the greater hydrophilicity and outward presentation of the anionic substituents in **DMP3**, promoting their localization at the nanoparticle–water interface, increasing surface charge density, and stabilizing self-assembly. Although **DMP4** carries five negative charges and **DMP3** carries only three, both exhibit nearly identical zeta potentials. This observation suggests that, during self-assembly, the glycopolymer adopts a morphology in which the sugar-based side chains orient outward, while the hydrophobic backbone and reducing-end GalNAc units are sequestered inward. As a result, the hydrophilicity and surface charge are dominated by the non-reducing end IdoA2/4S moieties, whose influence on the nanoparticles far exceeds that of the GalNAc4/6S units. All these physicochemical features above suggest that **DMP3** and **DMP4** may display superior biological activity [48,49].

Molecular docking indicated stronger binding of **DM3** and **DM4** to the spike RBD than **DM2** (Table S1). For **DM4**, the predicted interactions are dominated by hydrogen bonds with polar residues and electrostatic contacts with basic residues in the RBD. By contrast, **DM1** (unsulfated) and **DM2** (GalNAc C4/C6 sulfation) showed weak RBD affinity. Upon grafting the disaccharides onto the polymer backbone, the 'multivalent effect' potentially promotes further-enhanced protein binding [50,51].

Consistent with these predictions, SPR measurements against spike and ACE2 (Table 2) showed that **DMP4** bound spike with the greatest affinity ($K_D \approx 177$ nM), approximately an order of magnitude stronger than its binding to ACE2 ($K_D \approx 1088$ nM). Other glycopolymers also bound spike in the several-hundred-nanomolar range, with **DMP3** outperforming **DMP2**, underscoring the positional specificity of sulfation in GAG-mimetic oligosaccharides. These trends align with the nanoparticle characterization data (Figure 1d and Table 1). We also assessed the spike-binding properties of our previously synthesized glycopolymer **MMP**, which features 3,4,6-*O*-sulfated GalNAc motifs and is known for its antitumor activity [39]. **MMP** displayed the second-highest binding affinity following DMP4, despite its simpler structure. These results suggest that **MMP** holds strong potential for further development as a broad-spectrum antiviral agent, particularly for rapid deployment during public health emergencies.

Table 2. Binding kinetics of DS-mimetic glycopolymers to SARS-CoV-2 spike and ACE2 protein.

Compound and Protein	k_a ($M^{-1}s^{-1}$) [a]	k_d (1/s) [a]	K_D (M) [a]
DMP1-Spike	2.25×10^4	1.10×10^{-3}	4.89×10^{-7}
DMP2-Spike	1.09×10^4	3.90×10^{-3}	3.58×10^{-7}
DMP3-Spike	1.61×10^4	4.72×10^{-3}	2.92×10^{-7}
DMP4-Spike	2.27×10^4	4.00×10^{-3}	1.77×10^{-7}
MMP-Spike	1.78×10^4	4.75×10^{-3}	2.67×10^{-7}
DMP4-ACE2	4.41×10^3	4.80×10^{-3}	1.08×10^{-6}

[a] ka: Association rate constant; kd: dissociation rate constant; KD: apparent equilibrium dissociation constant.

SPR analysis confirmed the reliability of molecular docking for assessing the antiviral potential of GAG oligosaccharides. The results demonstrated that, once incorporated into a glycopolymer, the DS-mimetic disaccharides exhibited high-affinity binding to the viral spike protein, underscoring the promise of sulfated glycopolymers as antiviral candidates. Based on these findings, the safety and antiviral efficacy of the synthesized glycopolymers were then evaluated.

2.3. *In Vitro Antiviral Activity and Cellular Uptake of DS-Mimetic Glycopolymers*

Previous reported studies, including those by Linhardt and co-workers, have established that during SARS-CoV-2 infection, the viral spike protein first interacts with HS on the host cell surface, which facilitates subsequent engagement with the ACE2 receptor to trigger cellular entry [10,12,19,23,25]. The SPR analyses in this study have confirmed that DS-mimetic glycopolymers can bind both the spike protein and ACE2 (Figure 2 and Table 2). It is proposed that these glycopolymers competitively associate with the viral spike protein, thereby preventing the viral attachment to cell-surface HS, while exhibiting weaker, lower-toxicity interactions with ACE2 as well. This dual-binding behavior may effectively block the viral internalization pathway and enhance antiviral efficacy (Figure 3a).

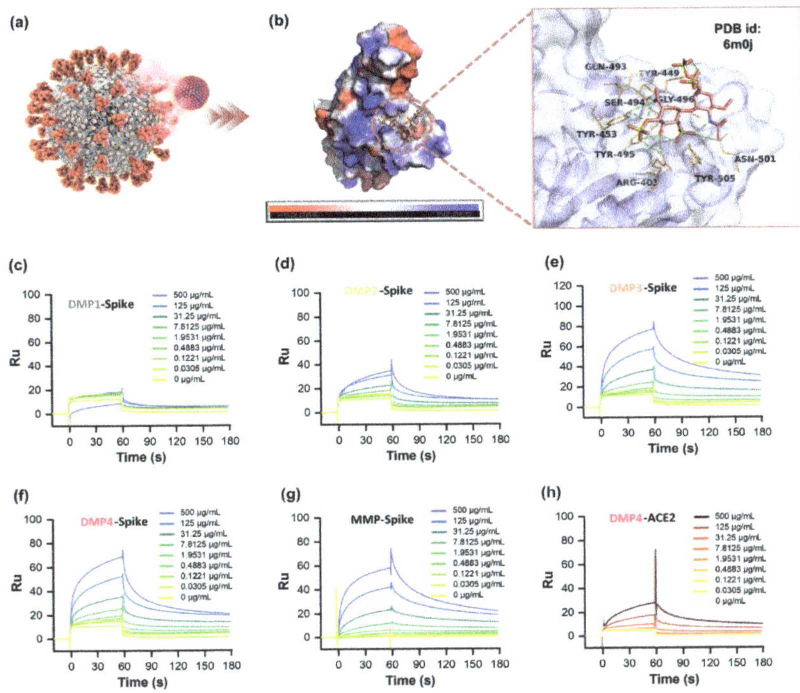

Figure 2. (**a**) Schematic diagram of glycopolymer nanoparticles inhibiting SARS-CoV-2. (**b**) Molecular docking of DS-mimetic disaccharides and spike protein. (**c**–**g**) SPR analysis of DS-mimetic glycopolymers with spike protein: (**c**) **DMP1**; (**d**) **DMP2**; (**e**) **DMP3**; (**f**) **DMP4**; (**g**) **MMP**. (**h**) SPR analysis of **DMP4** with ACE2 protein.

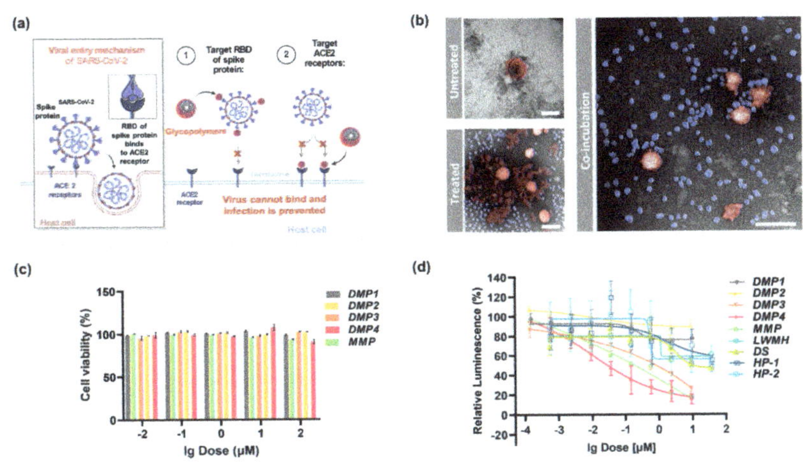

Figure 3. (**a**) Schematic diagram of DS-mimetic glycopolymer nanoparticles targeting viral particles and protecting host cells. (**b**) TEM images of pseudovirus before and after treatment with **DMP4**; scale bar, 100 nm; The pseudo-colors are added for visual clarity: red, pseudovirus particles and fragments; blue, glycopolymer nanoparticles. The original TEM image is provided in the Supporting Information (Figures S7–S9). Co-incubation: pseudovirus and glycopolymer were mixed and immediately processed for negative-stain TEM; Treated: samples prepared identically but incubated for 2 h at 37 °C before grid preparation. (**c**) Cytotoxicity assays of glycopolymers (mean ± SD, n = 3). (**d**) Pseudovirus infection assays of diverse sulfated glycopolymers (mean ± SD, n = 3).

TEM imaging revealed the morphology of SARS-CoV-2 pseudoviruses displaying surface spike proteins (highlighted in red in Figure 3b). TEM showed that **DMP4** glycopolymer nanoparticles (highlighted in blue in Figure 3b) adsorbed onto and aggregated on the pseudoviral surface upon co-incubation with the glycopolymers. Prolonged incubation caused pronounced structural damage to the pseudovirus. Numerous viral fragments (~50 nm) were observed, and intact particles shifted from a rough to a smooth surface, consistent with loss of spike proteins. These changes suggest that strong electrostatic interactions between the glycopolymers and the viral envelope destabilize and compromise pseudovirus integrity.

To further assess antiviral efficacy at the cellular level, we evaluated the ability of the glycopolymers to inhibit pseudovirus infection in 293T/17 cells. Prior to this, cytotoxicity was examined in 293 T/17 cells, where all glycopolymers demonstrated minimal toxicity, maintaining over 90% cell viability even at 100 μM (Figure 3c). After confirming their biocompatibility, we performed concentration-dependent assays to determine the half-maximal inhibitory concentration (IC_{50}) values against pseudovirus infection (Figure 3d). Among the tested compounds, **DMP4** exhibited the strongest inhibition (IC_{50} = 104 nM), followed by **MMP** (IC_{50} = 190 nM) and **DMP3** (IC_{50} = 1414 nM). These activities surpassed those of glycopolymers **DMP1** and **DMP2** as well as natural GAG polysaccharides (HP, LWMH, DS), aligning with the binding results observed at the protein level.

Building on the cellular assays and characterization of the self-assembled glycopolymer nanoparticles, we propose that these nanoparticles can enter host cells through endocytosis and subsequently release polysaccharide components via membrane flipping within endosomes (Figure 4c). This process may suppress intracellular replication of SARS-CoV-2 and inhibit key viral and host enzymes, including M^{pro} and HPSE, thereby achieving a coordinated and multi-targeted antiviral effect.

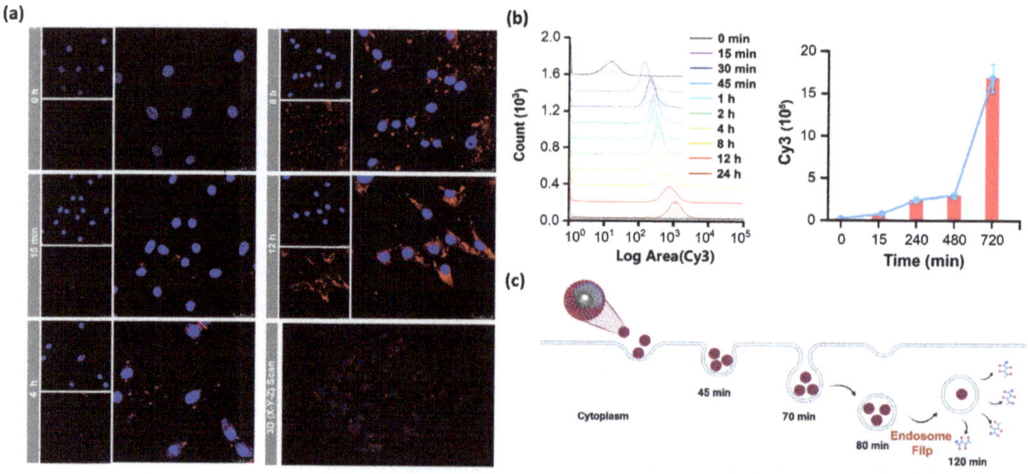

Figure 4. (**a**) Confocal images of Vero cells incubated with **Cy3-DMP4** (20 μg·mL^{-1}) for four hours. The scale bar indicates 5 μm. (**b**) Fluorescence intensity of Vero cells incubated with **Cy3-DMP4** obtained by laser scanning confocal microscopy. Flow cytometric analysis of fluorescence intensity in Vero cells incubated with **Cy3-DMP4** (20 μg·mL^{-1}) for different times. (**c**) Schematic diagram of entry of DS-mimetic glycopolymer nanoparticles into cells by endocytosis.

To verify the cellular internalization capability of the glycopolymer nanoparticles, **DMP4** was fluorescently labeled with sulfo-Cy3. Cellular uptake was then examined using confocal fluorescence microscopy (Figure 4a) and flow cytometry at various time points

(Figure 4b). The results demonstrated that the **DMP4** nanoparticles were efficiently internalized by Vero cells, with maximal uptake observed between 4 and 8 h post-incubation.

After confirming cellular internalization of the saccharide polymers as nanoparticles, we assessed their inhibitory activity against HPSE and M^{pro} in concentration-dependent assays. The results were consistent with both molecular docking predictions (Figure 5a,d) and antiviral activity measurements (Table 3). Among the tested polymers, **DMP4** exhibited the strongest inhibition of HPSE, with an IC_{50} comparable to that of natural heparin. In contrast, **DMP3** showed the most potent inhibition on M^{pro}, significantly exceeding that of natural GAGs, which is consistent with the docking analysis. These findings suggest that sulfation at the C2 and C4 positions of IdoA in the DS-mimetic disaccharides is critical for effective interaction with key residues in the active site of M^{pro} (Figure 5d).

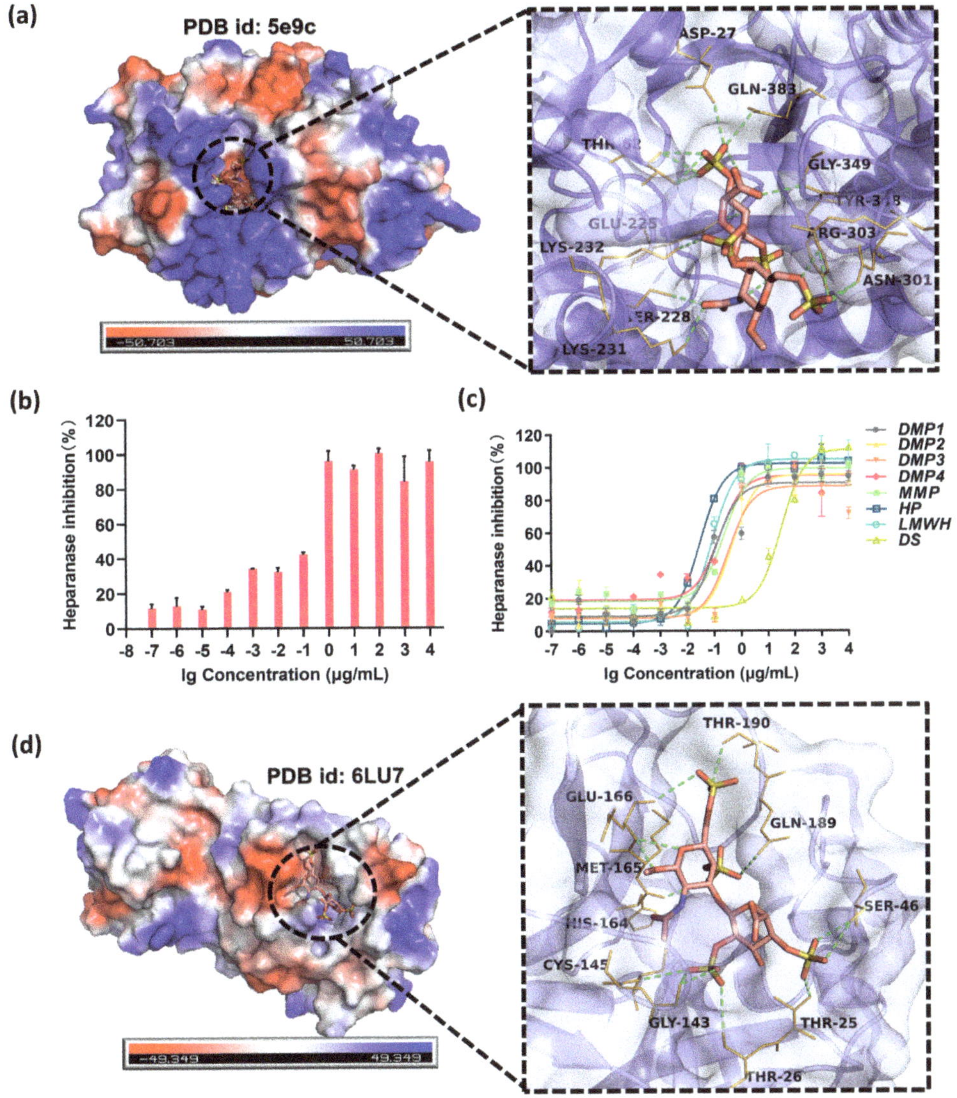

Figure 5. *Cont.*

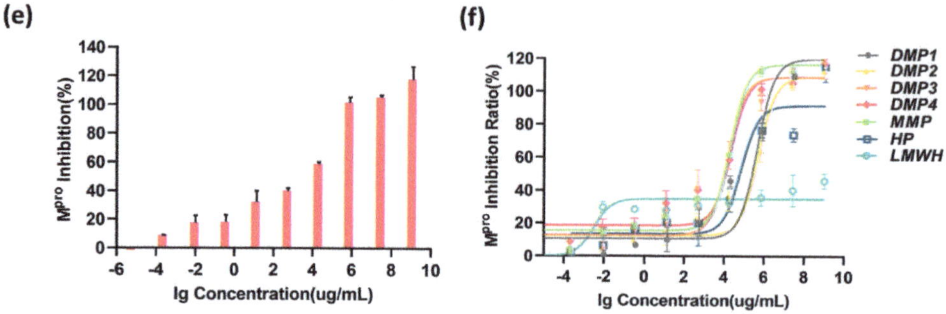

Figure 5. (**a**) Molecular docking of DS-mimetic disaccharides and heparanase protein. (**b**) Inhibition of heparanase by glycopolymer **DMP4** using a TR-FRET assay (mean ± SD, n = 3). (**c**) Inhibition of heparanase by diverse sulfated glycopolymers using a TR-FRET assay (n = 3). (**d**) Molecular docking of DS-mimetic disaccharides and Mpro protein. (**e**) Inhibition assay of Mpro by glycopolymer **DMP4** (n = 3). (**f**) Inhibition assay of Mpro by diverse sulfated glycopolymers (mean ± SD, n = 3).

Table 3. Inhibition of heparanase and M^{pro} by DS-mimetic glycopolymers.

Entry	Compounds	IC_{50}^{a} (nM)	IC_{50}^{a} (μg/mL)	IC_{50}^{b} (μM)	IC_{50}^{b} (μg/mL)
1	**DMP1**	5.48	0.18	2.01	66.33
2	**DMP2**	21.35	0.77	1.31	47.16
3	**DMP3**	8.12	0.25	0.47	14.57
4	**DMP4**	3.67	0.12	0.89	29.37
5	**MMP**	5.39	0.18	0.71	24.14
6	**DS**	1249	43.72	-	-
7	**LMWH** [c]	18.13	0.082	>1000	>4500
8	**Heparin**	3.74	0.056	8.97	134.55

[a] Inhibition of heparanase was assessed by in vitro TR-FRET assay against fluorescently tagged HS. [b] Inhibition of M^{pro} was assessed by in vitro fluorescence intensity assay against fluorogenic substrate MCA-AVLQSGFR-Lys (Dnp)-Lys-NH_2. [c] LMWH = low-molecular-weight heparin.

Both the molecular docking studies and the subsequent biological assays demonstrated that the DS-mimetic disaccharides effectively target the viral spike protein and inhibit the HPSE and M^{pro} enzymes. When formulated into nanoparticles, these disaccharide glycopolymers are efficiently internalized in Vero cells. The glycopolymers exert potent antiviral effects against SARS-CoV-2 by multi-targeted actions at the viral surface, cell membrane, and intracellular environment. These results highlight their promise as a new class of antiviral therapeutics.

3. Discussion

3.1. Strengths and Key Findings of the Study

In this study, the molecular docking and virtual screening were performed to assess the antiviral potential of sulfated GAG oligosaccharides against SARS-CoV-2 [20,38]. The focus is on key targets in the viral infection process, including the spike protein, as well as M^{pro} and HPSE enzymes involved in post-infection viral proliferation and further spread.

The screening identifies sulfated DS disaccharide units as promising candidates for antiviral drug development. These DS-mimetic disaccharides are synthesized through chemical methods and grafted onto a polymer backbone under mild and efficient conditions, forming distinct glycopolymers that enhance antiviral activity through multivalent effects [39,50]. SPR assays at the molecular level validate the docking prediction results, while in vitro cellular experiments demonstrate that the glycopolymer nanoparticles self-assembled under physiological conditions are effectively internalized by host cells. Additionally, the inhibitory effects of glycopolymers on M^{pro} and HPSE enzymes are evaluated in infected Vero cells. The surface DS-mimetic glycopolymers inhibit SARS-CoV-2 infection and replication through a multi-targeted mechanism (Figure 6), offering new insights into the development of broad-spectrum antiviral therapeutics based on GAG polysaccharide mimetics.

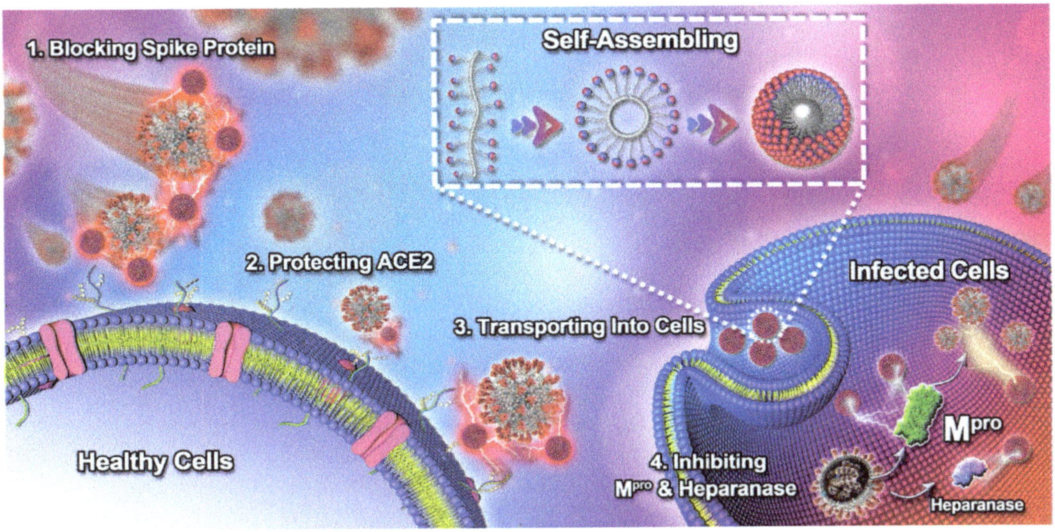

Figure 6. Proposed mechanism of action for DS-mimetic glycopolymers as multi-target antiviral agents against SARS-CoV-2: 1. Sulfated glycopolymers bind to the viral spike protein with high affinity. 2. Low-toxicity glycopolymers bind to and shield ACE2 on healthy cells, preventing the recognition between the viral spike protein and ACE2. 3. The glycopolymers self-assemble into stable nanoparticles, which are internalized by cells via endocytosis. 4. Inside infected cells, the glycopolymers inhibit HPSE and M^{pro} enzymes, suppressing viral replication and further infection.

3.2. Study Limitations and Outlooks

This insightful study still possesses several limitations. First, the antiviral activity of the DS-mimetic glycopolymers was evaluated only at the in vitro level. Due to constraints in synthesis scale and the relatively low yield of the chemical sulfation process, the amount of material obtained was insufficient for in vivo antiviral assessment in animal models. Similarly, the current quantities do not allow high-throughput screening against multiple coronavirus variants, limiting our ability to experimentally confirm the broad-spectrum antiviral potential of these glycopolymers. Moreover, the release behavior of the self-assembled glycopolymer nanoparticles requires further validation, particularly regarding the preservation of sulfated oligosaccharide integrity during cellular uptake, as sulfation patterns are critical for intracellular enzyme inhibition. Additionally, due to the structural complexity of GAGs and the diversity of possible sulfation motifs, the molecular docking model in this study did not encompass all structural variants. The DS disaccharide model used in this research does not include the structure with IdoA at the reducing end and GalNAc at the non-reducing end. Previous reports have also suggested that higher-ordered oligosaccharides, such as HS tetrasaccharides, exhibit stronger binding affinity toward M^{pro} [52]. Future studies should therefore extend the screening, synthesis, and biological evaluation to specific oligosaccharides with higher degrees of polymerization.

In our ongoing studies, we focus on the biomimetic synthesis of GAGs and sulfated polysaccharides derived from marine sources with structurally defined oligosaccharides and precise sulfation patterns. These efforts aim to further explore their antiviral activity against SARS-CoV-2, influenza virus, HSV, and other emerging viral pathogens, advancing the development of next-generation glycomimetic antiviral therapeutics.

4. Materials and Methods

4.1. Materials

Ethyl vinyl ether (EVE, 97%), N-(3-Dimethylaminopropyl)-N′-ethylcarbodiimide hydrochloride (EDC, 98%), and N-hydroxysuccinimide (98%, NHS) were purchased from Aladdin (Shanghai, China) and used without further purification. Nucleic acid dye DAPI and Grubbs-type catalysts (G 3rd) were purchased from Sigma Aldrich (St. Louis, MO, USA) and used directly. Other chemical reagents were purchased from Sinopharm Chemical Reagent Co., Ltd. (Shanghai, China) and used directly. SARS-CoV-2 spike Protein (S1 + S2 ECD, His-tag, cat No. 40589-V08B1) and Human Angiotensin-Converting Enzyme 2 (ACE2) Protein (His-Tag, HPLC-verified, cat No. 10108-H08B) were purchased from Sino Biological (Beijing, China). Minimum essential medium (MEM) was obtained from Gibco (Rockville, MD, USA). Fetal bovine serum (FBS) and trypsin were obtained from Gibco-Invitrogen (Grand Island, NY, USA). Cell proliferation/cytotoxicity assay kit (CCK8) was purchased from Dojindo (Tokyo, Japan). SARS-CoV-2 pseudovirus was purchased from PackGene Biotech (Guangzhou, China). Heparanase assay toolbox was purchased from Cisbio Assay (Codolet, France), and heparinase (human recombinant heparanase 7570-GH) was purchased from R&D systems (Minneapolis, MN, USA). Porcine intestinal heparin (Mw = 15 kDa) was obtained from Linhardt's laboratory (Troy, NY, USA). Low-molecular-weight heparin (LMWH, Enoxaparine, Mw $\approx$ 4.5 kDa) was purchased from China Resources Double-crane Pharmaceutical Co., Ltd. Dermatan sulfate ($\geq$90%, Mw $\approx$ 3.5 kDa) was purchased from Sigma Aldrich (St. Louis, MO, USA).

4.2. Synthesis of the Engineered Dermatan Sulfate–Mimetic Glycopolymers

4.2.1. General Procedure for the Preparation of Polymer Containing NHS Ester (30, DP = 50)

Compound **29** was synthesized based on our previously published procedure [39]. A solution of **29** (30 mg, 0.094 mmol) in DCM (1 mL) was stirred at −78 °C for 30 min with argon protection. A desirable amount of the Grubbs 3rd catalyst (1.42 mg, 0.0019 mmol, 2%) from the fresh-prepared stock solution in DCM (14.2 mg·mL^{-1}, 100 μL) was added to the reaction flask. The mixture was stirred vigorously at −78 °C for 20 min, protected from light, followed by warming up to room temperature. The resultant solution was stirred at room temperature for an additional 1 h, after which TLC indicated full conversion and it was quenched with excess ethyl vinyl ether (EVE). The mixture was stirred for 30 min, the excess Et_2O (×5 Volume) was added, and a light-brown precipitate was formed. The suspension was centrifuged and then the supernatant was discarded. The precipitate was washed by repeating the process of dissolving in DCM/Et_2O, centrifuging, and decanting until the supernatant appeared colorless to afford the final polynorbornyl NHS ester **30** (25 mg, DP = 50, 85%) as a gray solid. The polymer was stored at −20 °C and characterized by ^{1}H-NMR. ^{1}H NMR (500 MHz, DMF-*d7*) δ 7.70–7.36 (m, 5H), 6.12–5.54 (m, 125H).

4.2.2. General Procedure for Post-Modification of NHS-Containing Polymer with Sugar Units

Before coupling the NHS-activated polymer with the sugar units, the NHS-containing polymer (1.0 equiv., relative to monomer) was first dissolved in DMF (1.2 mL) to generate solution A. Separately, the terminal amine-functionalized disaccharide (1.2 equiv.) was dissolved in Milli-Q water (200 μL) to form solution B. Solution A was then added to solution B, followed immediately by triethylamine (5 equiv.). The reaction mixture was stirred vigorously at room temperature for 5 h, at which point TLC confirmed complete conversion.

The crude product was purified by dialysis against water for 48 h using a 3.5 kDa MWCO membrane. The resulting solution was lyophilized to afford the glycopolymer as a white powder. The purified materials were stored at −20 °C and characterized by ^{1}H NMR.

The degree of sugar substitution (DSS) was determined from ^{1}H NMR spectra by integrating the N-acetyl peaks of the grafted disaccharides relative to the backbone reference peaks (olefin protons of the ROMP scaffold).

4.2.3. General Procedure for Fluorescent Labeling of Glycopolymers by Post-Modification

To a solution of glycopolymers in PBS buffer (pH 7.4), EDC/NHS (2.0 equiv.) was added, which was then stirred at room temperature for 30 min. Sulfo-Cyanine3 amine (Sulfo-Cy3-NH_2) was then added, and the reaction was allowed to proceed for an additional 4 h in the absence of light. TLC analysis confirmed complete fluorescent labeling.

The reaction mixture was purified by dialysis against water for 48 h using a 3.5 kDa MWCO membrane, with protection from light maintained throughout. TLC analysis confirmed the absence of free Cy3 in the dialysate. The dialyzed solution was lyophilized to yield the Cy3-labeled glycopolymer as a pink powder. The final materials were stored at −20 °C in the dark.

4.3. *SPR Analysis*

4.3.1. Immobilization of Protein on a CM5 Sensor Chip

A CM5 chip was first set in a Biacore T200 to immobilize RBD and ACE2 protein for surface plasmon resonance (SPR) analysis. The carboxylate dextran matrix of the sensor chip was washed with PBS-P running buffer (1×, GE healthcare), and then activated with a mixture of 0.4 M EDC and 0.1 M NHS from the kit for 420 s at a flow rate of 10 µL/min. Afterwards, SARS-CoV-2 spike protein (pI 6.52) was immobilized at a concentration of 25 µg/mL in 10 mM sodium acetate (pH 5.0), and ACE2 protein (pI 5.60) was immobilized at a concentration of 25 µg/mL in 10 mM sodium acetate (pH 4.5) onto the chip surface. The remaining binding sites on the chip surface were blocked with 1 M ethanolamine (pH 8.5). The baseline was allowed to stabilize with PBS-P running buffer for at least 2 h before injecting test samples.

4.3.2. Kinetic Binding Affinity Assays

Varying concentrations (0.0305–500 µg/mL) of DS-mimetic glycopolymers were dissolved in the PBS-P running buffer and injected for 60 s at 30 µL/min, followed by a 300 s dissociation phase. Regeneration of the sensor chip after each analysis cycle was performed by injecting 0.5 mM NaOH for 5 s. The response was monitored as a function of time (sensorgram) at 25 °C and subtracted from the response of the reference surface. BIAevaluation software 4.1. was used to evaluate kinetic parameters (Ka: association rate constant; Kd: dissociation rate constant; KD: apparent equilibrium dissociation constant).

4.4. *Cell Viability Assay*

Vero cells (1 × 10^4 cells per well) were, respectively, cultured into a 96-well microplate overnight with MEM with 10% FBS and 1% Penicillin/Streptomycin. Then, varying concentrations (final working concentration 0.01–100 µM, in MEM) of glycopolymer stock solution were added to specific wells in triplicate and incubated for 24 h at 37 °C under 5% CO_2. Afterwards, the supernatant was replaced with fresh MEM with 10% CCK8 solution (Dojindo, Japan) and incubated for an additional 2 h, and quenched by adding 10 µL Stop solution. Eventually, OD 450 nm was measured by the microplate reader Tecan Spark

10 M, and the cell viability was calculated, normalized to the controls, and presented as a percentage as follows:

$$\text{Cell viability (\%)} = [\text{OD}_{450}(\text{sample})]/[\text{OD}_{450}(\text{control})] \times 100\%.$$

4.5. *SARS-CoV-2 Pseudovirus Neutralization Assay*

4.5.1. SARS-CoV-2 Pseudovirus Production and Transient Transfection of ACE2

293 T/17 cells were employed to pack the SARS-CoV-2 pseudoviral particles. Cells were cultured with DMEM supplemented (Coring, NY, USA, cat NO. 10-013-CVR) with 10% fetal bovine serum (ExCell, cat No. FND500) and 1% Penicillin Streptomycin solution (Coring, USA, cat No. 25-053-CI). Plasmid transfection was performed in 6-well plates by LipFiter 3.0 Reagent (HANBIO, cat No. HB-LF3-1000). The viral particle-containing supernatant was harvested at 48 h post-transfection and stored at −80 °C.

4.5.2. SARS-CoV-2 Pseudovirus Neutralization Assays

ACE2-pcDNA3.1 plasmid transfection was performed in 6-well plates by LipFiter 3.0 Reagent (HANBIO). The supernatant of 293 T/17 cells was abandoned, and cells were harvested by trypsinization, collected in a centrifuge tube, and centrifuged at 1000 rpm for 5 min, after which the supernatant was discarded, and the cells were resuspended with complete DMEM medium. Afterwards, 293 T/17-ACE2 cells (1.2 × 104 cells per well) was cultured into 96-well microplates (Corning 3917, NY, USA) for an additional 6–8 h at 37 °C under 5% CO2. Supernatant was replaced with complete medium (10% FBS, 1% Penicillin and Streptomycin) with varying concentration samples and incubated for 24 h. Then, the supernatant was replaced with fresh complete medium and incubated for an additional 48 h, and 15 µL Renilla luciferase reagent (Promega, cat lot #E2720) was added to the plate. The plates were placed on an orbital shaker for 2 min, followed by 10 min at room temperature to stabilize the luminescent signal. Eventually, the luminescent signal was measured by the microplate reader SpectraMax Paradigm. Relative light units (RLU) were calculated as follows:

$$\text{RLU (\%)} = [\text{RLU(sample)}/\text{RLU(DMSO)}] \times 100\%$$

Cell viability at various compound concentrations was calculated using Excel. The resulting data were then analyzed and plotted using GraphPad Prism 7.0 to generate dose–response curves and calculate the IC50 values.

4.6. *Confocal Microscopy for the Localization of Cellular Uptake of Glycopolymers*

4.6.1. Confocal Microscopy for Internalization of Vero Cell

Vero cells (8×10^4 cells per well) were cultured in 35 mm glass-bottomed Petri dishes (Nest, cat No. 801002-ZX) overnight with MEM (10% FBS, 1% Penicillin and Streptomycin). Afterwards, supernatant was replaced with fresh medium (1% Penicillin and Streptomycin) with 20 µg/mL **Cy3-DMP4** and incubated for 12 h at 37 °C under 5% CO_2. Then, cells were washed twice with PBS and fixed with 4% paraformaldehyde for 1 h, followed by washing away paraformaldehyde and staining with 200 µL of DAPI for an additional 10 min. Eventually, the supernatant was replaced with PBS and the cellular uptake of glycopolymer nanoparticles was imaged with a confocal microscope (Leica TCS SP8).

4.6.2. Confocal Microscopy for Internalization of Vero Cells at Different Time Points

Vero cells (8×10^4 cells per well) were cultured in 96-well microplate overnight with MEM with 10% FBS and 1% Penicillin/Streptomycin. Then, supernatant was replaced with fresh medium (1% Penicillin and Streptomycin) with 20 µg/mL Cy3-DMP4 and incubated for 15 min, 30 min, 45 min, 1 h, 2 h, 4 h, 8 h, 12 h, and 24 h, respectively. Afterwards, cells were washed twice with PBS and fixed with 4% paraformaldehyde for 1 h, followed by washing away paraformaldehyde and staining with 200 μL of DAPI for an additional 10 min. Eventually, the supernatant was replaced with PBS and the cellular uptake of glycopolymer nanoparticles was imaged with a confocal microscope (Leica TCS SP8). Fluorescence intensities were quantified by ImageJ 1.53c software.

4.7. Flow Cytometric Analysis of Cellular Uptake of the Glycopolymers

Vero cells (1×10^4 cells per well) were cultured in 35 mm glass-bottomed Petri dishes (Nest, cat No. 801002-ZX) overnight with MEM (10% FBS, 1% Penicillin and Streptomycin). Then, supernatant was replaced with fresh medium (1% Penicillin and Streptomycin) with 20 μg/mL Cy3-DMP4 and incubated for 15 min, 30 min, 45 min, 1 h, 2 h, 4 h, 8 h, 12 h, and 24 h, respectively. Then, the supernatant of Vero cells was abandoned, and the cells were digested with pancreatin, collected in a centrifuge tube, and centrifuged at 1000 rpm for 5 min, after which the supernatant was discarded, and the cells were washed twice with PBS and prepared in a single-cell suspension. Differential cell counting was performed by flow cytometry (Beckman MoFlo XDP).

4.8. TR-FRET Heparanase Inhibition Assay

Heparanase inhibition assays were performed using the heparanase assay toolbox (Cisbio) and human recombinant heparanase 7570-GH-005 (R&D, Lot. DCEM0218041). The homogenous time-resolved fluorescence (HTRF) signal (excitation 337 nm, emission 620 nm and 665 nm) was monitored with a microplate reader Tecan Spark 10 M.

The heparanase inhibition activity assays were performed in a 112-μL reaction (14 μL sample solution, 14 μL heparanase solution, 28 μL biotin-heparan sulphate-Eu cryptate substrate solution, 56 μL Streptavidin-XLent solution) to measure the inhibition constant IC_{50} for glycopolymers. In total, 14 μL varying concentrations (final working concentration 0.1 pg/mL–10 mg/mL) of glycopolymers and 14 μL 5.3 nM heparanase solution in pH 7.5 text buffer (20 mM Tris-HCl, 0.15 M NaCl, and 0.1% CHAPS) were added in a 384-well microplate (Greiner, #781080 384-well) in triplicate. Afterwards, the plate was incubated at 37 °C for 10 min. The enzyme reaction was initiated by adding 28 μL biotin-heparan sulphate-Eu cryptate (Cisbio, #61BHSKAA) substrate solution (0.7 μg/mL in 0.2 M $NaCH_3CO_2$ buffer, pH 5.5) and the plate was incubated at 37 °C for 1 h, followed by the addition of 56 μL Streptavidin-XLent (Cisbio, # 611SAXLA) solution (1.0 μg/mL in 0.1 M NaPO4, 0.8 M KF, 1 mg/mL heparin, 0.1% BSA buffer, pH 7.4) and incubation at 37 °C for 5 min. HTRF signals were monitored by microplate reader at $\lambda_{em1} = 620$ nm and $\lambda_{em2} = 665$ nm after 60 μs of excitation at $\lambda_{ex} = 337$ nm. Specific HTRF signal was expressed as percentage of delta F, and calculated as follows:

$$\text{Delta F (\%)} = \{[(F_{665}/F_{620})\ \text{sample} - (F_{665}/F_{620})\ \text{blank}]/(F_{665}/F_{620})\ \text{blank}\} \times 100\%.$$

4.9. In Vitro Activity Assays of the SARS-CoV-2 M^pro Inhibitors

4.9.1. SARS-CoV-2 M^{pro} Protein Expression In Vitro

Details and SDS-PAGE image can be found in the Supporting Information.

4.9.2. SARS-CoV-2 M^{pro} Inhibition Assay

The M^{pro} inhibitory activity assays were performed following established protocols from previous studies, with minor adjustments to suit our experimental setup [53]. All measurements were conducted within a 100 μL reaction volume (2 μL sample solution, 88 μL M^{pro} solution, 10 μL substrate solution). These setups were used to determine the inhibition constant (IC_{50}) of the glycopolymers. In total, 200 nM of M^{pro}, 20 μM of substrate, and varying concentrations (final working concentration 0.0274–540 μg/mL) of DS-mimetic glycopolymers were added into different wells in a black, clear-bottomed 96-well plate (Corning, NY, USA). Glycopolymers were dissolved in H_2O to prepare a stock solution and diluted in the assay buffer (50 mM Tris·HCl, 1 mM EDTA, pH 7.3) to the desired concentrations. In total, 2 μL of diluted glycopolymer solution was added to a solution of Mpro (228 nM) in assay buffer (88 μL), and then the mixture was incubated at room temperature for 30 min. The enzyme reaction was triggered by adding a solution of diluted substrate solution (200 μM) in assay buffer (10 μL). Fluorescence intensity (excitation 340 nm, emission 490 nm) was monitored by microplate reader once every 45 s. The initial reaction velocities (substrate cleaved/second) were calculated by fitting the linear portion of the curves (within the first 10 min of the progress curves) to a straight line using the software Origin Pro (Learning Edition, Version 2025b. OriginLab Corporation, Northampton, MA, USA.). Afterwards, the reaction velocity was converted to enzyme activity, and the inhibition rate was calculated as follows:

$$\text{Inhibition rate (\%)} = \{1 - [\text{Enzyme activity (compound)} - \text{Enzyme activity (blank)}]/[\text{Enzyme activity (control)} - \text{Enzyme activity (blank)}]\} \times 100\%$$

5. Conclusions

In summary, we developed a class of precision-engineered DS-mimetic glycopolymers that demonstrate multi-targeted inhibition of SARS-CoV-2. Based on the molecular docking and structure–activity analysis, regioselective sulfation at C2 and C4 positions of iduronic acid was identified as a key determinant of antiviral potency. These disaccharide modules, when covalently grafted onto a polymer scaffold via post-modification chemistry, self-assembled into uniform nanomicelles with enhanced colloidal stability and controlled surface charge. SPR analyses confirmed that the sulfated glycopolymers, particularly **DMP4**, bound to the viral spike protein with nanomolar affinity while exhibiting weaker and less toxic interactions with ACE2. Electron microscopy and pseudovirus infection assays revealed that these glycopolymers effectively prevented viral attachment through acting as molecular sentinels—adsorbing onto the viral surface and disrupting the integrity of the envelope. Cellular studies further demonstrated efficient endocytic uptake of the nanoparticles and subsequent inhibition of key viral and host enzymes, M^{pro} and HPSE, achieving synergistic antiviral activity across multiple biological targets.

Collectively, this study establishes a versatile platform for the rational design of glycosaminoglycan-mimetic therapeutics. The DS-mimetic glycopolymers combine structural precision, tunable sulfation, and favorable biocompatibility, offering a new strategy for broad-spectrum antiviral development beyond COVID-19. Their multivalent, multi-target mechanism provides a foundation for next-generation antiviral materials capable of addressing emerging viral threats with reduced resistance potential.

6. Patents

L.W., G.Y., and C.C. are co-inventors on a patent application describing sulfated glycosaminoglycan-mimetic polymer and the preparation method.

Supplementary Materials: The following supporting information can be downloaded at: https://www.mdpi.com/article/10.3390/md23120486/s1, Table S1. Predicted Binding Affinities of GAG-Mimetic Oligosaccharides with Target Proteins; Figure S1. 2D diagram of receptor-ligand interactions between SARS-CoV-2 RBD and GalNAc-346S (Table S1 Entry-1); Figure S2. 2D diagram of receptor-ligand interactions between SARS-CoV-2 RBD and DM1 (Table S1 Entry-16); Figure S3. 2D diagram of receptor-ligand interactions between SARS-CoV-2 RBD and DM2 (Table S1 Entry-18); Figure S4. 2D diagram of receptor-ligand interactions between SARS-CoV-2 RBD and DM3 (Table S1 Entry-

17); Figure S5. 2D diagram of receptor-ligand interactions between SARS-CoV-2 RBD and DM4 (Table S1 Entry-20); Figure S6. 2D diagram of receptor-ligand interactions between SARS-CoV-2 RBD and DS-2S-46S (Table S1 Entry-19); Scheme S1. Retrosynthetic route of DS-mimetic glycopolymers; Scheme S2. Synthesis of 6. Reagent and conditions; Scheme S3. Synthesis of 9. Reagent and conditions; Scheme S4. Synthesis of 12 and deprotection of 12.; Scheme S5. Synthesis of 15. Reagent and conditions; Scheme S6. Synthesis of 17; Scheme S7. Synthesis of 21, 24, 27, 29; Scheme S8. Synthesis of DS-mimetic glycopolymers; Figure S7. TEM images of pseudovirus; Figure S8. TEM images of co-incubation of the pseudovirus with DMP4 for 5 min at 37 °C; Figure S9. TEM images of co-incubation of the pseudovirus with DMP4 for 2 h at 37 °C; Figure S10. SDS-PAGE analysis of affinity chromatography-purified protein; Figure S11. Confocal images of cells incubated with Cy3-SS (20 $\mu g \cdot mL^{-1}$) for 12 h [54,55].

Author Contributions: Conceptualization, L.W., M.Y., J.S., L.Y., C.L. and C.C.; methodology, L.W., L.G., C.Y. and J.S.; compound synthesis, L.W., L.G. and M.Y.; SARS-CoV-2 pseudovirus production, J.S.; data curation, L.W. and C.Y.; discussion and writing, L.W., C.C., G.Y. and S.F.R.H.; project administration, G.Y. and C.C.; funding acquisition, G.Y. and C.C. All authors have read and agreed to the published version of the manuscript.

Funding: This research was financially supported by the National Natural Science Foundation of China (U21A20297), Taishan Scholar Climbing Project TSPD20210304, and the Young Project (TSQN202306099), the Fundamental Research Funds for the Central Universities (202461054).

Institutional Review Board Statement: Not applicable.

Data Availability Statement: The data are contained within the article or Supplementary Materials.

Acknowledgments: The BL21/pGEX4T1-Mpro strain was generously provided by Xin Wang (Ocean University of China). During the preparation of this manuscript/study, the author(s) used ChatGPT5 for the purpose of language refinement. The authors have reviewed and edited the output and take full responsibility for the content of this publication.

Conflicts of Interest: The authors declare no conflicts of interest.

Abbreviations

The following abbreviations are used in this manuscript:

SARS-CoV-2	Severe Acute Respiratory Syndrome-Related Coronavirus 2
COVID-19	Coronavirus Disease 2019
SARS-CoV	Severe Acute Respiratory Syndrome-Related Coronavirus
ACE2	Angiotensin-Converting Enzyme 2
GAG	Glycosaminoglycan
HS	Heparan Sulfate
DS	Dermatan Sulfate
HP	Heparin
RBD	Receptor Binding Domain
HPSE	Heparanase
HSPGs	Heparan Sulfate Proteoglycans
M^{pro}	Main Protease
Bn	Benzy
Cbz	Carbobenzyloxy
IdoA	Aldonic Acid
GalNAc	N-Acetylgalactosamine
TR-FRET	Time-Resolved Fluorescence Resonance Energy Transfer

References

1. World Health Organization. WHO Coronavirus (COVID-19) Dashboard. Available online: https://data.who.int/dashboards/covid19/more-resources (accessed on 10 November 2025).
2. Montcho, Y.; Amoussouvi, K.T.; Atchadé, M.N.; Salako, K.V.; Hounkonnou, M.N.; Wolkewitz, M.; Kakaï, R.G. Assessing the potential seasonality of COVID-19 dynamic in Africa: A mathematical modeling study. *Model. Earth Syst. Environ.* **2025**, *11*, 114. [CrossRef]
3. Anzalone, A.J.; Vest, M.T.; Schissel, M.E.; Price, B.; Hillegass, W.B.; Horswell, R.; Chu, S.; Rosen, C.J.; Miele, L.; Santangelo, S.L.; et al. Higher mortality following SARS-CoV-2 infection in rural versus urban dwellers persists for two years post-infection. *Nat. Commun.* **2025**, *16*, 8933. [CrossRef]
4. Al Huraimel, K.; Alhosani, M.; Kunhabdulla, S.; Stietiya, M.H. SARS-CoV-2 in the environment: Modes of transmission, early detection and potential role of pollutions. *Sci. Total Environ.* **2020**, *744*, 140946. [CrossRef] [PubMed]
5. Callaway, E. Could new COVID variants undermine vaccines? Labs scramble to find out. *Nature* **2021**, *589*, 177–178. [CrossRef] [PubMed]
6. Lavine, J.S.; Bjornstad, O.N.; Antia, R. Immunological characteristics govern the transition of COVID-19 to endemicity. *Science* **2021**, *371*, 741–745. [CrossRef]
7. Ibarrondo, F.J.; Fulcher, J.A.; Goodman-Meza, D.; Elliott, J.; Hofmann, C.; Hausner, M.A.; Ferbas, K.G.; Tobin, N.H.; Aldrovandi, G.M.; Yang, O.O. Rapid decay of anti–SARS-CoV-2 antibodies in persons with mild COVID-19. *N. Engl. J. Med.* **2020**, *383*, 1085–1087. [CrossRef]
8. Liu, Y.; Li, D.; Han, J. COVID-19 vaccines and beyond. *Cell. Mol. Immunol.* **2024**, *21*, 207–209. [CrossRef] [PubMed]
9. Cui, T.; Su, X.; Sun, J.; Liu, S.; Huang, M.; Li, W.; Luo, C.; Cheng, L.; Wei, R.; Song, T.; et al. Dynamic immune landscape in vaccinated-BA.5-XBB.1.9.1 reinfections revealed a 5-month protection-duration against XBB infection and a shift in immune imprinting. *Ebiomedicine* **2024**, *99*, 104903. [CrossRef]
10. Lang, J.; Yang, N.; Deng, J.; Liu, K.; Yang, P.; Zhang, G.; Jiang, C. Inhibition of SARS pseudovirus cell entry by lactoferrin binding to heparan sulfate proteoglycans. *PLoS ONE* **2011**, *6*, e23710. [CrossRef]
11. Lan, J.; Ge, J.; Yu, J.; Shan, S.; Zhou, H.; Fan, S.; Zhang, Q.; Shi, X.; Wang, Q.; Zhang, L.; et al. Structure of the SARS-CoV-2 spike receptor-binding domain bound to the ACE2 receptor. *Nature* **2020**, *581*, 215–220. [CrossRef]
12. Hoffmann, M.; Kleine-Weber, H.; Schroeder, S.; Krüger, N.; Herrler, T.; Erichsen, S.; Schiergens, T.S.; Herrler, G.; Wu, N.-H.; Nitsche, A.; et al. SARS-CoV-2 cell entry depends on ACE2 and TMPRSS2 and is blocked by a clinically proven protease inhibitor. *Cell* **2020**, *181*, 271–280.e8. [CrossRef]
13. Ju, X.; Wang, Z.; Wang, P.; Ren, W.; Yu, Y.; Yu, Y.; Yuan, B.; Song, J.; Zhang, X.; Zhang, Y.; et al. SARS-CoV-2 main protease cleaves MAGED2 to antagonize host antiviral defense. *mBio* **2023**, *14*, e01373-23. [CrossRef]
14. VK, P.; Rath, S.P.; Abraham, P. Computational designing of a peptide that potentially blocks the entry of SARS-CoV, SARS-CoV-2 and MERS-CoV. *PLoS ONE* **2021**, *16*, e0251913.
15. Yamasaki, K.; Adachi, N.; Tun, M.M.N.; Ikeda, A.; Moriya, T.; Kawasaki, M.; Yamasaki, T.; Kubota, T.; Nagashima, I.; Shimizu, H.; et al. Core fucose-specific pholiota squarrosa lectin (PhoSL) as a potent broad-spectrum inhibitor of SARS-CoV-2 infection. *FEBS J.* **2023**, *290*, 412–427. [CrossRef]
16. Chang, Y.-J.; Le, U.N.P.; Liu, J.-J.; Li, S.-R.; Chao, S.-T.; Lai, H.-C.; Lin, Y.-F.; Hsu, K.-C.; Lu, C.-H.; Lin, C.-W. Combining virtual screening with *cis-/trans*-cleavage enzymatic assays effectively reveals broad-spectrum inhibitors that target the main proteases of SARS-CoV-2 and MERS-CoV. *Antivir. Res.* **2023**, *216*, 105653. [CrossRef] [PubMed]
17. Varki, A.; Cummings, R.D.; Esko, J.D.; Stanley, P.; Hart, G.W.; Aebi, M.; Mohnen, D.; Kinoshita, T.; Packer, N.H.; Prestegard, J.H.; et al. (Eds.) *Essentials of Glycobiology*; Cold Spring Harbor Laboratory Press: Cold Spring Harbor, NY, USA, 2022.
18. Clausen, T.M.; Sandoval, D.R.; Spliid, C.B.; Pihl, J.; Perrett, H.R.; Painter, C.D.; Narayanan, A.; Majowicz, S.A.; Kwong, E.M.; McVicar, R.N.; et al. SARS-CoV-2 infection depends on cellular heparan sulfate and ACE2. *Cell* **2020**, *183*, 1043–1057.e15. [CrossRef]
19. Kim, S.Y.; Jin, W.; Sood, A.; Montgomery, D.W.; Grant, O.C.; Fuster, M.M.; Fu, L.; Dordick, J.S.; Woods, R.J.; Zhang, F.; et al. Characterization of heparin and severe acute respiratory syndrome-related coronavirus 2 (SARS-CoV-2) spike glycoprotein binding interactions. *Antivir. Res.* **2020**, *181*, 104873. [CrossRef] [PubMed]
20. Kwon, P.S.; Oh, H.; Kwon, S.-J.; Jin, W.; Zhang, F.; Fraser, K.; Hong, J.J.; Linhardt, R.J.; Dordick, J.S. Sulfated polysaccharides effectively inhibit SARS-CoV-2 in vitro. *Cell Discov.* **2020**, *6*, 50. [CrossRef]
21. Liu, L.; Chopra, P.; Li, X.; Bouwman, K.M.; Tompkins, S.M.; Wolfert, M.A.; de Vries, R.P.; Boons, G.-J. Heparan sulfate proteoglycans as attachment factor for SARS-CoV-2. *ACS Cent. Sci.* **2021**, *7*, 1009–1018. [CrossRef] [PubMed]
22. Dwivedi, R.; Farrag, M.; Sharma, P.; Shi, D.; Shami, A.A.; Misra, S.K.; Ray, P.; Shukla, J.; Zhang, F.; Linhardt, R.J.; et al. The sea cucumber thyonella gemmata contains a low anticoagulant sulfated fucan with high anti-SARS-CoV-2 actions against wild-type and delta variants. *J. Nat. Prod.* **2023**, *86*, 1463–1475. [CrossRef]

23. Pomin, V.H.; Zhang, F.; Dordick, J.S. Role, binding properties, and potential therapeutical use of glycosaminoglycans and mimetics in SARS-CoV-2 infection. In memory of dr. Robert linhardt (1953–2025). *Carbohydr. Polym.* **2025**, *362*, 123703. [CrossRef] [PubMed]
24. Tree, J.A.; Turnbull, J.E.; Buttigieg, K.R.; Elmore, M.J.; Coombes, N.; Hogwood, J.; Mycroft-West, C.J.; Lima, M.A.; Skidmore, M.A.; Karlsson, R.; et al. Unfractionated heparin inhibits live wild type SARS-CoV-2 cell infectivity at therapeutically relevant concentrations. *Br. J. Pharmacol.* **2021**, *178*, 626–635. [CrossRef]
25. Tandon, R.; Sharp, J.S.; Zhang, F.; Pomin, V.H.; Ashpole, N.M.; Mitra, D.; McCandless, M.G.; Jin, W.; Liu, H.; Sharma, P.; et al. Effective inhibition of SARS-CoV-2 entry by heparin and enoxaparin derivatives. *J. Virol.* **2021**, *95*, e01987-20. [CrossRef] [PubMed]
26. Mycroft-West, C.J.; Su, D.; Pagani, I.; Rudd, T.R.; Elli, S.; Gandhi, N.S.; Guimond, S.E.; Miller, G.J.; Meneghetti, M.C.Z.; Nader, H.B.; et al. Heparin inhibits cellular invasion by SARS-CoV-2: Structural dependence of the interaction of the spike S1 receptor-binding domain with heparin. *Thromb. Haemost.* **2020**, *120*, 1700–1715. [CrossRef]
27. Ustyuzhanina, N.E.; Bilan, M.I.; Dmitrenok, A.S.; Tsvetkova, E.A.; Nifantiev, N.E.; Usov, A.I. Oversulfated dermatan sulfate and heparinoid in the starfish *lysastrosoma anthosticta*: Structures and anticoagulant activity. *Carbohydr. Polym.* **2021**, *261*, 117867. [CrossRef]
28. Habuchi, O. Functions of chondroitin/dermatan sulfate containing GalNAc4,6-disulfate. *Glycobiology* **2022**, *32*, 664–678. [CrossRef]
29. Wei, L.; Xu, Y.; Du, M.; Fan, Y.; Zou, R.; Xu, X.; Zhang, Q.; Zhang, Y.-Z.; Wang, W.; Li, F. A novel 4-*O*-endosulfatase with high potential for the structure-function studies of chondroitin sulfate/dermatan sulfate. *Carbohydr. Polym.* **2023**, *305*, 120508. [CrossRef]
30. Inubushi, T.; Nag, P.; Sasaki, J.-I.; Shiraishi, Y.; Yamashiro, T. The significant role of glycosaminoglycans in tooth development. *Glycobiology* **2024**, *34*, cwae024. [CrossRef]
31. Yu, Y.; Williams, A.; Zhang, X.; Fu, L.; Xia, K.; Xu, Y.; Zhang, F.; Liu, J.; Koffas, M.; Linhardt, R.J. Specificity and action pattern of heparanase bp, a β-glucuronidase from burkholderia pseudomallei. *Glycobiology* **2019**, *29*, 572–581. [CrossRef] [PubMed]
32. Rangarajan, S.; Richter, J.R.; Richter, R.P.; Bandari, S.K.; Tripathi, K.; Vlodavsky, I.; Sanderson, R.D. Heparanase-enhanced shedding of syndecan-1 and its role in driving disease pathogenesis and progression. *J. Histochem. Cytochem.* **2020**, *68*, 823–840. [CrossRef]
33. Agelidis, A.; Shukla, D. *Heparanase: From Basic Research to Clinical Applications*; Vlodavsky, I., Sanderson, R.D., Ilan, N., Eds.; Springer International Publishing: Cham, Switzerland, 2020; pp. 759–770.
34. Xiang, J.; Lu, M.; Shi, M.; Cheng, X.; Kwakwa, K.A.; Davis, J.L.; Su, X.; Bakewell, S.J.; Zhang, Y.; Fontana, F.; et al. Heparanase blockade as a novel dual-targeting therapy for COVID-19. *J. Virol.* **2022**, *96*, e00057-22. [CrossRef] [PubMed]
35. Sugimoto, A.; Koike, T.; Kuboki, Y.; Komaba, S.; Kosono, S.; Aswathy, M.; Anzai, I.; Watanabe, T.; Toshima, K.; Takahashi, D. Synthesis of low-molecular-weight fucoidan analogue and its inhibitory activities against heparanase and SARS-CoV-2 infection. *Angew. Chem. Int. Ed.* **2025**, *64*, e202411760. [CrossRef]
36. Greinacher, A.; Farner, B.; Kroll, H.; Kohlmann, T.; Warkentin, T.E.; Eichler, P. Clinical features of heparin-induced thrombocytopenia including risk factors for thrombosis. *Thromb. Haemost.* **2017**, *94*, 132–135.
37. Nie, C.; Pouyan, P.; Lauster, D.; Trimpert, J.; Kerkhoff, Y.; Szekeres, G.P.; Wallert, M.; Block, S.; Sahoo, A.K.; Dernedde, J.; et al. Polysulfates block SARS-CoV-2 uptake through electrostatic interactions. *Angew. Chem. Int. Ed.* **2021**, *60*, 15870–15878. [CrossRef]
38. Abdulsalam, H.; Li, J.; Loka, R.S.; Sletten, E.T.; Nguyen, H.M. Heparan sulfate-mimicking glycopolymers bind SARS-CoV-2 spike protein in a length- and sulfation pattern-dependent manner. *ACS Med. Chem. Lett.* **2023**, *14*, 1411–1418. [CrossRef]
39. Yang, C.; Gao, L.; Shao, M.; Cai, C.; Wang, L.; Chen, Y.; Li, J.; Fan, F.; Han, Y.; Liu, M.; et al. End-functionalised glycopolymers as glycosaminoglycan mimetics inhibit HeLa cell proliferation. *Polym. Chem.* **2020**, *11*, 4714–4722. [CrossRef]
40. Grant, O.C.; Wentworth, D.; Holmes, S.G.; Kandel, R.; Sehnal, D.; Wang, X.; Xiao, Y.; Sheppard, P.; Grelsson, T.; Coulter, A.; et al. Generating 3D models of carbohydrates with GLYCAM-web. *bioRxiv* **2025**. [CrossRef]
41. Nivedha, A.K.; Thieker, D.F.; Hu, H.; Woods, R.J. Vina-carb: Improving glycosidic angles during carbohydrate docking. *J. Chem. Theory Comput.* **2016**, *12*, 892–901. [CrossRef]
42. Hemker, H.C. A century of heparin: Past, present and future. *J. Thromb. Haemost.* **2016**, *14*, 2329–2338. [CrossRef]
43. Hogwood, J.; Mulloy, B.; Lever, R.; Gray, E.; Page, C.P. Pharmacology of heparin and related drugs: An update. *Pharmacol. Rev.* **2023**, *75*, 328–379. [CrossRef] [PubMed]
44. Gómez, S.A.; Rojas-Valencia, N.; Gómez, S.; Lans, I.; Restrepo, A. Initial recognition and attachment of the zika virus to host cells: A molecular dynamics and quantum interaction approach. *Chembiochem* **2022**, *23*, e202200351. [CrossRef]
45. Trowbridge, J.M.; Gallo, R.L. Dermatan sulfate: New functions from an old glycosaminoglycan. *Glycobiology* **2002**, *12*, 117R–125R. [CrossRef]
46. Lohman, G.J.S.; Hunt, D.K.; Högermeier, J.A.; Seeberger, P.H. Synthesis of Iduronic Acid Building Blocks for the Modular Assembly of Glycosaminoglycans. *J. Org. Chem.* **2003**, *68*, 7559–7561. [CrossRef]

47. Yeap, S.P.; Lim, J.; Ngang, H.P.; Ooi, B.S.; Ahmad, A.L. Role of particle–particle interaction towards effective interpretation of Z-average and particle size distributions from dynamic light scattering (DLS) analysis. *J. Nanosci. Nanotechnol.* **2018**, *18*, 6957–6964. [CrossRef]
48. Miura, Y.; Yasuda, K.; Yamamoto, K.; Koike, M.; Nishida, Y.; Kobayashi, K. Inhibition of alzheimer amyloid aggregation with sulfated glycopolymers. *Biomacromolecules* **2007**, *8*, 2129–2134. [CrossRef] [PubMed]
49. Koide, H.; Yoshimatsu, K.; Hoshino, Y.; Lee, S.-H.; Okajima, A.; Ariizumi, S.; Narita, Y.; Yonamine, Y.; Weisman, A.C.; Nishimura, Y.; et al. A polymer nanoparticle with engineered affinity for a vascular endothelial growth factor (VEGF165). *Nat. Chem.* **2017**, *9*, 715–722. [CrossRef] [PubMed]
50. Yoshiko, M.; Yu, H.; Hirokazu, S. Glycopolymer Nanobiotechnology. *Chem. Rev.* **2016**, *116*, 1673–1692.
51. Müller, C.; Despras, G.; Lindhorst, T.K. Organizing multivalency in carbohydrate recognition. *Chem. Soc. Rev.* **2016**, *45*, 3275–3302. [CrossRef]
52. Li, J.; Zhang, Y.; Pang, H.; Li, S.J. Heparin interacts with the main protease of SARS-CoV-2 and inhibits its activity. *Spectrochim. Acta Part A* **2022**, *267*, 120595. [CrossRef] [PubMed]
53. Li, Z.; Li, X.; Huang, Y.-Y.; Wu, Y.; Liu, R.; Zhou, L.; Lin, Y.; Wu, D.; Zhang, L.; Liu, H.; et al. Identify potent SARS-CoV-2 main protease inhibitors via accelerated free energy perturbation-based virtual screening of existing drugs. *Proc. Natl. Acad. Sci. USA* **2020**, *117*, 27381–27387. [CrossRef]
54. Kong, F. Recent studies on reaction pathways and applications of sugar orthoesters in synthesis of oligosaccharides. *Carbohydr. Res.* **2007**, *342*, 345–373. [CrossRef]
55. Castelli, R.; Overkleeft, H.S.; van der Marel, G.A.; Codée, J.D.C. 2,2-dimethyl-4-(4-methoxy-phenoxy) butanoate and 2,2-dimethyl-4-azido butanoate: Two new pivaloate-ester-like protecting groups. *Org. Lett.* **2013**, *15*, 2270–2273. [CrossRef] [PubMed]

MDPI AG
Grosspeteranlage 5
4052 Basel
Switzerland
Tel.: +41 61 683 77 34

Marine Drugs Editorial Office
E-mail: marinedrugs@mdpi.com
www.mdpi.com/journal/marinedrugs

www.ingramcontent.com/pod-product-compliance
Lightning Source LLC
Chambersburg PA
CBHW061614210926
51850CB00009B/2315
* 9 7 8 3 7 2 5 8 6 6 3 4 2 *